THE MIDWIFE–MOTHER RELATIONSHIP

The Midwife–Mother Relationship

2nd Edition

Edited by

Mavis Kirkham

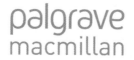

First published 2010 by
PALGRAVE MACMILLAN

Palgrave Macmillan in the UK is an imprint of Macmillan Publishers Limited,
registered in England, company number 785998, of Houndmills, Basingstoke,
Hampshire RG21 6XS.

Palgrave Macmillan in the US is a division of St Martin's Press LLC,
175 Fifth Avenue, New York, NY 10010.

Palgrave Macmillan is the global academic imprint of the above companies
and has companies and representatives throughout the world.

Palgrave® and Macmillan® are registered trademarks in the United States,
the United Kingdom, Europe and other countries

ISBN 978–0–230–57736-7

This book is printed on paper suitable for recycling and made from fully
managed and sustained forest sources. Logging, pulping and manufacturing
processes are expected to conform to the environmental regulations of the
country of origin.

A catalogue record for this book is available from the British Library.

A catalog record for this book is available from the Library of Congress.

10   9   8   7   6   5   4   3   2   1
19   18   17   16   15   14   13   12   11   10

Printed and bound in China

Contents

Notes on contributors

Tricia Anderson
A the time of writing her chapter, Tricia was a lecturer in Midwifery Studies at the Institute of Health and Community Studies, Bournemouth University and an independent midwife. She trained as a midwife in Dorset, where she worked in both community and hospital settings before commencing independent midwifery practice in 1997. She was formerly editor of the *MIDIRS Midwifery Digest*, co-editor of the *Informed Choice Initiative* and associate editor of *The Practising Midwife*. At Bournemouth University she pioneered student midwife case-holding as a model for midwifery education. Her research interests included the second stage of labour and breastfeeding peer support. Sadly, after two years of living with a brain tumour, Tricia died in October 2007.

Marie Berg PhD, MPH, MNSc, RN, RM
Marie Berg is Associate Professor in Health Care Sciences in the Sahlgrenska Academy at the University of Gothenburg. She is head of the midwifery programme and Master's modules in midwifery science and also teaches research modules. Her research aims at developing person-centred care supporting well-being in mothers and their partners/families. Central theoretical standpoints for her research are lifeworld theory and salutogenesis. The research is encompassed in two extensive programmes of work: motherhood and diabetes; and intrapartum care. Her main international projects are the BfiN network for developing qualitative research in childbearing in Nordic and other European countries; COST action for creating a dynamic EU framework for optimal maternity care; and the support for developing nursing and midwifery care in and education in Kivu province, Democratic Republic of Congo. Marie has published widely in Swedish and in English.

Chris Bewley
Chris Bewley is currently Head of Department for Midwifery, Child Health and Primary Care at Middlesex University. Chris's interests are in all aspects of interpersonal skills and communication. She was also involved in developing professional guidelines for various groups on supporting women experiencing domestic violence, particularly during

pregnancy. Chris also writes on working with pregnant women who have medical disorders, with the emphasis on providing individualized care.

Kuldip Bharj OBE, PhD, MSc, BSc(Hons), RM, RN, MTD, DN (London), IHSM Cert, RSA Counselling skills

Kuldip Bharj is Senior Lecturer in Midwifery and Lead Midwife for Education at the University of Leeds. Kuldip has 34 years' experience of midwifery education, research and practice, including ten years in NHS public appointments. She is dedicated to excellence in the provision and delivery of services in education and practice. Successfully leading on issues of equal opportunities has equipped her with the knowledge and skills necessary to facilitate the generation of culturally sensitive and appropriate health care for service users. Kuldip serves on the editorial board of the *British Journal of Midwifery*; is a registrant member of the Nursing and Midwifery Council; and currently serves on the Prime Minister's Commission on the Future of Nursing and Midwifery.

Margaret Chesney

Margaret began nursing in 1974 and has been a midwife since 1980. Her clinical background is in community midwifery, as a midwife then a manager. She made eight working trips to Pakistan to work in a Red Crescent Maternity Hospital in Sahiwal. For her PhD she studied home birth for some women in Pakistan. Until her retirement she was Senior Midwifery Lecturer and Associate Head of the School of Health Professions (Research), University of Salford. Whilst working in education, she carried a small caseload of women, with students, providing continuity of care. Since her retirement, she has worked for two years as a Hospice Education Co-ordinator and been made a Fellow of the RCM.

Mary Cronk

Mary Cronk is a mature midwife who has been in clinical practice, mostly in the community, for practically all her professional life. She started off as a domiciliary midwife employed by a county council and then a community midwife employed by the NHS. Since 1990 Mary has been in independent practice. She was elected to the English National Board for Nursing, Midwifery and Health Visiting (ENB) in 1983, and was a member of its Midwifery and Investigating Committees until 1987, when she was elected as a Midwife Member of the United Kingdom Central Council for Nursing, Midwifery and Health Visiting (UKCC). She served on the Midwifery and Professional Conduct Committees of the UKCC until 1998 when her term of office finished. Until September 2008 she was an appointed practitioner member of the Midwifery and Preliminary Proceedings Committees of the NMC.

Ruth Deery

Ruth Deery is Reader in Midwifery at the University of Huddersfield. Her key interest at doctoral level was in applying sociological theory and action research methodology to the organizational culture of midwifery in the National Health Service (NHS) in England. Since then her main work has been in the maternity services and women's health in the new NHS, with particular interests in organizational change, public policy and emotions and care. Her work has been widely published in refereed journals.

Nadine Edwards

Nadine Edwards became interested in the politics of birth following the births of her own three children. She joined AIMS and is currently the Vice Chair, and then trained as a birth educator. She completed a PhD on women's experiences of home birth in Scotland (Birthing Autonomy). Her current research interests include public involvement through Maternity Services Liaison Committees and unassisted birth. She is one of the Directors at the Pregnancy and Parents Centre in Edinburgh and runs yoga for pregnancy sessions there.

Anna Gaudion

Anna has an academic background in anthropology, museum ethnography/anthropology of art and refugee studies. She has an eclectic career pathway which weaves through the arts and maternity services, working at the weekend as a midwife on the 'bank' at Guys and St Thomas' NHS Trust during her studies and career as a curator in the ethnographic department of the British Museum, arts critic and lecturer in the anthropological aspects of women's health at King's College. In 2004 she directed and made the film *Florence: The Experience of Becoming a Mother in Exile*. More recently she has gained experience in accessing and consulting vulnerable groups about maternity services: a Health Equity Audit of access to maternity services in SE London (Maternity Matters Early Adopter site) and a Needs Assessment concerning the specific needs of asylum seekers and refugees (Brunel University). She is currently the Project Lead for the Centering Pregnancy Pilot at King's College Hospital, London and the researcher and designer for The Polyanna Project.

Claire Elizabeth Homeyard

Claire has been employed as a consultant midwife in public health at Barking, Havering and Redbridge University Hospitals NHS Trust since 2001. In addition she is a lead professional adviser at the NMC, on projects related to public health and EU and international work, and is director of The Polyanna Project. Claire has represented midwifery at a number of regional and national forums, including membership of the clinical working group for the Healthcare for London Maternity and Newborn Care Pathway and Midwifery 2020. She has an MSc in Public Health from the London School of Hygiene and Tropical Medicine and was appointed Honorary Fellow at London South Bank University in 2003. She has presented and published in midwifery and health-related journals both nationally and internationally. She has a particular interest in influencing policy and practice to meet the needs of women and families who are vulnerable.

Billie Hunter

Billie Hunter is the first Midwifery Professor in Wales, UK, based in the Institute for Health Research, Swansea University. She is a Visiting Professor at the University of Surrey, Chair of the Iolanthe Midwifery Trust and Chair of the All Wales Midwifery and Reproductive Health Research Forum. Billie has been a midwife for 30 years, working in NHS, voluntary sector and independent midwifery settings, before moving into midwifery education and research in 1996. Her PhD investigated the emotion work of midwives and was awarded by the University of Wales in 2002. Billie leads a research programme which uses qualitative approaches to investigate the culture of maternity care and the work of midwives, including the effects on the quality of care and women's experiences. She is particularly interested in the role of relationships and emotions in maternity care. Billie has published widely and is a regular speaker at both UK and international conferences.

Mavis Kirkham

Mavis is Emeritus Professor of Midwifery, Sheffield Hallam University. She has 40 years' experience as a clinical midwife and a researcher. She still does some research, has research students and attends a few home births as an independent midwife.

Nicky Leap RM, MSc, DMid

For over 30 years, Nicky Leap has been engaged in midwifery practice, education and research in a variety of roles in both the UK and Australia.

This has included extensive writing about practice, in particular the development of community-based midwifery, continuity of care and issues related to engaging with women around pain in labour. Nicky is an Adjunct Professor of Midwifery in the Centre for Midwifery, Child and Family Health at the University of Technology, Sydney and is a Visiting Senior Research Fellow at King's College London.

Sally Pairman MNZM, DMid, MA, BA, RM, RGON
Sally is Head of the School of Midwifery and the Health and Community Group Manager at Otago Polytechnic, Dunedin, New Zealand; Inaugural Chair of the Midwifery Council of New Zealand; honorary member, previous president and founder member of the New Zealand College of Midwives; co-chair of the International Confederation of Midwives Regulation Standing Committee and Regulation Taskforce; co-author with Karen Guilliland, of *Midwifery Partnership: A Model for Practice*, a monograph describing a theoretical model of midwifery as a partnership between the woman and the midwife; and co-editor of the midwifery text-book *Midwifery: Preparation for Practice*. In 2008 Sally was made a Member of the Order of New Zealand for her services to midwifery and women's health.

Meg Taylor
During Meg's first degree in social psychology and her Master's in psychopathology the work of Klaus and Kennell, on the interaction of mothers with their newborn babies, touched her deeply. Then, in the mid-1970s, there was much discussion about the medicalization of child-birth, increasing induction rates and the demise of direct-entry midwifery training, and the Association of Radical Midwives was formed. These influences came together and Meg wondered if, since early relationships were vital in their influence on later mental health, good midwifery could be a kind of preventive psychotherapy. She took a direct-entry midwifery course, qualified in 1980 and practised for seven years, in hospital and community. In 1987 she gave birth to her first son and decided that statutory maternity leave was incompatible with the kind of care she wished to give him. She had been training as a psychotherapist and, after a diagnosis of multiple sclerosis in 1985, undertook the unique counselling training at South West London College. She worked for two years as district staff counsellor to Tower Hamlets Health District and nine years in private practice as a psychotherapist. She is now retired as a result of the multiple sclerosis. She has two sons, both born at home.

Ruth Wilkins

Ruth first became aware of the unique relationship between midwife and mother when she experienced it at first hand. It shifted her axis of understanding from that of 'self/other' to that of being 'in relationship', one with the other. In this way the limitations of being 'professional' were exposed in the same glimpse of understanding that revealed the importance of empathy, experience and personal connectedness to midwifery practice, aspects completely eclipsed by the subject/object divide which underwrote conventional professional discourse. Ruth went on to pursue a career in commercial law, but the insights gained from her experiences of midwifery practice endured. Formerly a trustee of a healing sanctuary, she is now a trustee of the United Kingdom Council for Psychotherapy (UKCP) and is also a qualified spiritual counsellor.

Introduction

I am delighted to introduce this second edition of *The Midwife–Mother Relationship* and even more delighted that sufficient midwives and mothers have felt the subject important enough to merit buying the book, thus leading the publishers to commission this edition.

The midwife–mother relationship is the foundation of maternity services. For many women that relationship is the service, and from it can spring self-care and the confidence to ask for appropriate care from family and friends. For others, complex webs of specialist services and technical provisions support and are made human and intelligible by the woman's relationship with her midwife. As midwives from several countries stated in 2008:

> ...maternity care is a tapestry, in which the weft threads are the visible factors such as clinical outcomes, technologies, policies and protocols. Relationships are the warp threads that hold it all together, but which are hidden in the final work. The visibility of the weft threads, means that these become the focus of our attention: measurement of outcomes, achievement of targets, introduction of new technologies and production of protocols become synonymous with achieving excellence... this focus ignores the warp threads – relationships – and thus misses the point entirely.
>
> Without the existence of strong warp threads, a tapestry would disintegrate; any snagging or disruption of the warp threatens the integrity of the whole. In a similar way, without good-quality relationships, the tapestry of maternity care is compromised and weakened and it is highly unlikely that any new interventions, policies or systems will be effective or sustainable, or that high-quality care will be provided. We urgently need to pay real attention to the significance of relationships, and consider how best these can be developed, nurtured and sustained. (Hunter *et al.*, 2008:136)

This book seeks to pay just that attention to the fundamental midwife–mother relationship.

Though continuity of midwifery care and ongoing relationships feature in healthcare policy much more than was the case in 2000, when the first edition of this book was published, many women experience fragmented care and many midwives try to relate to women they meet only once. It is, therefore, important to consider relationships where there is conventional, fragmented care and where there is continuity.

This book is very different to the first edition. It has been hard to decide what chapters from the first edition to leave out. None has been left out because of its quality, only because more recent work in the same area merits inclusion or space prevents more than one chapter exploring similar areas. It would have been easy to produce a book twice as long as this.

I particularly regret the omission from this book of Jean Davies' waterboatman theory of women coping in poverty and adversity:

> To stop and ponder would invite trouble; survival meant keeping on top, moving on the surface. To stop was to sink, so like waterboatmen on a pond, staying on top was not to stay anywhere for long. (Davies, 2000: 129)

Jean Davies is long retired and Anna Gaudion and Claire Homeyard are now working with women in poverty (see Chapter 8). Yet, whenever I see a removal van in a poor area or hear a skittering pattern of speech – checking many things but staying nowhere long – I think of the waterboatman theory. Thank you for your insight, Jean.

Only two chapters remain unchanged from the first edition. Tricia Anderson's lucid chapter stands in memory of her. Her death in 2007 was a great loss to midwifery. Her chapter is as relevant today as it was in 2000. Ruth Wilkins' chapter comes from research inspired by her use of maternity services. She returned to her original, very different area of work, but her insights remain; her chapter was much cited and no similar work that I know replaces it. It has therefore been reproduced here.

Other authors who also contributed to the first edition have revised or completely rewritten their chapters. Kuldip Bharj has joined Margaret Chesney to produce a new chapter on Pakistani Muslim women, now using Kuldip's recent research alongside Margaret's. Seven new authors have joined us and four completely new chapters have been added.

It has been a great pleasure to work on this book with 15 women who are deeply concerned with the nature of the midwife–mother relationship. Thirteen of the contributors are midwives, as I am myself; four of us are retired but maintain close links with midwifery. Two, Nadine Edwards and Ruth Wilkins, write from the mother's perspective. They report research that arose from a wish to understand their own and other women's experience. Both have close, continuing involvement in women's health. Most of the chapters report research on various aspects of the midwife–mother relationship in England, Wales, Scotland, Sweden, Pakistan, Australia and New Zealand.

In Chapter 1 I have sought to examine the context of maternity services, looking at the situation in England and pulling out the tensions and dilemmas in modern public services which strongly influence relationships between midwives and mothers in many countries. In Chapter 2 Nicky Leap uses research from England and Australia to reflect on the philosophy of 'the less you do the more you give' as a midwife. She sees midwives as being 'alongside women', embracing uncertainty together as women: 'take up the power that will enable them to lead fulfilling lives as individuals and mothers and motivating the woman's friendship group to be there for her'.

In Chapter 3, Ruth Deery and Billie Hunter bring sociological interpretation to research data and professional reflection in order to examine how emotions may be experienced and potentially managed by midwives in their relationships with mothers. They see reciprocity as the 'central ingredient' in positive relationships and examine the settings in which reciprocity can be fostered. Two important concepts are introduced in Chapter 3: emotion work and social capital.

Chapter 4 is written by Mary Cronk, our most experienced midwife contributor. She describes her role as that of a 'professional servant'. This is a highly rhetorical chapter, which challenges midwives to revise the way we see and speak to mothers in order to correct power imbalances and enable women to feel more confident and more responsible as parents.

Chapters 5 and 6 focus on childbearing women's experience. Both look at their relationship with community midwives. Ruth Wilkins describes the 'professional paradigm' and its 'profound lack of fit' with the mothers' viewpoint and the way in which the dominance of that paradigm alienates midwives from their own experience. Nevertheless, her sample of mothers describes a special relationship with their community midwives. This research was conducted some time ago and there have been organizational changes since then, but the findings of the next chapter are very similar. Nadine Edwards researched how women planning home births saw their relationship with midwives and writes from this research, together with women's ongoing experiences at the Edinburgh Pregnancy and Parents Centre. Relationships are seen as fundamental to the building of trust, confidence and safety, yet the political context inhibits relationship building for both mothers and midwives.

Tricia Anderson analysed a key point in the midwife–mother relationship: the second stage of labour. The tensions of trust and control are sharply focused in the title of Chapter 7: 'Feeling safe enough to let go'. The midwife's power to support or undermine is central and has an important influence on the woman's relationship with her body.

Chapters 8, 9 and 10 look at relationships in circumstances where the cultural gap between midwife and mother is likely to be wide. In Chapter 8, Anna Gaudion and Claire Homeyard look at the midwife–mother relationship where there is poverty and disadvantage. They examine these women's need to be listened to and their need for support and respect. They report that many midwives feel overwhelmed when confronted with the complex, interconnected issues arising from poverty and disadvantage in pregnancy. This can lead to stereotyping, which fuels the women's feeling of being ignored or rejected. Yet kindness and respect could mean so much to these women and they greatly appreciated the midwives who treated them humanely.

In Chapter 9, Kuldip Bharj and Margaret Chesney look at Pakistani Muslim women's relationships with their midwives, drawing on two research studies considering these women's childbearing experiences in England and in Pakistan. Their findings reflect work with many other populations of childbearing women. The women saw 'good' midwives as those who were approachable, understanding and who treated them with respect. Some midwives, however, were seen as 'too busy' to relate in this way. Margaret Chesney recalls, with remarkable honesty, her 'bad care days' when she was too rushed to listen, a phenomenon seen in many other settings. The 'three-way relationship' with an interpreter alters the balance of power and the time taken for communication, requiring further skills to maximize the positive potential of the midwife–mother relationship.

In Chapter 10, Marie Berg examines midwifery relationships with women whose childbearing carries increased medical risks for mother or baby. Here again, the mothers expressed their need to be accepted and affirmed as individuals and as mothers and to be listened to. Where these needs were not met they 'were discouraged and did not trust themselves or their capacity for giving birth'. Marie Berg draws on her several research studies, conducted in Sweden, to produce an elegant midwifery model of care for childbearing women at high risk which could fruitfully be used with all mothers. Her concept of 'genuine care' in caring for 'the genuine' within the mother highlights the need to balance 'the medical and the natural'. This can be hard, but can transform women's experience in settings which prioritize medical issues over individuals' concerns.

In Chapter 11 Chris Bewley draws on her several research studies on how midwives' own experiences of pregnancy-related losses affect their relationships with women in their care. Parents often ask whether the midwife is herself a mother, when seeking to discover whether she is empathic and emotionally trustworthy. This creates real problems and considerable emotion work for midwives in sublimating their own emotional needs and judging when it is appropriate to conceal or reveal their own situation or even create a fictitious family. Colleague support is very important and potentially supportive strategies are outlined.

The New Zealand model of midwifery partnership is examined by Sally Pairman in Chapter 12. A close alliance of childbearing women and midwives brought about the legislative changes which reinstated midwifery autonomy in New Zealand. This alliance also forged a 'new professionalism' based on reciprocal and equitable relationships between professional and client. This model of a one-to-one relationship, with the conscious aim of balancing the power of the midwife and the mother, is seen as important to midwives in many other countries. The chapter includes recent work on outcomes of midwifery care in New Zealand.

In Chapter 13 Meg Taylor, a retired midwife and psychotherapist, uses her psychoanalytical knowledge to reflect on 'the midwife as container'. She highlights 'parallel processes' and suggests that 'the midwife–mother relationship is in some ways parallel to that of the mother and child'. In the postnatal period the midwife, who demonstrates that she accepts and trusts her client, 'metaphorically holds the mother so that she can both literally and metaphorically hold her baby'.

Common threads can be seen through the chapters, though they speak of very different places and use different theoretical approaches. Women's need to be listened to, and for respect, kindness and trust, is reported many times, as is the need for time to develop relationships. The satisfaction midwives derive from meeting women's needs is clear. Yet there are considerable political barriers to meeting these fundamental needs. In Chapter 14 I attempt to draw some conclusions.

I am grateful to all the chapter authors for fitting this work into their busy lives. Anna Fielder's insights have improved Chapters 1 and 13. Helen Shallow has supported me with Chapter 1. Jo Murphy-Lawless stimulated my thoughts on safe space whilst supporting me on another project. Nadine Edwards tracked down the last page reference and helped my thinking in many ways. Thank you all.

I trust that what is offered here will make a substantial contribution to the now considerable literature on a subject fundamental to our practice as midwives.

References

Davies, J. (2000) Being with women who are economically without, in Kirkham, M. (ed.), *The Midwife–Mother Relationship*, 1st edn, Basingstoke: Palgrave.

Hunter, B., Berg, M., Lundgren, I., Olafsdottir, O.A. and Kirkham, M. (2008) Relationships: The hidden threads in the tapestry of maternity care, *Midwifery* 24: 132–7.

CHAPTER 1

The Maternity Services Context

MAVIS KIRKHAM

Any relationship is very much influenced by its context and this is certainly true for the midwife–mother relationship. The social context of those involved, their values, beliefs and social obligations, affect what the two parties bring to their relationship. For the mother this context includes the wider society's values concerning birth and the childbearing experiences of her friends and family. These factors have an impact on the midwife too. She is also influenced by her commitments as a professional and as an employee. The immediate organizational context of the maternity services greatly influences the relationships within it and this organizational context is the main subject of this chapter. As I have had a career in midwifery in England, this chapter considers the English organizational context, but the same major influences apply in many other countries.

We live in a highly technologized society, where problems are defined and solved by experts with specialist knowledge. For birth, and most of life's rites of passage, the technical specialists are medical. Many issues are now classified as medical problems which in former years, or other contemporary societies, would have been seen as spiritual, educational, family or community issues. Midwifery has been greatly influenced by medical values. Indeed, the 1902 Midwives Act, which achieved the first state licensing of midwives in England, would never have been passed without the support of some medical practitioners. They thus achieved relief from 'tiresome and un-remunerative work' (HMSO, 1892: 22) in maternity care, which many of the aristocrats of British medicine at the time saw as 'an occupation degrading to a gentleman' (Smith, 1979: 23). The 1902 Act established the statutory body, the Central Midwives Board, whose members were mostly doctors, not midwives. Thus we have a long tradition of midwifery taking on tasks cast off by medicine or seen

1

by medicine as essential but inappropriate or too time-consuming for doctors to do themselves. This can be traced from the 1892 House of Commons Select Committee (HMSO, 1892) to the implementation of the European Working Time Directive (European Union, 1993) and beyond.

With medicalization came hospitalization: the centralization of medical expertise and equipment for maximum efficiency. It is over 30 years since English midwifery services moved out of local government public health services and into NHS Trusts, usually ones providing acute hospital services. Within hospitals, the relationships between midwives and mothers became closely supervised and divided up into specialized fragments. They were in the presence of 'a hierarchy of institutional expertise' (Freidson, 1970: 137) in which the position of midwives was nearly as low as that of mothers.

English community midwifery services continue, though the numbers of antenatal and postnatal meetings of midwives and mothers have been reduced on grounds of efficiency. In recent years maternity care support workers have increased in number and been used to ease the midwifery workload in hospital and community. This can be very helpful for all concerned (e.g. Walker, 2003), but can cause some unease where midwives do not feel involved in the choice of work to be delegated and may feel that some aspects of the relationship with mothers have been delegated whilst midwives retain technical and clerical tasks.

In recent years midwives have been involved in some innovative community development projects such as Sure Start. This programme was launched in 1998 in deprived areas in order to combat child poverty. It had similarities to Head Start in the United States (US Department of Health and Human Services, 2009) and is also comparable to initiatives in Australia and Ontario, Canada. Local Sure Starts had a considerable degree of autonomy and user involvement and some involved really innovative midwifery roles focusing on the development of supportive relationships for mothers and the growth of social capital in deprived areas. The policy document *Every Child Matters* (Department of Children, Schools and Families, 2003) started a switch from Sure Start local programmes to Sure Start Children's Centres, which are controlled by local authorities and will be provided in all areas. The midwifery input has been largely absorbed into mainstream maternity services. Despite some local lobbying, I do not know of any Children's Centres which are linked with birth centres.

Partly as a result of Sure Start projects and partly as a result of a Department of Health initiative (Dykes, 2003), voluntary breastfeeding peer support projects are now widespread and effective in supporting breastfeeding mothers in areas where the local culture is one of bottle feeding. Such projects can be enabling for the mothers involved and their training with or by local midwives can greatly enhance the relationships between them. However, some studies have noted problematic relations between peer supporters and community midwives not closely involved with these projects (e.g. Curtis *et al.*, 2007), who may have felt their authority and professional role being encroached on.

Thus community developments in recent years have provided new opportunities for developing relationships between mothers and midwives, as well as some occasions for complexities in these relationships. Meanwhile, most midwives continue to work in hospitals where the growth in obstetric technology has enabled information to be gathered and problems to be defined and dealt with directly from the bodies of the mother and foetus, rather than from communication with the mother. This has profoundly changed all the relationships concerned.

High technology, thus, draws in its wake a hierarchical distribution of knowledge and social authority that reflects the equally hierarchical social position of birth attendants in medicalised settings. (Jordan, 1987: 39)

Childbearing women became patients and later 'consumers' of maternity services, still a relatively passive role for life's most creative act. Many surveys of their views contain graphic descriptions of being on a conveyor belt, not a place where relationships flourish. This industrial model of care profoundly changed midwives' relationships too and priority had to be given to pleasing power-holders within the institution rather than mothers, who passed through it relatively rapidly.

The organization of maternity services on an industrial model and the centralization of services have proceeded apace throughout the industrial world. This process has been speeded up by the introduction of market values (Pollock, 2004) rather than guardianship values (Jacobs, 1992) into health care. Centralization is particularly seen in England, where many large cities now have one maternity unit with an annual delivery rate far greater than anything in this country in the past or elsewhere in Europe at present (Thornton, 2006). The primary argument for this is the same as that used for hospitalization: bringing the childbearing women to the experts, in this case consultant obstetricians (RCOG *et al.*, 2007). The closure of small maternity units has been going on for many years and units now seen to be so small as to merit closure were viewed as large only a decade ago. I am unaware whether the economies of scale which are stressed before small units are closed have ever been proven after the event. There has been no systematic evaluation of the relationship between the size of maternity units and the quality of their care or their users' experience (Macfarlane, 2007). Nevertheless, the pressures towards centralization make small midwifery units and birth centres very vulnerable. Their running costs are obvious areas of potential saving in times of financial stringency.

It is ironic that industrialization, which had such an impact on the organization of public services, also led to the commodification of those services. Thus childbearing women are defined in relation to the service they use, rather than by their social role as new mothers. The commodification of maternity services has led to concepts of customer choice, and informed choice has become a big issue in maternity care (Kirkham, 2004). Yet the service provider controls the menu; with centralization ensuring only one service provider in most areas, and the powerful professional concept of the 'right choice', options are limited for many women (Kirkham and Stapleton, 2001). There are very impressive exceptions to this trend and midwives who work tirelessly to extend women's choice, examples of which are discussed in this book.

Standardization of services is another key factor in modern maternity care and is manifest in the proliferation of policies, protocols and clinical guidelines. Two major factors have fuelled the standardization of practice. First, this has developed from efforts to provide clinical care which is based on research evidence (Sackett *et al.*, 1997). Secondly, standardization has followed the growing emphasis on risk management in the NHS, especially in maternity care where litigation can be very costly. The requirements of the Clinical Negligence Scheme for Trusts (NHS Litigation Authority, 2008) link guidelines to costs and add a further economic imperative to the many pressures to standardize care.

Standardization of services proceeds by means of proceduralization: having a written procedure for every eventuality. Such procedures, ideally based on research evidence, lead to expectations of standardized behaviour and a 'right way' for clinicians to act in any situation, which reflects the culture of the local service and may pay little heed to individual circumstances, needs and expectations (Kirkham and Stapleton, 2001). Behaving in the 'right way' gives staff the security afforded by risk management, but can be seen as protecting the organization rather than its users or clinicians, for whom it can increase risk (Edwards, 2005). Such rule-following is described by an insightful colleague as 'Teflon-coated management', to which neither blame nor responsibility can adhere.

Tensions within the context

Standardization has come to be equated with safety in the management of high-risk births (*Practising Midwife*, 2009a). There is, however, a real tension between the desire to craft systems which seek safety through uniform management of patients and the desire of clinicians to craft relationships with individuals in their care (Sennett, 2008). Complete standardization of care would make relationships peripheral, since the midwife's actions would always be as laid down by protocols rather than in response to individual women. This tension is one of many within modern health care which merit public debate and is especially important around childbirth, where most women are healthy and relationships are all important (Hunter *et al.*, 2008), greatly valued by childbearing women (as much of this book demonstrates) and central to midwives' job satisfaction (Kirkham *et al.*, 2006; Kirkham and Morgan, 2006).

There is a parallel major tension within the NHS and modern public services: that between service management and individual clinicians' desire for self-management. Management posts have increased in recent years and are seen as essential in achieving good service outcomes. There are midwifery managers who see their role as facilitating midwives' autonomy, just as there are midwives who see their role as facilitating their clients' autonomy; but both these approaches are unusual. Where autonomous action is seen as 'deviation' from the pathway laid down, and in need of careful written justification (Griffiths, 2009), managers tend to work by ensuring that the 'right' course of action is both laid down and followed. Yet autonomy at work is central to any worker's job satisfaction (Marmot, 2004) and is particularly important to midwives (Kirkham *et al.*, 2006; Kirkham and Morgan, 2006). For midwives, autonomy enables them to exercise their clinical skills appropriate to each woman's circumstances and to forge the relationships with women which are also essential to good care and job satisfaction.

Safety is clearly of key importance in maternity care. It is, however, ironic that when childbirth has never been safer in terms of mortality, fear of birth is growing amongst mothers (Green, 2002) and fear is an important factor in the professional culture around birth (Kirkham and Stapleton, 2004). Fear leads to rigidity and a need to control, and fear of litigation is certainly one factor leading to standardization of care.

Equating safety with a proscribed 'right' clinical decision assumes a narrow professional definition of safety: ensuring a live mother and baby at the end of a defined period of care. Yet Nadine Edwards (2005) demonstrated how childbearing women have a much wider view of safety which has relationships at its centre and involves the continuing physical and mental well-being of their entire family. The 1993 Department of Health Report 'Changing Childbirth' also stated:

> Safety is not an absolute concept. It is part of a greater picture encompassing all aspects of health and wellbeing. Each woman should be approached as an individual, and given clear and unbiased information on the options which are available to her, and in this way helped to balance the risks and benefits for herself and her baby.
>
> We believe that safety, encompassing as it does the emotional and physical wellbeing of the mother and baby, must remain the foundation of good maternity care. (Department of Health, 1993: 10)

Treating women as individuals has to be done in a relationship and helping them balance risks and benefits is best done where there is a relationship of trust. Sadly, this is one of many aspects of that report which go largely unimplemented and it demonstrates clearly the current gap between policy and practice.

Resources

In an era in which economic efficiency is required of public services and health care is seen as a market service, resources are crucial. In Nadine Edwards' view:

> The documented but seemingly invisible quality of care that can be provided by midwives is difficult to promote in the neoliberal market place because midwifery is labour, skill and time intensive and much of what it achieves remains hidden, and is therefore inefficient in terms of monetary profit. (Edwards, 2008a: 465)

This creates a situation where – even when hospitals have their full staffing establishment, and this is rarely the case – midwives on the ground experience a shortage of staff. Midwives certainly think that a shortage of midwives and of other resources makes maternity care less safe in England (Kirkham et al., 2006; Kirkham and Morgan 2006; Smith et al., 2009). Midwifery vacancy rates are rising at the time of writing (Practising Midwife, 2009b). The RCM annual survey of UK heads of midwifery services (quoted in RCOG et al., 2007: 5) shows that a growing majority hold the view that the number of funded midwifery posts in their trust is not adequate for the level of work undertaken. This situation is exacerbated by extra government funding for maternity services and for increasing the number of midwives not being specifically earmarked (Smith *et al.*, 2009) and often not reaching those services (*Guardian*, 2009).

Payment by Results (PBR) is still being developed as the system for funding maternity care in England (O'Sullivan and Tyler, 2009). This tariff pays significantly more for births with technical interventions, which are costly but must always be available options, and this has been a great concern to those providing services such as birth centres where the emphasis is on relationships rather than technology (Jowitt, 2009). Efforts to support and promote normal birth inevitably encounter perverse economic incentives under this system.

Recent work by three obstetricians (Budhaa *et al.*, 2009) shows that their Trust is claiming significantly less than it is entitled to under PBR because not all data is being entered on the appropriate forms. To rectify this they 'are now looking at ways to deliver a short compulsory teaching session to all the midwives as well as convince the powers to provide us with more clerical staff to deal with routine paperwork' (Budhhaa *et al.*, 2009: 809). This is a well-conducted piece of work that was worth doing in financial terms. It also demonstrates the values of the system within which we work, where each new organizational development creates a fresh opportunity for clinicians to be discovered as negligent in record keeping and therefore trained and exhorted to do more clerical work.

The pressure for midwives to capture every task they perform so that it can be coded and paid for defines the service as a set of tasks. This may lead service commissioners to examine 'tasks' and question whether in fact a midwife is needed to perform particular tasks. As 'relationship' doesn't have a tariff *per se* (although one-to-one care in labour is now embedded as an aspiration and is being monitored), the midwife is at risk of being be 'tasked' out of business as health-care assistants or maternity assistants are seen as perfectly able to do many tasks at less cost.

The policy context

In 1992 the House of Commons *Health Select Committee Maternity Report* (House of Commons, 1992) concluded that a medical model of care should no longer drive maternity services. This ushered in an era of increased policy influence for consumers. The subsequent document *Changing Childbirth* (Department of Health, 1993) marked something of a watershed in Department of Health policy documents. The Expert Maternity Group, which wrote the report, included the president of the National Childbirth Trust, a management consultant and a health authority chief executive, alongside an obstetrician, a paediatrician, a GP and a midwife. It was clearly informed by the views of consumer groups and had a real emphasis on relationships in maternity care. Its remit was, however, much narrower than that of the Select Committee Report which informed it (House of Commons, 1992), which had a more social focus, raising key social issues affecting childbearing outcomes, such as poverty.

The recommendations of *Changing Childbirth* (Department of Health, 1993) addressed the individuality of women's needs, their need for information, involvement and choice in the planning of their care, continuity of care within an ongoing relationship with a lead professional, accessibility of services and privacy in labour and postnatally. Support within an ongoing relationship with a midwife was emphasized. The aims were to be achieved within five years, including the ambitious aim that 'at least 75% of women should know the person who cares for them during their delivery' (Department of Health, 1993: 70). A number of highly innovative pilot schemes followed, most seeking to achieve continuity of care, a considerable number of which were funded by Department of Health grants. Despite excellent evaluations in many cases, most of these pilot schemes ended when their funding finished. There was no requirement that service providers implement *Changing Childbirth* and it faded into history, leaving many midwives and childbirth campaigners disillusioned. It did, however, influence subsequent policy documents and more recent policy statements have built on the foundation laid in *Changing Childbirth*.

Maternity Matters (Department of Health, 2007) is the current policy document at the time of writing. It builds on and puts into policy terms the National Services Framework for Children, Young People and Maternity Services (Department of Health, 2004). In the foreword to *Maternity Matters* the Secretary of State for Health stresses the aims of 'positive experiences for everyone', 'a wider choice in maternity care' and 'the need for flexible services with a focus on the needs of the individual' (p. 2). It is also cheering to see specific mention of these issues as applied to childbearing women from 'our most deprived communities'. This document lays down 'choice guarantees' to be achieved by the end of 2009 (p. 5). In addition to choice of how to access maternity care, type of antenatal care, place of birth and postnatal care, it is stated that 'every woman will be supported by a midwife she knows and trusts throughout her pregnancy and after birth' (p. 5). This statement has profound implications for the mother–midwife relationship, since it speaks of a continuing relationship which allows time for the midwife and mother to get to know each other and for trust to be developed.

Maternity Matters was written to be implemented and for that implementation to be monitored; a monitoring framework is part of the document (Department of Health, 2007: 26). Early signs of preparation for such monitoring are highly encouraging and open up the possibility of new developments in the midwife–mother relationship. It is, however, important not to underestimate the changes that would be needed just to bring about the choice of place of birth for all women.

Maternity care policy statements echo the general themes of policy statements covering the whole NHS. The Darzi Report says little about maternity care specifically, but what it does say is significant: 'women want high quality personal care with greater choice over place of birth and care provided by a named midwife' (Darzi, 2008: 18). The document stresses the need for the most effective care throughout the NHS, both clinically and in terms of costs, seeing quality as consisting of good clinical outcomes plus a positive patient experience with appropriate monitoring and outcomes available to the public. The two themes of efficiency and consumer empowerment are closely meshed throughout the report, together with putting front-line staff in control, empowering staff and supporting NHS staff to deliver high-quality care.

As policy aims, there can be tensions between efficiency and consumer empowerment. This is especially likely when the empowered professionals are making decisions, such as centralization of services, on grounds of greater economic efficiency and more efficient use of their own services. Clearly, much will depend on the importance attached to patient experiences and how those experiences are monitored.

The National Institute for Health and Clinical Excellence Clinical Guideline on intrapartum care (NICE, 2007) has considerable implications for the midwife–mother relationship, not least in relation to the clear statement of the need for 'supportive one-to-one care'(p. 7). 'This guideline offers best practice advice' (p. 6) and opens with the statement that 'women and their families should always be treated with kindness, respect and dignity'. It goes on to stress that women and families' views concerning their care should be 'sought and respected' and stresses the importance of informed decision making, good communication and involving the woman in flexible care. The guidance given is clear and detailed and helpful to midwives, especially with regard to outmoded practices. Nevertheless, guidelines can come to be seen as rules. For instance, the frequency of auscultation of the foetal heart (FH) in labour is derived from research studies comparing different methods of FH monitoring, not seeking to determine the ideal frequency of auscultation, yet these frequencies came to be accepted as professional opinion and were then incorporated into guidelines; midwives now have to justify any deviation from these 'rules'. The 'best-practice' title of such guidelines carries great authority, despite the rhetoric of consumer choice.

Normality and safety

At a time of increasing medicalization and technical interventions in maternity care and a generally increased preoccupation with risk in our society, safety and normality have become major themes in policy documents. The rising rate of caesarean sections (24.6 per cent in 2007–08) and other technical interventions in childbirth (Information Centre for Health and Social Care, 2009) is widely felt to be unacceptable, especially since there has been little concurrent improvement in clinical outcomes. This has led to considerable work around supporting normal birth, as can be seen on the websites for the Royal Colleges involved with birth and the NHS Institute for Innovations and Improvements. A very clear consensus statement was issued by the Royal Colleges of Obstetrics and of Midwifery together with the National Childbirth Trust, with an impressive number of supporting organizations. The statement (NCT *et al.*, 2007) gives an agreed definition of normal birth and makes useful recommendations, including 'the chance for women to get to know their midwife prior to labour', one-to-one support in labour, choice of place of birth and the implementation of NICE Guidelines. Thus we see again the rhetoric of relationship and choice alongside the stress on standardization of services. One very interesting recommendation is 'Revision of Payment by Results tariffs in England, as a matter of urgency, to remove the current perverse incentive to maintain high intervention rates' (p. 2), which could, if implemented, have a really positive impact on the finances of midwife-led units.

The detection of abnormality is highly valued in our risk-conscious and medicalized society. Monitoring and surveillance have proliferated in maternity care, thus defining all women, not merely those with apparent problems, as needing medical procedures (Arney, 1982). Whilst the NICE Guidelines have usefully highlighted occasions when maximum monitoring is not recommended (NICE, 2007: 28), the assumption is now established that normality has to be continually proved. This assumption has greatly added to the work of midwives. Such monitoring and fears concerning safety now extend to social as well as clinical risk and require midwives to monitor for risks such as domestic violence or potential child abuse. This monitoring can undermine the midwife–mother relationship, especially if trust has not already been established and the mother feels that the midwife is prying. There is also the potential for midwives to be blamed if they did not detect social risks, in a way which previously was only experienced by social workers (Robinson, 2009).

Safer Childbirth (RCOG *et al.*, 2007) was produced by the four Royal Colleges involved with maternity care and sets minimum standards for the organization and delivery of care in labour. Good communication between professionals and with care users is stressed repeatedly and much that is laid down with regard to staffing would improve the time midwives have available to forge and maintain relationships with women. The document is balanced in its approach and its wording. It is the only official document I have read which requires women to be told, prior to booking, the risks of hospital birth as well as the risks of birth in other settings. The complexity of the many standards set reflects the complex structures involved in maternity care. These standards carry a lot of weight because of their source, but no standards can fit all circumstances or always be observed as is demonstrated in the report (RCOG *et al.*, 2007, Appendix 1) on the implementation of the recommendations of the previous report, *Towards Safer Childbirth* (RCOG and RCM, 1999).

The King's Fund Report *Safe Births* calls for just the 'single set of evidence-based guidelines that are backed by professional organisations, NICE and other organisations' (2008: 62) that the Royal Colleges have endeavoured to provide (see above). The review in the *Association for Improvements in Maternity Services Journal* states that this report does an 'excellent job of pointing out that the "safety" women may be coerced into accepting is both relative and limited' (Edwards, 2008b: 18). It commends the report for being meticulous in setting out 'technologically to best protect women and babies who suffer major incidents during childbearing'. But 'the report does not get to grips with the underlying problems of different ideologies surrounding birth, where safety might be defined differently depending on one's beliefs, values and circumstances' (Edwards, 2008b: 19). Fundamental to all the professional documents on safety lies the professional definition of safety, despite the inclusion of consumerist statements on choice.

Conclusion

Improved and sustained midwife–mother relationships have now been supported by Department of Health policy for 17 years. There are excellent examples of projects where midwives give real continuity of care and relationships are fostered (e.g. McCourt and Stevens, 2009). Yet the majority of women having babies in England experience a very fragmented service, with little opportunity to get to know 'their' midwife. Some women come to trust their community midwife. But with staff rotation, reduced antenatal consultations, fewer postnatal visits and few arrangements whereby community midwives can attend 'their' mothers in labour (except for home births), many women do not get to know, or even identify, 'their' community midwife.

Meanwhile, working in an underresourced service, and often feeling they lack autonomy, wears midwives down (Kirkham *et al.*, 2006; Kirkham and Morgan, 2006). Midwives value the relationships with women in which much of their job satisfaction is rooted. When they feel that these relationships are threatened or undermined or they cannot practise midwifery as they would wish, some become disillusioned and some leave (Ball *et al.*, 2002). Those who stay have to adjust to a frustrating situation. This adjustment and the expectations of the service within which they work can lead to the development of coping mechanisms, such as bullying (Kirkham, 2007) or professional dissociation (Garrett, 2008), which are very damaging to all concerned in the long term. Despite policy exhortations to good relationships and good communication, it is very difficult to behave in a caring manner and foster relationships within a fragmented service, run on an industrial model and understaffed. It is perhaps not surprising that midwives' behaviour can be seen as characterized by 'obedience and conformity' (Hollins Martin and Bull, 2008) or experienced as uncaring (Eliasson *et al.*, 2009).

There is much reason for optimism in current policy documents, which, if actually implemented, could transform practice, given sufficient midwives. The bodies producing statements and toolkits demonstrate a real degree of consensus about the problems. The proposed means of achieving change, however, tend to be rooted in targets rather than relationships. The main changes in practice currently continue to standardize care and the documents that call for care to be personalized also call for the guidelines which standardize it. This leads Nadine Edwards to conclude:

The best that can be done in this under-resourced climate is to attempt to make care technically safe in settings that reduce safety, through standardisation of practice. (Edwards, 2008a: 466)

Midwives can, of course, be exhorted to do more, and many do. Debby Gould, in a recent editorial in the *British Journal of Midwifery*, stated:

> ...'quality' care is much more than a set of processes, and although having systems in place may help improve quality, they can never guarantee it... a collective focus on narrow quality targets could have unforeseen negative effects, whereby some people may avoid responsibility for their individual actions and behaviours...
>
> Quality care is elusive and immensely variable because the perception of quality care must inevitably reside within the individual delivering that care and the individual receiving it. No matter what we say or do, it will always remain within the individual carer's gift to enhance basic care or undermine it at the point of delivery. Thus true quality care becomes a reality, not through bureaucratic processes, but by understanding the hidden personal drivers of individuals which cause them to choose one over the other. (Gould, 2009: 210)

Gould goes on to suggest that we develop a fatalistic attitude when we believe things are out of our control and that this is a logical response to a proceduralized work setting delivering standardized care. She calls for a sense of meaning to restore a 'sense of personal control and direction'. I think that she has identified the heart of the problem, but midwives are leaving midwifery because they lack autonomy at work and cannot relate to women as they would wish (Ball *et al.*, 2002). These midwives accurately 'sense' the priorities of their employers, within a public service which is increasingly target driven. It is hard, and can be personally damaging, to change one's own perceptions in the absence of organizational change.

Midwives know that childbearing women flourish when they are trusted; confidence is infectious but can easily be undermined. Midwives also flourish when they are trusted (e.g. Jones, 2000; Hunter, 2003). Our policy framework now contains the rhetoric of relationship, which could be achieved with patterns of work which allow midwives a degree of autonomy and ongoing relationships with women. This same policy carries the internal contradiction of requiring the standardization which limits both autonomy and relationship, and can produce the fear of getting something wrong which undermines confidence. To improve the midwife–mother relationship for all childbearing women, that relationship needs to be seen as important. Whilst midwives must make skilled efforts to relate, organizational change is required in order to foster relationships and end fragmented care. More midwives are needed for this to be achieved. Organization for relationship is possible and it is happening in some places, albeit slowly. We could learn from places as far apart as Torbay (Leyshon, 2004), Australia (Homer *et al.*, 2001, 2008) and New Zealand (see Chapter 12), where real moves are being made to develop the midwife–mother relationship.

References

Arney, W.R. (1982) *Power and the Profession of Obstetrics*, Chicago: University of Chicago Press.

Ball, L., Curtis, P. and Kirkham, M. (2002) *Why Do Midwives Leave?* London: Royal Collage of Midwives.

Budhaa, L., Sanjeevib, A. and Navaneethamc, N. (2009) What happened to our money? *British Journal of Midwifery* 16(12): 806–9.

Curtis, P., Woodhill, R. and Stapleton, H. (2007) The peer–professional interface in a community-based, breastfeeding peer support project, *Midwifery* 23(2): 146–56.

Darzi, Lord (2008) *High Quality Care for All.* London: HMSO

Department of Children, Schools and Families (2003) *Every Child Matters*, London: Department of Children, Schools and Families.

Department of Health (1993) *Changing Childbirth: Report of the Expert Maternity Group*, London: HMSO.

Department of Health (2004) *National Services Framework for Children, Young People and Maternity Services:* London, Department of Health.

Department of Health (2007) *Maternity Matters: Choice, Access and Continuity of Care in a Safe Service*, London: Department of Health.

Dykes, F. (2003) *Infant Feeding Initiative: A Report Evaluating the Breastfeeding Practice Projects 1999–2002*, London: Department of Health.

Edwards, N. (2005) *Birthing Autonomy*, Abingdon: Routledge.

Edwards, N. (2008a) Safety in birth: The contextual conundrums faced by women in a 'risk society', driven by neoliberal policies, *MIDIRS Midwifery Digest* 18(4): 463–70.

Edwards, N. (2008b) Safe births: Everybody's business, *AIMS Journal* 20(3): 18–19.

Eliasson, M., Kainz, G. and von Post, I. (2009) Uncaring midwives, *MIDIRS Midwifery Digest* 19(1): 29–35.

European Union (1993) Council Directive 93/104/EC of 23 November 1993, www.incomesdata.co.uk/information/worktimedirective.htm, accessed March 2010.

Freidson, E. (1970) *Professional Dominance: The Social Structure of Medical Care*, Chicago: Aldine.

Garrett, E.F. (2008) The childbearing experiences of survivors of childhood sexual abuse, PhD thesis, Sheffield Hallam University.

Gould, D. (2009) Quality care is more than a set of processes, *British Journal of Midwifery* 17(4): 210.

Green, J.M. (2002) Verbal presentation of findings of the Greater Expectations Study,

Sheffield: University of Sheffield, Society for Reproductive and Infant Psychology Conference.

Griffiths, R. (2009) Maternity care pathways and the law, *British Journal of Midwifery* 17(5): 324–5.

Guardian (2009) Funding gap puts maternity reform at risk, *Guardian* 22 December: 1.

HMSO (1892) *Report from the Select Committee on the Registration of Midwives, House of Commons,* London: HMSO.

Hollins Martin, C.J. and Bull, P. (2008) Obedience and conformity in clinical practice, *British Journal of Midwifery* 16(8): 504–9.

Homer, C., Brodie, P. and Leap, N. (2001) *Establishing Models of Continuity of Midwifery Care in Australia: A Resource for Midwives,* Sydney: University of Technology Sydney, Centre for Family Health and Midwifery.

Homer, C., Brodie, P. and Leap, N. (2008) *Midwifery Continuity of Care,* Sydney: Churchill Livingstone/Elsevier.

House of Commons (1992) *Health Committee Second Report, Session 1991–2: Maternity Services,* London: HMSO.

Hunter, B., Berg, M., Lundgren, I., Olafsdottir, O.A. and Kirkham, M. (2008) Relationships: The hidden threads in the tapestry of maternity care, *Midwifery* 24(2): 132–7.

Hunter, M. (2003) Autonomy, clinical freedom and responsibility, in Kirkham, M. (ed.), *Birth Centres: A Social Model for Maternity Care,* Oxford: Elsevier Science.

Information Centre for Health and Social Care (2009) *NHS Maternity Statistics, England 2007–8,* London: NHS.

Jacobs, J. (1992) *Systems of Survival,* London: Hodder and Stoughton.

Jones, O. (2000) Supervision in a midwife managed birth centre, in Kirkham, M. (ed.) *Developments in the Supervision of Midwives,* Manchester: Books for Midwives.

Jordan, B. (1987) The hut and the hospital: Information, power and symbolism in the artefacts of birth, *Birth* 14(1): 36–40.

Jowitt, M. (2009) Maternity services funding, *Midwifery Matters* 121(Summer): 28.

King's Fund (2008) *Safe Birth,* London: King's Fund.

Kirkham, M. (ed.) (2004) *Informed Choice in Maternity Care,* Basingstoke: Palgrave.

Kirkham, M. (2007) Traumatised midwives, *AIMS Journal* 19(1): 12–13.

Kirkham, M. and Morgan, R.K. (2006) *Why Midwives Return and their Subsequent Experience,* London: Department of Health (www.nhsemployers.org and www.rcm. org, accessed March 2010).

Kirkham, M. and Stapleton, H. (eds) (2001) *Informed Choice in Maternity Care: An Evaluation of Evidence Based Leaflets,* York: NHS Centre for Reviews and Dissemination.

Kirkham, M. and Stapleton, H. (2004) The culture of the maternity services in Wales and England as a barrier to informed choice, in Kirkham, M. (ed.), *Informed Choice in Maternity Care,* Basingstoke: Palgrave Macmillan.

Kirkham, M., Morgan, R.K. and Davies, C. (2006) *Why Midwives Stay,* London: Department of Health (www.nhsemployers.org and www.rcm.org, accessed March 2010).

Leyshon, L. (2004) Integrating caseloads across a whole service: The Torbay model, *MIDIRS Midwifery Digest,* 14(1, Supplement 1): S9–S11.

Macfarlane, A. (2007) Reconfiguration of maternity units – what is the evidence? *Radical Statistics* 96: 77–86.

Marmot, M. (2004) *Status Syndrome,* London: Bloomsbury.

McCourt, C. and Stevens, T. (2009) Relationships and reciprocity in caseload midwifery, in Hunter, B. and Deery, R. (eds), *Emotions in Midwifery and Reproduction,* Basingstoke: Palgrave.

National Childbirh Trust, Royal College of Midwives and Royal College of Obstetricians and Gynaecologists (2007) *Making Normal Birth a Reality: Consensus Statement from the Maternity Care Working Party,* London: NCT.

NHS Litigation Authority (2008) *Clinical Negligence Scheme for Trusts. Clinical Risk Management Standards for Maternity Care,* London: Willis.

National Institute for Health and Clinical Excellence (2007) *Clinical Guideline 55. Intrapartum Care,* London: NICE.

O'Sullivan, S. and Tyler, S. (2009) New arrangements for payment by results, *Midwives* June/July: 36–7.

Pollock, A.M. (2004) *NHS plc,* London: Verso.

Practising Midwife (2009a) Editorial: Computer systems could manage high-risk births, *Practising Midwife* 12(1): 8.

Practising Midwife (2009b) News item: Midwifery vacancy rates rise, *Practising Midwife* 12(8): 10.

Robinson, J. (2009) Whose baby? *AIMS Journal,* 21(2): 3.

Royal College of Obstetricians and Gynaecologists and Royal College of Midwives (1999) *Towards Safer Childbirth: Minimum Standards for the Organisation of Labour Wards,* London: RCOG Press.

Royal College of Obstetricians and Gynaecologists, Royal College of Midwives, Royal College of Anaesthetists and Royal College of Paediatrics and Child Health (2007) *Safer Childbirth: Minimum Standards for the Organisation and Delivery of Care in Labour,* London: RCOG Press.

Sackett, D.L., Richardson, W.S., Rosenberg, W. and Haynes, R.B. (1997) *Evidence Based Medicine: How to Practise and Teach EBM,* London: Churchill, Livingstone.

Sennett, R. (2008) *The Craftsman,* London: Yale University Press.

Smith, A.H.K., Dixon, A.L. and Page, L.A. (2009) Health care professionals' views about safety in maternity services, *Midwifery* 25(1): 21–31.

Smith, F.B. (1979) T*he People's Health,* London: Croom Helm.

Thornton, J. (2006) *Maternity Unit Mergers in the NHS,* www.igreens.org.uk/maternity_unit_mergers_in_the_nh.htm, accessed March 2010.

US Department of Health and Human Services (2009) *Head Start Impact Study and Follow-up 2000–2009,* Administration for Children and Families, Office of Planning, Research and Evaluation, www.acf.hhs.gov/programs/opre/hs/impact_study/, accessed March 2010.

Walker, J. (2003) Midwifery assistants: A place for non-midwives in a midwifery service, in Kirkham, M. (ed.), *Birth Centres: A Social Model for Maternity Care,* Oxford: Elsevier Science.

CHAPTER 2

The Less We Do the More We Give

NICKY LEAP

In this chapter I shall use the first person in order to acknowledge and own the subjectivity of the ideas I shall be exploring. Feminists, such as Christine Webb (1992), have advocated this technique for some time when presenting a personal evaluation or critique. The thoughts expressed in this chapter have arisen from my midwifery practice over three decades in Britain and Australia and are not necessarily based on standard 'research-based evidence'. The chapter therefore contributes to a growing body of opinion arguing that knowledge arising from experience and understandings of physiology and contexts should not be discounted in the drive to develop evidence-based practice, particularly around decision making regarding individualized care and reflection on practice (Fahy, 2008; Mantzoukas, 2007).

Although I am a mother, I am writing this chapter from the perspective of a midwife. Therefore, when I use the collective pronoun it will usually be in order to generalize about how we, as midwives, engage with women. This is not to deny the important contribution to my thinking that several midwives played in my life on the occasions when I became a new mother, or the insights that arise from being on the other side of the midwife–mother partnership.

The concept of the less we do, the more we give

In life there is the potential to stumble across a phrase that pulls us up short, often a simple truth that will resonate through our core beliefs and values, heralding a profound impact on how we approach life thereafter. So it was for me when I was a newly qualified midwife and independent midwife Hazel Smith said, in an almost throwaway aside, 'You know, in midwifery, it's often true that the less we do, the more we give.' At that time these words may have reflected Hazel's interest in Zen or her passion for reflecting on life and midwifery, but for me it was a gift. It altered the way I practised and became part of a midwifery philosophy at the very heart of how I see the role of the midwife.

During my midwifery training, I had learnt a lot about 'doing things'. I had learnt that when you are thrown together with a labouring woman whom you have never met before, you work hard at building rapport and gaining her trust. This would involve a lot of talking, finding common ground, jokes, massage, eye contact, loving attention, sitting beside her throughout labour, encouraging her with the sponge and iced water constantly poised. This is what I thought being 'with woman' was all about.

Midwives like Hazel Smith started showing me another way. I saw these midwives checking that all was well when a woman was labouring at home and then going to lie down in another room – or even going home if the woman was happy with that arrangement. I saw them sitting in a corner of a room in watchful anticipation during labour, but on the whole they were very quiet and non-directive. I saw women who were undisturbed withdraw into the state of consciousness that is associated with the release of endogenous opiates. I saw that where women were asking for physical support, the people doing all the eye contact, massage and loving attention were the people the woman had chosen to be there for her. The people who would have the ongoing relationship with the woman and her baby were the key players, not the midwives who would move on after the first month or so of the baby's life.

Slowly, over the years, a different underlying philosophy of care emerged as I had the privilege of working in the relatively untrammelled world of home birth practice. I learnt about the potential for women to become empowered through an approach that:

• minimizes disturbance, direction, authority and intervention
• maximizes the potential for physiology, common sense and instinctive behaviour to prevail
• places trust in the expertise of the childbearing woman
• shifts power towards the woman.

I am not saying that this approach can only happen where midwives are able to provide home birth services, only that it is easier to develop in the woman's own environment, particularly where midwives and women have a chance to get to know each other. When a woman labours in her own home, she tends to slip, undisturbed, into the productive, altered state of consciousness that takes over when the physiology of labour is swirling; neither she nor the midwife has to worry about the niceties of establishing rapport and trust. Even if they have hardly met before, the midwife views the woman in the context and culture of her own environment, surrounded by her own familiarity. The midwife does not have to negotiate a foreign terrain for the woman and this enables a dynamic that affects the interactions of all who are present. In a woman's home, it is usually relatively easy to simply 'be' alongside the labouring woman in mindful anticipation. The challenge for midwives who attend women who are labouring in out-of-home situations is to orchestrate an environment that minimizes disturbance and enhances the woman's belief in her ability to labour and give birth (Brodie and Leap, 2008). This requires an alert understanding of how power dynamics affect situations we find ourselves in on a daily basis in both our working and social lives (Leap, 2006).

The concept of 'the less we do, the more we give' is directly related to the feminist notion of empowerment. The word 'empowerment' is bandied around liberally, and I often hear midwives talk about how 'we need to empower women'. There is an inherent contradiction in such a statement. None of us can 'empower' another person or indeed give women power. By its very nature, power is not given but taken. At every stage of our interactions with childbearing women, as midwives, we should be adopting behaviours that will maximize the potential for women to take up the power that will enable them to lead fulfilling lives as individuals and as mothers. This process of empowerment may have far-reaching consequences in terms of women's feelings of self-worth and confidence.

In this chapter, I shall explore some examples of how the philosophy of enabling women to take their power relates to midwifery practice. In particular, I shall consider how midwives can engage with women in ways that avoid dependency and enable the potential for women to learn from each other and build supportive networks in the community. First, it may be useful to consider the overall nature of the midwifery relationship that we refer to as being 'with woman', the term derived from the Anglo-Saxon *mid wyf*.

The particular nature of the 'with woman' relationship

The relationship that develops between the woman and the midwife is at the core of human caring and may provide the basis of the professional body of knowledge that encapsulates midwifery. (Siddiqui, 1999: 111)

As has been articulated so well by midwifery leaders in New Zealand (Guilliland and Pairman, 1995), the relationship between a woman and her midwife is based on mutual respect, trust and the potential for both parties to learn from each other as they engage in partnership. Through their interactions, there is the potential for both the woman and her midwife to be enriched by exploring the inherent possibilities that are within the self (Leap and Pairman, 2006). Much has been written about midwives facilitating the empowerment of women through their experience of childbirth, but this midwifery skill depends on the midwife being self-aware and 'in touch' with herself (Hunter, 2002; Siddiqui, 1999). Furthermore, it cannot happen where midwives themselves are disempowered, a situation that can lead to disengagement and disparate relationships between women and their midwives (Thompson, 2004).

Within the concept of continuity of care, this relationship is different from any other relationship that involves health-care workers. Having a baby can be seen as a rite of passage. In many situations throughout the world, there is the potential for a woman to engage a 'midwife' to be alongside her as she explores how the experience of childbirth has impacts on all elements of her life. This includes the emotional, physical, spiritual, intellectual and social challenges and ramifications as she journeys through pregnancy, childbirth and new motherhood. The 'midwifery overview' is maintained, ensuring that all these interwoven elements of the woman's life are kept in relief, whatever the events that unfold. The midwife works with the woman and her community, collaborating with other health professionals if necessary, to ensure that everything is done to ensure a safe and supported transition to new motherhood, taking into consideration the woman's individual circumstances and wishes.

With occasional exceptions to be found in the field of palliative care, there is no other example of a person engaging a health-care worker to be alongside them in this way throughout a life event, or 'episode of care' (a reductionist term often used by health-care economists). The midwifery relationship is therefore intrinsically different from the relationships with clients that develop in, for example, nursing and medicine. This is not to deny the important and potentially emancipatory nature of other health professionals' relationships with clients. Old-fashioned rhetoric about midwifery being different from nursing and medicine because it adopts a 'wellness', holistic approach is no longer useful in a culture where primary health-care philosophy and politics have permeated the education and working environment of all health-care workers. Furthermore, in many western countries there is a move to ensure that access to midwifery continuity of care is not restricted to women considered to be 'well' or 'low risk'; indeed, some midwifery group practices are developed specifically to address the needs of women who are most vulnerable to poverty and ill-health (Byrom and Downe, 2007; Homer *et al.*, 2008). It is therefore important to articulate how the unique nature of midwifery is based in the relationship between the midwife and the woman across cultures and contexts.

Embracing uncertainty together

One of the essential elements of the midwifery process of being 'with woman' can be seen as the embracing of uncertainty together. This notion is at odds with the dominant paradigm of certainty as the goal of modern science (Downe and McCourt, 2008). The uncomfortable fact is that no amount of screening and information giving can give pregnant women and new parents the complete certainty they seek or, indeed, the ability to make 'the right choice' (Leap and Edwards, 2006). The question marks of pregnancy are the beginning of a process of grappling with the uncertainty and decision making that will persist throughout the experience of raising a child. In the early days of this process, engaging with uncertainty involves profound learning for each individual woman and her midwife in a way that is reciprocal and unique. To describe the relationship between the two as one of 'equals', however, denies an inherent power imbalance. Women ask midwives to join with them in order to draw on our expertise, our experience and our knowledge. They are asking us to provide them with a safety net, a point of reference that they can choose to use as a resource in a world where there are more questions than answers.

Recognizing and owning our midwifery expertise is an important step in understanding the power dynamics of this situation. Equally important is an understanding of the limitations of our expertise. There is a fragile element within the notion we call 'informed choice'. Apart from the potential for decision making that is biased by the person who is doing the informing, there are many situations where no amount of information will clarify the decision process for women (Kirkham, 2004; Leap and Edwards, 2006). As identified by Robin Gregg (1995: 114):

> We need to develop a more nuanced view of choice, one that recognises how historical and present patterns of oppression construct and constrain women's choices, but also acknowledges women's agency and capacity for self-determination.

Instead of giving women lists of possibilities and options to choose from, a 'wait and see/keep your options open' policy is arguably more useful. In antenatal groups and with individual women I have found that in many situations, raising the notion of 'uncertainty' has led to more fruitful discussion than pursuing the idea of 'informed choice'. Sometimes, embracing uncertainty brings a sense of calm, a sense that what will be, will be. This is not about engendering a passive fatalism, more about enabling women to learn to trust that they will cope with whatever comes their way. Working through these issues is particularly important in a culture that privileges the notion of 'choice' and continues to design policy documents accordingly (Department of Health, 1993, 2007).

Believing in women

Our expertise as midwives rests in our ability to watch, to listen and to respond to any given situation with all of our senses. This will include the conscious and subconscious 'knowing' that has been generated from our experience and learning. It also involves a 'cluefulness' as we respond to the overt and covert clues from women and their worlds. The skill lies in knowing when to inform, suggest, act, seek help and, most importantly, when to be still or when to withdraw and remove ourselves. Our belief in a woman's inherent ability to be her own and her baby's expert should underpin all of these responses.

If we believe that women have within themselves everything that is needed for the physiological processes of childbirth, we are bound to ask questions about the need to employ 'complementary therapies' as a matter of course. The very act of suggesting their use in a normal process can suggest that we think women cannot manage without them or that women's bodies are in some way deficient. If, at the end of the day, after an uncomplicated pregnancy and labour, a woman feels that she could not have managed without the aid of (for example) homoeopathy, acupuncture, aromatherapy, hypnotherapy or indeed the midwife, then at some level she is giving away her power. She has invested in something outside of herself and this can perhaps subtly diminish her sense of achievement and triumph.

Ever since the wealth of publications from the alternative birth movement of 1970s North America, there has been a tendency for midwives to feel that, in the tradition of 'wise women', they should work out the deep psychological processes affecting the women they care for. The message within this literature was that midwives should engage in psychotherapeutic interventions; in other words, they should identify and help women get rid of the 'baggage' that might impede the process of childbirth.

Anne Oakley (1980) has identified and questioned a process where physiological problems of childbirth are sometimes identified as psychosomatic defences and psychological maladjustments. In a similar vein, Diane Gosden and Ann Saul (1999) have expressed concern about the potentially disempowering effects that can arise if there is a shift in the midwife's role 'from empathetic listener to a more interventionist psychological role'. Drawing on interviews with women conducted in the course of a research study on home birth in Australia (Gosden, 1996), they describe the sense of intrusion and loss of autonomy in determining their own pace of personal growth felt by women when midwives openly engage in this form of 'psychotherapy'. They cite, for example, a woman's feelings of vulnerability, self-blame and low self-esteem when the midwife suggested that she was holding on to her baby in an 'overdue' pregnancy because she was too scared to give birth (Gosden, 1996: 150).

In my own study regarding midwives' attitudes to being with women in pain during labour (Leap, 1997), midwives discussed the fallacy of predicting how women would 'be' in labour. They described a culture where midwives still tend to make these predictions in private, based on ill-founded 'psychological' value judgements and in spite of the apparent unreliability of such predictions. The place of psychotherapy philosophies in midwifery practice needs further exploration, especially in terms of the implications for power dynamics and the relationships between women and midwives.

As midwives we need to believe in women even when, or maybe especially when, it seems as though the psychosocial odds are stacked against them. This means being clear that we have confidence in their potential to be able to:

- monitor their baby's development and well-being in pregnancy
- find a way through pain in labour
- give birth in spite of any fears or previous traumas in their life
- nurture their baby and monitor the baby's well-being and development
- listen to their baby's needs and respond appropriately according to instinct and common sense
- make wise decisions in the face of uncertainty, upheaval and exhaustion.

This process of inspiring confidence in women by our confidence in their abilities is often more based in asking questions than in giving answers.

Asking women how their baby has been moving – and making it clear that there is no clinical or predictive value in us listening in to the baby's heart routinely in pregnancy (NICE, 2007) – makes it clear that we recognize the supremacy of their expertise in monitoring their baby's well-being. Thus we can encourage women's awareness and sense of independence and responsibility. We can also avoid the 'separation from self' and enforced dependency described by Emily Martin (1984: 1202):

> ...my doctor gave me the heartbeat. It's like he took it away from me because he said, 'Here's the heartbeat...' and I sort of felt like, well this is my baby's heartbeat but I can't hear it unless he does it for me... I felt funny about the fact we had to rely on him.

Similarly in the postnatal period, asking the woman how her baby 'is' and listening carefully to the answer rests in a far more empowering model of care than 'strip searching' her baby. The new mother has more knowledge of her baby than the midwife and any concerns can be followed up carefully (Gunn, 2006). The same applies for tasks that were once routine around the woman's body in the postnatal period. The process of 'top-to-toe' examination with the undignified 'checking the pad and the perineum' are no longer being advocated as routine procedures in midwifery education. Midwives are now being taught to listen to women and only perform such tasks at the invitation of a woman if she has expressed concern (Dixon, 2006).

Putting our faith in women gives them powerful messages, especially during labour where the quiet 'midwifery muttering' – 'You can do it' – when a woman is saying words to the contrary is often all it takes to get women through the aptly named 'transition' phase of labour. These are the 'whispered words of wisdom' of 'letting it be' (Lennon and McCartney, 1970). Sheila Kitzinger (1988: 18) has described the skill of helping a woman in labour to have confidence in herself and the 'power of her uterus' in terms of 'patience and the willingness to wait for the unfolding of life'. Similarly, Holly Powell Kennedy and Maureen Shannon (2004) have identified the quiet reassurance that midwives give by creating a safe space in which a woman can labour and tap into her personal strength. Midwives in their study described learning to 'sit' with a labouring woman and give quiet reassurance, sometimes by knitting:

> ...everyone thinks, OK, she's knitting, things have to be *OK*, otherwise she'd be doing. So I sit and knit. (Powell Kennedy and Shannon, 2004: 557)

Time and again I have heard women reflecting on their labours and saying, 'I didn't think I could do it, but the midwife said I could do it, so I thought, "If she thinks I can do it, then maybe I can".' Creating an environment where this level of calm and reassurance can prevail is about understanding the importance of women's individual needs for intimacy, respect and patience, most easily achieved where continuity of carer has fostered a relationship of trust (Huber and Sandall, 2009). This skill has been described in terms of 'midwifery guardianship' and is linked to the protection of all the intricacies of the psychological, spiritual and neuro-hormonal processes that promote straightforward, undisturbed birth (Fahy *et al.*, 2008).

An important key to these skills of creative patience is the ability to be with women in pain and resist the urge to try to take away the pain. Many midwives recognize the important role pain can play in labour (Leap and Vague, 2006). This is not just in terms of its place within the inter-related hormonal cascades that enable a physiological process to occur and at the same time stimulate the release of the woman's endogenous opiates. Experienced midwives will hold back from offering the 'pain relief menu' in a normal labour, knowing that where women give birth without having pain taken away from them, their sense of triumph may have far-reaching consequences (Leap and Anderson, 2004). The notion of triumph, however, does not belong only to the realm of 'normal' birth. Where women need to give birth with all the support of modern technology and surgical intervention, our expressed appreciation of the woman's courage and endurance may play an important role during the experience and in the potentially empowering process of active reflection together in the early postnatal period.

The fourth 'C': Community

> When you combine continuity of care with social support from other women, you have a powerful recipe for improving physical and psychosocial outcomes during pregnancy and childbirth for women, children and their partners. (Sandall, 1996: 621)

Starting with the groundbreaking document *Changing Childbirth* (Department of Health, 1993), maternity care policy in western countries has tended to concentrate on placing women at the centre of care by addressing the three Cs: 'Choice, Control and Continuity'. In the South East London Midwifery Group Practice (SELMGP) – a group of self-employed midwives who worked within the NHS in the 1990s with predominantly disadvantaged women – we came to believe that the three Cs should hinge on a fourth: 'Community'. We developed a 'philosophy in action' which concentrates on motivating the pregnant woman's own friendship group to be there for her, putting her in touch with other pregnant women and new mothers who will become her lifeline in the early months of her baby's life. The friendships thus formed often endure for many years, as identified by one of the women in a video that was made about the groups in Deptford, southeast London: 'I think it's most probably friends you'll have for life really' (Leap, 1992).

The SELMGP became the Albany Midwifery Group Practice and is one of several midwifery group practices that have been developed within King's Health Care, a large London teaching hospital (Reed, 2002a, 2002b). The Albany midwives continue to work within this 'philosophy in action' from community-based premises in Peckham, southeast London. Women, their families and friends are given clear messages that reinforce their own role in taking responsibility and control around their experience of childbirth. Conversely, the midwives minimize their own role. They recognize that they are invited guests in people's lives for a short while and do not delude themselves that they can change the underlying social conditions that often make life so difficult for women and their families. The aim, however, is to instil the confidence and sense of independence that can change lives. The bottom line has to be: 'You can do this.' Although the midwives end up spending more time with women where medical problems arise, in this situation they still attempt to activate the main source of support from within the woman's family and community.

A study of approximately 2000 women who have received care from the Albany midwives over ten years showed that this model of care leads to reduced interventions and improved outcomes, including a significant reduction in perinatal mortality rates when local comparisons are made (Reed and Sandall, 2008). There are probably multiple reasons why this particular midwifery group practice has sustained such impressive outcomes, but increasingly there is strong evidence to support the idea that all women should be offered midwifery continuity of care (Hatem *et al.*, 2008). It is possible that there are long-term, positive effects on women's lives of having a trusting relationship with midwives who provide support and a 'listening ear' as women face the challenges of pregnancy and new motherhood (Oakley *et al.*, 1996).

I would not want to diminish in any way the positive repercussions of our input at this crisis time in a woman's life. I would suggest, however, that we need to be mindful of the potential dangers of creating mutual dependencies if continuity of care leads to exclusive, special relationships between individual women and their midwives. There is something very worrying if a situation of 'friendship' or 'companionship' between a woman and her midwife leads to a scenario where, at a last visit, the two sit having a final cup of tea feeling overwhelmed by a sense of loss because the relationship has to end there. Luckily, this does not happen that often because most women are so absorbed by their new relationship with their baby that the strong ties with the midwife that can develop in pregnancy are already loosened into realistic proportions.

There will always be some enduring friendships that emerge between women and midwives. Such friendships are often responsible for effective political action where women and midwives work together to change systems in the interests of childbearing women. However, it is possible that our most important contribution to the long-term well-being of women and their children lies in our role in activating support and networks within the woman's community. In supporting this notion, Soo Downe (1997: 43) writes:

> Perhaps in the end the best model for women is one in which the midwife's role is not, to paraphrase a Christian Aid slogan, to 'give a woman support in childbirth and she'll be happy for a day' but 'teach a woman and her family how to tap into support systems and they'll be happy for life'.

Midwives in the SELMGP recognized that strategies to promote community support and minimize dependency also contribute to the avoidance of 'burn-out' (Leap, 1996a; Sandall, 1997). We were increasingly motivated to address these issues as we moved from the independent midwifery model that some of us had come from into a public health service (NHS) model with its incumbent pressures of increased caseload. Two important strategies that we developed within our 'philosophy in action' were the development of the 36-week home visit with the woman's supporters and the provision of antenatal and postnatal groups. These strategies became the nucleus of the midwifery group practice. We became increasingly aware that, as suggested by Mavis Kirkham (1986: 47), 'linking women with others makes them stronger'.

Moving from classes to groups

The basic structures of the antenatal group are simple and can be summarized as follows:

- Women can come to the antenatal group at any stage of their pregnancy.
- The group is there every week and is facilitated by a midwife.
- There is no fixed agenda; it evolves during the course of each session.
- Every week the facilitator co-ordinates a round where each group member in turn says their name, when their baby is due, where they are having their baby, whether it is their first baby or not, where they live, anything else they may wish to say or ask about.
- Each week somebody returns to the group with a new baby and tells their birth story. This forms a trigger for discussion and information sharing and a rich source of learning and support.

The original postnatal group grew out of a situation where women kept coming back to the antenatal group after they had had their babies. The midwives concerned hired another room and started running a postnatal group with the same structure of starting with a round so that everyone gets introduced and has a chance to say something. Again, responding to requests from women, another antenatal group was set up in the evening so that men could attend as well as women who worked during the day. The women asked for the women-only group to continue in the afternoon, as they identified that the discussion and support had a different quality at that session.

Helping You to Make Your Own Decisions: Antenatal and Postnatal Groups in Deptford, South East London (Leap, 1992) is a video that was made by women who felt passionately that they wanted to tell people about how important the groups had been to their lives:

The group has been absolutely crucial to my pregnancy.

It means that you're not there as an island trying to cope on your own with a new baby. You can ring someone up and say 'I'm feeling like throwing the baby over the balcony. Have you ever felt like that?' And they'll say, 'Right what you need to do is this…' And it might not work but that doesn't matter, it's just the fact that you've been able to have a conversation with someone in the middle of the night. You know that you're not the only one.

I would have been very isolated otherwise. Like a lot of West Indian women who work, I didn't know many women in the area.

The model for running these groups is very simple. Although we ran our groups in a community centre for many years, the model has been adapted to several settings such as:

- health centres, GPs' surgeries, midwifery group practice premises
- hospital clinics
- a maternity hospital ward for inpatients and women attending a risk assessment unit
- midwives' own homes
- a swimming pool following aquanatal swimming sessions.

The groups are not run on a 'drop-in' basis. They start and finish at a set time. Therefore we found it essential to offer a crèche to those women who had toddlers in tow. The groups run for about an hour and a half and consideration needs to be given to the timing so that the group finishes before women have to collect children from school.

The women are able to learn from each other in a way that is relevant to their lives. The midwife is not setting the agenda. She is not the central focus of the group, since the bulk of the learning comes from the sharing of ideas and experiences by women in the group:

> We were all seen as having our own expertise really. It wasn't like, 'Experts/Novices... Midwives/Us'. We were all seen as having a valuable contribution to make. That meant we took more risks, we shared more and we formed really deep friendships.

> It wasn't abstract information that you were getting. It stayed in my head because it was attached to real people. Therefore it got absorbed differently. Information came up in a sort of organic way. So that, as a woman was telling about the birth she's had last week and how the baby got stuck, the midwife picked up a pelvis and baby [doll] and showed how that happened.

One woman in the video compares the group to the antenatal classes offered in the local health centre:

> Clinic classes, the ones I went to, you were taught at a certain level, which wasn't a very high level so it was rather patronising. This group deals with the more social aspects of things. It's made me feel more comfortable with the whole attitude of being pregnant.

The advantages for midwives of working in this way are manifold. Once the structure has been set up, there is never the uncomfortable first session of a new group where the midwife has to worry about 'breaking the ice' and getting the group established. Women who have been coming for many weeks are relaxed, set the tone for newcomers and explain to them how the group operates. Since women set the agenda for the topics that are discussed each week (usually triggered by somebody's story about birth and new motherhood), the midwife does not need to prepare information, as she would do if she were running classes. The answers to any questions that arise lie within the group and the midwife facilitating can ensure that this happens by deflecting back to the group, for example: 'What do the rest of you think about this?' or: 'Has anyone else had this experience?' The midwife is not expected to have all the answers. If she does not know the answer to a complex clinical question, her response can be: 'Shall we look up what the latest thinking is about that?' – either with appropriate resources to hand or with a promise to return next week with the information.

For midwives, the group provides an illuminating forum for hearing women's stories of their experiences. Hearing them tell other women has a different quality to the reflection that happens postnatally between a woman and her midwife. It is the best situation to learn from women that I know of. There are also practical advantages in organization around continuity of carer. Where midwives work in group practices with individual caseloads, women can be invited to attend other midwives' groups if they feel it is important to them to meet the other midwives in the practice. Thus, the onus is on the woman and antenatal care does not have to be fragmented in order to 'meet the other midwives'.

The philosophical base for this way of providing community-based education and support for women – groups rather than classes – is in line with theory about adult learning (Knowles, 1975, 1978), which includes the following principles:

- An adult learner's self-concept moves from dependency to self-direction.
- Life experiences are an increasing resource for learning.
- Readiness to learn is oriented to developmental tasks and social roles.
- Learning is problem centred.
- Adults respond to a friendly, informal environment.
- The process of learning is a shared experience between teacher and learner.

In recent years, in both Australia and the UK, I have been involved in the introduction of another model that recognizes the importance of providing situations in which pregnant women can support each other and share ideas and information. Developed by midwife Sharon Schindler and rising in the early 1990s in Connecticut, CenteringPregnancy® combines antenatal care with education and support and is now offered in over 50 sites across North America, with increasing interest in other countries. Women who are due to give birth at around the same time receive all their antenatal care at the usual scheduled times, but within two-hour, structured group sessions, with continuity of facilitators – usually two midwives and/or other health professionals. This allows for dynamic learning opportunities and the development of friendship networks. Evaluations of CenteringPregnancy® have consistently demonstrated that this model is very popular with women; in marginalized and vulnerable communities in the US, it has also been linked with increased birth weight and gestational age for mothers who give birth prematurely (Baldwin, 2006; Grady and Bloom, 2004; Ickovics *et al.*, 2003; Ickovics *et al.*, 2007; Massey *et al.*, 2006).

The 36-week 'birth talk'

Another important strategy to promote community support, which was first described by the SELMGP midwives (Leap, 1996b), is the 36-week home visit. Although it became known as the 'birth talk', this session in the woman's home brings together anyone in the woman's family and friendship group who may be involved in supporting her in the early postnatal period as well as during labour. Where the woman has no support, the midwife will draw on her own contacts within the community, often women who have been through the group. The purpose of this meeting can be outlined thus:

• It provides an opportunity for the midwives to explore various choices the woman might like to make around her labour. Details are discussed such as whether she wants photographs, what she wants to do with her placenta, whether she has any particular wishes that are dictated by her culture or religion or beliefs.
• Childcare for other children can be explored and, if the children are likely to be involved during the labour, appropriate arrangements can be made for their support.
• The woman's friends can meet the midwives, determine their perspectives and be reassured that they are not going to have to negotiate on

the woman's behalf 'against' the midwives. Where people meet for the first time when a woman is in labour, much energy can be wasted in building up the trust that does not come easily on first acquaintance.

- Everyone has a chance to be clear about his or her roles. The midwives can explain that they will be there at appropriate times during the labour as a 'safety net', but that they will not be the people providing all the tender loving care. That is the job of the people who will have the ongoing relationship with the woman and her child.
- Birth photographs provide an excellent resource for talking about what to expect, particularly in terms of noise and pain. The midwives can explain that they are not being cruel if they are not offering 'pain relief' and can explain the purpose and nature of pain in labour.
- Discussion can take place about the place of birth. Many women and their supporters need to be reassured that the option to make a final decision in labour and stay at home if all is well is a safe option where midwives carry full emergency equipment with them at all times.
- The midwives can reassure everyone that all the midwives in the practice have the same philosophy of care, should someone else be their midwife during labour.
- Practical support in the early weeks following birth can be arranged. Rotas can be suggested for visiting friends to take responsibility for one pre-arranged evening each, where they will come in and cook, clean, shop or take away washing.

During this meeting, particular attention can be given to talking through the concept of 'pre-labour', also known as the 'latent phase of labour'. This can lead to realistic expectations, particularly if it is a first baby, as well as the avoidance of early hospitalization. The support group can have confidence in their ability to support the woman and not phone the midwife until labour is well established (unless they are worried). Discussion also includes clarification about what to do if the baby arrives before the midwife. Bullet points in the maternity notes can reinforce these messages by listing situations that warrant calling the midwife, as well as a simple list of instructions detailing what to do if the baby is arriving in a hurry.

In a study of the role of the 36-week birth talk in caseload midwifery practice, Joy Kemp and Jane Sandall (2008) concluded that the effectiveness of these birth talks cannot be separated from the philosophy and continuity offered by the midwives. The authors observed midwives communicating an underpinning philosophy that birth is both normal and transformational and that it is a social and cultural event. The expertise and experience of the midwives contributed to the communication of authoritative knowledge and a sense of coherence that reinforced these messages. This study described many of the issues discussed in this chapter in terms of midwifery 'philosophy in action' and approaches that enrich both women and midwives.

The midwife/woman relationship: A metaphor

When considering the 'less we do, the more we give' philosophy, it may be useful to think in terms of a metaphor. Pregnancy, birth and the early weeks of a baby's life can be seen as a journey. The midwife provides a map for the woman if she needs one, warning her at the same time that the journey includes uncharted landscapes for which there can be no planning. She points out the signposts for various alternative routes. She warns of hazards to avoid or obstacles that can be circumvented or surmounted. Most importantly, she puts the woman in touch with other women who have recently explored the same terrain, as well as those who will be making similar journeys and may wish to share resources and support each other along the way.

The midwife may be there for part of the journey if it is particularly rocky, for usually she knows the terrain well. Where she does not, she makes sure that the woman is put in touch with those who will consider the safety issues involved by offering their technical expertise and specialist knowledge of complicated landscapes. The midwife knows that for most of the journey, the woman will manage with the support of her chosen travelling companions, so she gives these people various tools that may be useful along the way. She will have prepared them all to keep an open mind about the many unforeseeable adventures they may have ahead. She will have been at pains to instil confidence and to give them the message that she believes them all to have the stamina and courage to handle anything that comes their way.

At the end of the journey, the midwife will enjoy celebrating the woman's sense of triumph and achievement as she sets off with her friends on her next journey. The midwife says goodbye and enjoys a quiet satisfaction. She knows that the woman has discovered her independence. Whatever the unplanned events of the next phase of her life, the woman will be able to rely on her inner strengths, her new knowledge, her common sense and her instinctive responses. A new-found awareness of these skills will get her through all the crucial decisions and responses she will have to make in this next journey.

Conclusion

The words of the *Tao Te Ching*, written over 2500 years ago (cited in Heider, 1986), summarize the concepts that have been explored in this chapter:

> The wise leader does not intervene unnecessarily. The leader's presence is felt, but often the group runs itself...
>
> Remember that you are facilitating another person's process. It is not your process. Do not intrude. Do not control. Do not force your own needs and insights into the foreground.
>
> If you do not trust a person's process, that person will not trust you.
>
> Imagine that you are a midwife: You are assisting at someone else's birth. Do good without show or fuss. Facilitate what is happening rather than what you think ought to be happening. If you must take the lead, lead so that the mother is helped, yet still free and in charge.
>
> When the baby is born, the mother will rightly say, 'We did it ourselves!'

References

Baldwin, K. (2006) Comparison of selected outcomes of CenteringPregnancy versus traditional prenatal care, *Journal of Midwifery and Women's Health* 51(4): 256–72.

Brodie, P. and Leap, N. (2008) From ideal to real: The interface between birth territory and the maternity service organisation, in Fahy, K., Foureur, M. and Hastie, C. (eds), *Birth Territory and Midwifery Guardianship*, Edinburgh: Butterworth Heinemann/ Elsevier.

Byrom, S. and Downe, S. (2007) Narratives from the Blackburn West caseholding team: Setting up, *British Journal of Midwifery* 15(4): 225–7.

Department of Health (1993) *Changing Childbirth*, London: Department of Health/HMSO.

Department of Health (2007) *Maternity Matters: Choice, Access and Continuity of Care in a Safe Service*, London: Department of Health.

Dixon, L. (2006) Supporting women becoming mothers, in Pairman, S., Pincombe, J., Thorogood, C. and Tracy, S. (eds), *Midwifery: Preparation for Practice*, Sydney: Elsevier.

Downe S (1997) The less we do, the more we give, *British Journal of Midwifery* 5(1): 43.

Downe, S. and McCourt, C. (2008) From being to becoming: Reconstructing childbirth knowledges, in Downe, S. (ed.), *Normal Childbirth: Evidence and Debate*, 2nd edn, Edinburgh: Churchill Livingstone/Elsevier.

Fahy, K. (2008) Evidence-based midwifery and power/knowledge, *Women and Birth* 21(1): 1–2.

Fahy, K., Foureur, M. and Hastie, C. (2008) *Birth Territory and Midwifery Guardianship: Creating Birth Space*, Oxford: Elsevier.

Gosden, D. (1996) Dissenting Voices: Conflict and Complexity in the Home Birth Movement in Australia. MA Honours thesis. Anthropology Department, Maquarie University, Sydney.

Gosden, D. and Saul, A. (1999) Reflections on the use of psychotherapy in midwifery, *British Journal of Midwifery*, 7(9): 543–6

Grady, M. and Bloom, K. (2004) Pregnancy outcomes of adolescents enrolled in a Centering Pregnancy program, *Journal of Midwifery and Women's Health* 49(5): 412–20.

Gregg, R. (1995) *Pregnancy in a High-Tech Age: Paradoxes of Choice*, New York: New York University Press.

Guilliland, K. and Pairman, S. (1995) *The Midwifery Partnership: A Model for Practice*, Wellington, New Zealand: Department of Nursing and Midwifery Monograph Series, Victoria University.

Gunn, J. (2006) Supporting the newborn infant, in Pairman, S., Pincombe, J., Thorogood, C. and Tracy, S. (eds), *Midwifery: Preparation for Practice*, Sydney: Elsevier.

Hatem, M., Sandall, J., Devane, D., Soltani, H. and Gates, S. (2008) Midwife-led versus other models of care for childbearing women, *Cochrane Database of Systematic Reviews* (Issue 4. Art. No.: CD004667. DOI: 10.1002/14651858.CD004667.pub2).

Heider, J. (1986) *The Tao of Leadership*, Aldershot: Wildwood House.

Homer, C., Brodie, P. and Leap, N. (2008) Midwifery continuity of care for specific communities, in Homer, C., Brodie, P. and Leap, N. (eds), *Midwifery Continuity of Care: A Practical Guide*, Sydney: Churchill Livingstone/Elsevier.

Huber, U. and Sandall, J. (2009) A qualitative exploration of the creation of calm in a continuity of care model of maternity care in London, *Midwifery* 25(6): 613–21.

Hunter, B. (2002) Being with woman: A guiding concept for the care of labouring women, *Journal of Obstetric, Gynecologic and Neonatal Nursing* 31: 650–57.

Ickovics, J., Kershaw, T., Westdahl, C., Magriples, U., Massey, Z., Reynolds, H. and Schindler Rising, S. (2007) Group prenatal care and perinatal outcomes: A randomized controlled trial, *Obstetrics and Gynecology* 110(2): 330–39.

Ickovics, J., Kershaw, T., Westdahl, C., Rising, S.S., Klima, C., Reynolds, H. and Magriples, U. (2003) Group prenatal care and preterm birth weight: Results from a two-site matched cohort study, *Obstetrics and Gynecology* 102: 1051–7.

Kemp, J. and Sandall, J. (2008) Normal birth, magical birth: The role of the 36-week birth talk in midwifery practice, *Midwifery*, doi:10.1016/j.midw.2008.1007.1002.

Kirkham, M. (1986) A feminist perspective in midwifery, in Webb, C. (ed.), *Feminist Practice in Women's Health*, Chichester: John Wiley & Sons.

Kirkham, M. (ed.) (2004) *Informed Choice in Maternity Care*, London: Macmillan.

Kitzinger, S. (ed.) (1988) *The Midwife Challenge*, London: Pandora.

Knowles, M.S. (1975) *Self-Directed Learning: A Guide for Learners and Teachers*, Chicago: Follett.

Knowles, M.S. (1978) *The Adult Learner: A Neglected Species*, London: Gulf.

Leap, N. (1992) *Helping You to Make Your Own Decisions: Antenatal and Postnatal Groups in Deptford SE London*, VHS Video, available from Birth International, www.birthinternational.com.au, accessed March 2010.

Leap, N. (1996a) Caseload practice: A recipe for burnout? *British Journal of Midwifery* 4(6): 329.

Leap, N. (1996b) Woman-led midwifery: The development of a new midwifery philosophy in Britain, in Murray, S. (ed.), *Baby Friendly Mother Friendly*, London: Mosby.

Leap, N. (1997) A Midwifery Perspective on Pain in Labour, unpublished MSc dissertation, South Bank University, London.

Leap, N. (2006) Promoting physiological birth, in Pairman, S., Pincombe, J., Thorogood, C. and Tracy, M. (eds), *Midwifery: Preparation for Practice,* Sydney: Elsevier.

Leap, N. and Anderson, T. (2004) The role of pain and the empowerment of women, in Downe, S. (ed.), *Normal Childbirth: Evidence and Debate,* Edinburgh: Churchill Livingstone.

Leap, N. and Edwards, N. (2006) The politics of involving women in decision making, in Page, L.A. and Campbell, R. (eds), *The New Midwifery: Science and Sensitivity in Practice,* 2nd edn, London: Churchill Livingstone/Elsevier.

Leap, N. and Pairman, S. (2006) Working in partnership, in Pairman, S., Pincombe, J., Thorogood, C. and Tracy, S. (eds), *Midwifery: Preparation for Practice,* Sydney: Elsevier.

Leap, N. and Vague, S. (2006) Working with pain in labour, in Pairman, S., Pincombe, J., Thorogood, C. and Tracy, S. (eds), *Midwifery: Preparation for Practice,* Sydney: Elsevier.

Lennon, J. and McCartney, P. (1970) *Let It Be (lyrics),* London: Northern Songs.

Mantzoukas, S. (2007) A review of evidence-based practice, nursing research and reflection: Levelling the hierarchy, *Journal of Clinical Nursing* 17(2): 214–23.

Martin, E. (1984) Pregnancy, labor and body image in the United States, *Science and Medicine* 19(11): 1201–6.

Massey, Z., Rising, S. and Ickovics, J. (2006) Centering Pregnancy group prenatal care: Promoting relationship-centred care, *Journal of Obstetric, Gynecologic and Neonatal Nursing* 35(2): 286–94.

NICE (2007) *Intrapartum Care: Care of Healthy Women and Their Babies During Childbirth,* London: RCOG Press.

Oakley, A. (1980) *Women Confined: Towards a Sociology of Childbirth,* Oxford: Martin Robertson.

Oakley, A., Hickey, D., Rajan, L. and Grant, A. (1996) Social support in pregnancy: Does it have long term effects? *Journal of Reproductive Health and Infant Psychology* 14: 7–22.

Powell Kennedy, H. and Shannon, M. (2004) Keeping birth normal: Research findings on midwifery care during labour, *Journal of Obstetric, Gynecologic and Neonatal Nursing* 33(5): 554–60.

Reed, B. (2002a) The Albany Midwifery Practice (1), *MIDIRS Midwifery Digest* 12(1): 118–21.

Reed, B. (2002b) The Albany Midwifery Practice (2), *MIDIRS Midwifery Digest* 12(3): 261–4.

Reed, B. and Sandall, J. (2008) The 2000 Study: Albany Midwives Practice Statistics over 10 years, paper presented at the International Confederation of Midwives 28th Triennial Congress, Glasgow.

Sandall, J. (1996) Moving towards caseload practice: What evidence do we have? *British Journal of Midwifery* 4: 620–21.

Sandall, J. (1997) Midwives' burnout and continuity of care, *British Journal of Midwifery* 5(2): 106–11.

Siddiqui, J. (1999) The therapeutic relationship in midwifery, *British Journal of Midwifery* 7(2): 111–14.

Thompson, F. (2004) *Mothers and Midwives: The Ethical Journey,* Edinburgh: Books for Midwives.

Webb, C. (1992) The use of the first person in academic writing: Objectivity, language and gatekeeping, *Journal of Advanced Nursing* 17: 747–52.

CHAPTER 3

Emotion Work and Relationships in Midwifery: Enhancing or Challenging?

RUTH DEERY AND BILLIE HUNTER

Relationships between midwives and women require emotion work; that is, the management of personal emotions and the emotions of others. We now have an increasing body of literature in midwifery (see Hunter and Deery, 2009; Kirkham, 2000) showing us that emotions, and their subsequent effects, are a fundamental part of midwifery work that cannot be ignored. Midwives need to manage their own feelings so that they are appropriate for the situation they are in, and so do women, although we also need to acknowledge that this is not always possible. In any interaction between a woman and a midwife, whether this is short-lived and transitory or a sustained connection over the whole childbirth period, there will be emotion work, with some emotions being concealed and others emphasized or even 'acted out'. In this chapter, we will explore the nature of this emotion work and how it can be experienced, and potentially managed, by midwives.

There are many aspects of the midwife–woman relationship that can generate emotions, whether these are positive (e.g. joy, calm, affection, humour) or negative (e.g. frustration, sadness, fear, anger). Interactions between midwives and women are social encounters that take place in a variety of public and private contexts. They may involve many 'out of the ordinary' experiences, for example intimate 'body work' (Twigg, 2006), disclosure and discussion of personal information and working with women experiencing pain. At times both midwives and women are required to deal with the intense emotions of loss, bereavement and fear. While for most women the childbirth experience is usually a relatively infrequent life event and thus 'out of the ordinary', for midwives it is the very essence of their day-to-day work. This may set up tensions between both sets of experiences.

As we know from many studies, encounters between midwives and women have the potential to be mutually rewarding and enriching (Anderson, 2002; Berg *et al.*, 1996). However, this is not always the case. Women have described 'uncaring encounters' with midwives within research studies (Berg *et al.*, 1996; Halldorsdottir and Karlsdottir, 1996) and in surveys conducted as part of maternity service reports and reviews (Healthcare Commission, 2008; Redshaw *et al.*, 2007). In these situations midwives have been likened to 'caring robots' (McCourt and Stevens, 2009) or described as being 'absently present' (Berg *et al.*, 1996) or even hostile (Robinson, 2000). As one woman in Berg *et al.*'s study evocatively described: 'But I felt as she always came just two minutes too late... I felt as if half of her was still in the other room' (Berg *et al.*, 1996: 13).

The result is a distressing experience that may be remembered by women for a lifetime (Leap and Hunter, 1993; Simkin, 1991). Midwives too can experience negative interactions with women. Frustration might be experienced when women decline or are unreceptive to midwifery advice, or when women appear to have unrealistic expectations of what the midwife can offer (Hunter, 2006). Negative experiences are also frequently the result of midwives being unable to provide the quality of care and attention that they wish to, usually because of organizational demands and constraints (Hunter and Deery, 2005; Hunter and Deery, 2009).

In this chapter we explore how the relationship between the midwife and the woman is experienced on an emotional level by both and consider the implications this may have for practice. Drawing on theoretical and research-based literature, we analyse why the relationship can be a source of emotional satisfaction or, conversely, of emotional difficulty. We argue that the central ingredient is the presence of reciprocity. Where there is reciprocity, even if the connection is short-lived, the evidence suggests that it will be meaningful and mutually satisfying (Hunter, 2006; McCourt and Stevens, 2009; Sandall, 1997). Context is all important in facilitating reciprocal relationships; some contexts (birth centres, one-to-one care) enhance reciprocity, whilst in others reciprocity is not always possible (e.g. large maternity units where care is fragmented and a busy, industrialized system dominates).

We begin by illustrating the significance of context and reciprocal relationships for the emotional experiences of midwives and mothers, using two different accounts. One is based on data from an ethnographic study (Billie Hunter) and the other is based around experiences in clinical practice (Ruth Deery).

Research account: 'It was so perfect I could cry even now'

This narrative is taken from a focus group held as part of an ethnographic study of the emotion work of midwives (Hunter, 2002, 2004) and describes a situation which appeared to be mutually satisfying for all concerned. The speaker, Ann, was working within a community-based team approach which aimed to offer continuity of care to women. This was an emotional account, both for the speaker and the other members of the focus group. It appeared to represent an ideal for all concerned, whereby the individual needs of the woman were recognized and facilitated and the midwife felt that she had been able to 'make a difference'. There is a strong sense of connection and mutual trust. As will be seen, it contrasts sharply with Ruth's account.

> ***Ann***: The mother was very sort of anxious and guarded and worried. We hadn't met before, and it came out that she'd had quite bad post natal depression after the first one, and she was really scared about having this baby, more so because of the emotion of it. So, I thought that she would benefit by some continuity, so I said 'would you like me maybe to come and see you at home next week and, perhaps there's a possibility I could be with you, and you'd know the person that delivers you', 'cause I mean there's a lot of research to support that continuity has a good effect for postnatal depression. So, we did that. And it just so happened that when she went into labour I was on duty. So I went in, she had an epidural, and she knew me and I was glad to be there, and I wanted to support her. So with her epidural – she'd been fully (dilated) for an hour, and then I got her to start to push. And nothing much was happening. And she just had this urge, and at the same time I thought it would be a really good idea if she'd just get up. I said 'well how do your legs feel? If we support you, what about...?', and she said 'well I'd really like to stand!' And she got up, and she just delivered this baby (...) and I thought 'oh, he's huge! Oh my goodness me! How are his shoulders going to come out?' And he just slid down my arm. (*Appreciative noises and laughter from group*) And when we weighed him he was eleven pounds ten ounces. (*Voices: Oh my God.*) Massive! And he was gorgeous, and it was perfect. It was so perfect I could cry even now. I really could. She went home, and I did her care at home. And it was just so wonderful and she didn't develop postnatal depression, and she just kept saying, 'This is just so wonderful, this is just so lovely'. I was just so glad that I saw her when I did, and recognised what she needed, and I was able to fulfill that need. So that for

me, that was really satisfying. (Focus Group, Integrated team midwives in Hunter, 2002: 177)

Clinical practice account: The cost of being 'absently present'

In this contrasting account, Ruth Deery reflects on a clinical shift; a shift that was, as usual, busy and relentless and where she cared for two women for most of the time.

It is not my intention to be negative in this account. Rather, I think as midwives we can learn by critically engaging with clinical practice experiences in order to think differently or help change the status quo. During this particular shift I could not be 'with woman' because I was spending most of my time running from room to room, completing paper records and computer records, answering the door bell, answering the telephone and other women's buzzers – I was 'absently present' and always had 'half of [me]... in the other room' (Berg *et al.*,1996: 13). A familiar tale I feel sure to most midwives who work in large, busy maternity units, but for some reason yesterday I felt ground down as the reality hit me that, for most of the time, to be a midwife in the British National Health Service meant that I could rarely be 'with woman'. During the course of the shift I had also been reminded of my mandatory training requirements, most of them now computer based, as well as two study days to attend. My technical competence as a midwife seemed much more important than engaging with women in the birth process. I was becoming increasingly aware of how difficult it was for me to just 'be a midwife' – I felt worn out and in need of a recharge (see also Deery and Kirkham, 2007). How could I possibly engage in a meaningful relationship with a woman when I had no quality time to spend with her? We were both being denied the development of a personally energizing, reciprocal relationship (see Deery, 2009). On reflection I feel sure that my 'busyness' and lack of engagement stopped the women from asking me any questions. Similarly, Bone (2002) found that nurses often presented a detached demeanour to prevent clients from making requests that they did not have time to complete. The constant stream of paperwork, form filling, lack of resources and shortage of midwives only served to reiterate that the system was more committed to the outcome of childbirth and industrialized obstetrics than the dynamics within the midwife–mother relationship. Bone (2002), in an American study, has also reported that nurses experience constant tensions between being the nurse they want to be and who the system wants them to be. I looked around me at the way we were working and wondered how much longer we could sustain this way of working without going into emotional meltdown.

Discussion

As we can see from these accounts, the midwife–woman relationship has the potential to be emotionally satisfying for both mothers and midwives, but also the potential to be emotionally frustrating and distressing. Challenging emotional experiences for women and midwives are extremely significant, not just for the individuals concerned, but also for the wider community. They can contribute to women's unhappiness, resulting in feelings of trauma and depression (Nilsson and Lundgren, 2009) that may last for years. They also have an impact on the emotional well-being of the whole family unit and can affect health outcomes (Varcoe *et al.*, 2003). The concept of social capital could be usefully applied when considering the dynamics within the midwife–mother relationship. As Putnam (1995: 67) has stated, '…"social capital" refers to features of social organization such as networks, norms, and social trust that facilitate coordination and cooperation for mutual benefit'. However, complex, fragmented and rapidly changing neoliberal organizations such as the NHS are not conducive to social relatedness and could be 'inimical to enhancing social capital' (Edmondson, 2003: 1723), as was seen in Ruth Deery's reflective account. On the other hand, Walsh's ethnographic study of a free-standing birth centre describes the existence of collaboration and solidarity amongst staff who sought to 'comfort and protect' women in labour (Walsh, 2006: 237). Therefore, 'connections among individuals – social networks and the norms of reciprocity and trustworthiness that arise from them' (Putnam, 2000: 19) are important resources for developing meaningful relationships.

When social capital levels are low, caring for women becomes more of a prescribed 'human relations' approach rather than an authentic engagement. Being instructed to 'greet the women with a smile', as in recent NICE guidance (2007), is an example of this type of approach, arguably more appropriate for the scripts given to sales assistants than for healthcare practitioners. In such situations workers may be aware of a lack of authenticity and sincerity. A midwife with whom Ruth recently worked a clinical shift described this situation as 'not being real'. Deery (2003) found evidence of this lack of engagement when studying community midwives' work, identifying how detachment helped the midwives 'make conscious choices based on their emotional needs and on their understanding of what they can handle at a particular time' (Carmack, 1997: 141). Rather than engaging with women in ways that could enhance social capital, the midwives in her study frequently detached themselves either technically or emotionally. *Technical detachment* involved fragmenting the woman's care into manageable tasks in order to maximize the midwife's control over clinical decision making. *Emotional detachment* protected against overinvolvement with women, and appeared to be of short-term benefit in times of heightened anxiety (Deery, 2003). These strategies, however, may lead to a routine and depersonalized approach to midwifery work, low morale, stress and burn-out (Deery, 2005; Deery and Kirkham, 2007; Hunter, 2004; Sandall 1997, 1998), and eventual decisions to leave the profession (Ball *et al.*, 2002). Even from a purely pragmatic point of view this is unacceptable; the economic costs to the health service resulting from client complaints, staff sickness and workforce shortages should alone make it imperative that these issues are addressed as a matter of urgency.

We also know the converse: that relationships with women are crucial for midwives' job satisfaction. Relationships which have meaning and authenticity contribute to midwives' sense of self, so that they feel they are 'a person not a role' (McCourt and Stevens, 2009). There are similar findings in many other recent studies (Hunter, 2006; Walsh, 2007).

So how can we optimize the potential for emotionally positive experiences within the midwife–woman relationship? In the next section we explore the circumstances that enhance – or militate against – mutually rewarding experiences.

Enhancing experiences

When a meaningful relationship can be created, emotion work is not experienced as hard work but as something akin to a 'gift' (Bolton, 2000). Supporting a woman through a long, hard labour can certainly be emotionally demanding, but if the circumstances are facilitative and the midwife is able to establish an authentic connection with the woman, then the midwife feels a sense of satisfaction, as in the following account:

> I had a lovely normal delivery with a primip, had an intact perineum and I felt – even though it was draining, because it was a positive draining, you feel different about it. You feel it's OK to be drained in a posi-

tive way. (*Group agreement*) It's back to this normal thing, it's not the same as looking after somebody with all the works and ending up in theatre, that kind of draining – then you go home and you don't know where you are. (FG 10 E and F grade hospital midwives [the equivalent of band 5 and 6 now] in Hunter, 2002: 199)

Even in extremely distressing experiences, such as when a baby is stillborn, where it has been possible to establish a supportive relationship built on mutuality and trust it is possible for both woman and midwife to feel that the situation was 'as good as it could have been' (Hunter, 2002).

The idea that emotion work can be rewarding – a 'positive draining' – differs from earlier studies of emotion management in health care, which emphasized its 'sorrowful and difficult' nature (James, 1989: 9). In contrast, there is evidence in several studies of midwives doing 'over and above the call of duty' by choice, for example working extra hours, doing home visits in off-duty time, calling into birth centres when on holiday to make contact with colleagues and clients (Deery, 2003; Hunter, 2002; Walsh, 2007). The motivation for this appears to be altruistic; there is something in this autonomous use of the self that is pleasurable and satisfying in itself.

As Benner and Wrubel (1989: 373) observe: 'It is a peculiarly modern mistake to think that caring is the cause of burnout, and that the cure is to protect oneself from caring to prevent the disease called burnout. Rather the loss of caring is the sickness, and the return to caring is the recovery.'

So if the crux of the matter is the potential to create a meaningful relationship, how can this be achieved? How is it that a meaningful relationship can be developed in some contexts at some times and not in others? We can consider this from both a micro level (i.e. interpersonal) and on a macro level (i.e. taking into account the broader context, including the effects of policy, models of service delivery and politics).

On a micro level, there are likely to be a number of influencing factors. For example, personalities come into play: we do not respond similarly to all individuals we meet. There are people with whom we 'click' and where rapport is easily established, and others where this is not the case and we have to work on our emotions to establish connection. In Billie Hunter's study of the emotion work of midwives, focus group participants discussed the formation of 'rapport' and how crucial it was to midwifery care:

I can think of a girl from another team (caseload) who I'd never met before in my life. I looked after her – not for hours and hours and hours, but *oo there was something*. And it was lovely going back to see her afterwards, it was like we'd known each other for years and years and years, and we really liked each other, you know? It was lovely. And then others of your own (caseload), perhaps that you'd looked after all the way through, it's nice, but it's, yeah... (*trails off*). (Focus Group G grade team midwives in Hunter, 2002)

However, even if this strong sense of connection does not exist, midwives can draw on self-awareness and communication skills to establish rapport, as in the following:

...I don't worry about how I'm going to get on with women now and I know I have a good relationship with 99.9% of them... there's always a clash with one in a thousand... but I think my relationships are good and I've just become a better communicator with experience and a bit of awareness... (Community midwife in Deery, 2003)

It is also the case that individuals differ in their ability to communicate effectively, both verbally and non-verbally, and that their capacity for empathy and trust also varies. All of these factors inevitably contribute to the quality and meaning of interactions for all involved.

We know little, however, about how to optimize these factors. For example, it is difficult to anticipate whether affinities are likely to develop between individual midwives and women, and most of our current models of care do not value or support such connections. Indeed, midwives report that it is often frowned on for a 'special bond' to be forged; hospital-based care in particular emphasizes the need for midwives to be interchangeable and to avoid 'getting too close'. As the community midwife above states, in many ways it is a matter of luck when such a 'click' is experienced. It is possible that schemes which facilitate continuity of carer, such as one-to-one caseloading (Stevens and McCourt, 2002), will assist the development of rapport. They may also allow for expression of personal preference, with women being able to choose midwives with whom they feel a sense of connection. However, as the midwife above describes, this way of working does not guarantee affinity. Developing rapport is considered by many midwives to be an integral feature of the artistry of practice (Kennedy, 1995) and an area worthy of more research exploration.

It should be more possible to enhance interpersonal skills. However, we currently know little about how best to develop maternity care practitioners' communication skills and capacity for empathy (Hunter *et al.*,

2008), despite the fact that research evidence suggests that communication within maternity care leaves much room for improvement (Deery, 2003, 2005; Kirkham *et al.*, 2002; Rowe *et al.*, 2002). It is all too often evident that women report that their midwives were 'too busy to listen' or that they 'jolly' women along the childbirth trajectory without authenticity or engagement, as in this extract from Nadine Edwards' study of women choosing home births:

> They [midwives] were very helpful, but one thing I would say [...] is that they seem to have been trained how to treat people and the sorts of problems people have and the sorts of anxieties people have. And when they're faced with you [...] you're an individual [...] and I didn't sometimes think that I was being heard [...] and, do you know, I didn't feel there was a dialogue. I felt a little bit invisible. It was a bit smiley and a bit formulaic. (Edwards, 2005: 174)

This tendency for midwives to provide 'formulaic' responses that lack authenticity is hardly surprising, given the evidence that midwives also struggle with honest and forthright communication within their collegial relationships. Deery's (2003, 2005) research found that midwives feared hurting each other through clumsy communication. In their efforts to save each other from emotional discomfort, midwives reported dealing with work-related issues superficially, sometimes manipulatively, often destructively, and in a manner that often sabotaged their good intentions. This behaviour was described by one of the research participants as being akin to a 'ladylike saboteur'. In a paper examining the culture of midwifery, Kirkham (1999: 737) also reports that midwives 'engineer changes by a process of subtle manipulation'. Clearly then, relational work generates a vast amount of emotion work, which includes 'soothing tempers, boosting confidence, fuelling pride, preventing frictions and mending ego wounds' (Calhoun, 1992: 118).

At a macro level, our knowledge base is stronger. We are developing a body of research which identifies the circumstances facilitating the formation of meaningful relationships. Put simply, it is smallness of scale that is crucial (Kirkham, 2003). Whether this is the literal small size of a midwife-led birth centre, as described in Denis Walsh's ethnographic study (Walsh, 2007), or the smallness of scale afforded by one-to-one caseload midwifery (Stevens and McCourt, 2002), it seems that small is beautiful. In both these models of care, small numbers of midwives interact with small numbers of women. There is the potential for each to really know the other, and it is this 'knowing and being known' (McCourt and

Stevens, 2009: 18) that is crucial for the development of trust and mutual respect.

Central to 'knowing and being known' is reciprocity. That is, where there is mutual 'give and take' in the relationship, both midwife and woman feel valued and affirmed (Hunter, 2006). This contrasts sharply with experiences of midwives working in large-scale organizations, as exemplified in Ruth's clinical practice account. In such settings, midwives describe how they feel objectified, a 'thing' which has no selfhood or other identity, someone who is valued only for their physical labour and ability to complete organizational tasks. In the following account, a caseload midwife provides a vivid comparison of her experience of working for a day with the maternity unit, where she was moved around to meet organizational demands, with her regular experience of working within a community-based model where the development of reciprocal relationships was supported:

> You're running in and out of rooms, taking babies and things. And you're completely invisible, you run in, take the baby, come out, or you may suture their perineum. (...) you're just so used to working the way we have been we become so used to this sort of family atmosphere, that at the end of whatever you've done you expect them to say, oh (*applauds, laughter*) – but they're not interested. Cos you're just a thing that came in did them up a bit, and then disappeared again. So that's what the core (hospital) staff have all the time. (*group agreement*) They don't have this great sense of fulfilment. (Focus Group F grade team midwives in Hunter, 2002: 259)

Reciprocal relationships mean that midwives feel valued not only for their professional skills and knowledge but also for themselves as people; they are not just a 'faceless professional' (Edwards, 2005: 163). In the studies by Stevens and McCourt (2002), Walsh (1999) and Hunter (2006), there are very similar accounts of the personal interest that mothers have in their midwives and the support that they can offer:

> *Jane*: They often pop in and see you – cos they know where I am in clinic on a Tuesday, so if they've got anything they often ring up for a chat so that's nice – but they're often the ones who keep you going – just little things like when she rang up and said 'oh I'm really disappointed you haven't seen my daughter today' and it was just little things like that that actually ooh! That's nice.

BH: Yes... so it makes you feel sort of valued?

Jane: Yes it does yes. (Interview 4, team midwife in Hunter, 2002)

It is not that there is no emotion work within a meaningful and reciprocal relationship. Rather, it is that the emotion work that is needed to establish and sustain this relationship is a shared endeavour, and one which is experienced positively. As one team midwife in Billie Hunter's study neatly put it: 'So from an emotional point of view – you give more but you get more!' (Interview 1 in Hunter, 2002)

Challenging experiences

However, when the needs of the system outweigh the ability of the midwife just to 'be a midwife', relationships suffer. As one of the community midwife's in Deery's (2003) study stated:

> I don't think you include yourself in women's needs... I think we see ourselves as... I try to respond to the needs of the service if you like... so we make ourselves available... you're so busy now... that personal touch is lost...

This is especially so in large maternity units where some midwives have become obedient technicians in order to cope with whatever the working day throws at them (see Deery, 2005, 2009; Hollins Martin and Bull, 2008). Obedient technicians (Deery, 2003) have no control over their working environment because they have to engage in production line work (Dykes, 2005), which means increasing workloads (Lipsky, 1980) and time demands (Deery, 2005). Emotions in this context can only usually be experienced as 'matter out of place' because they impede the smooth running of the 'conveyor belt' within the service if they leak out (Deery and Kirkham, 2007: 81).

Lipsky (1980) provides important insights into the occupational culture described above. In a sociological study he describes how, as a result of their inability to carry out their work as they would like, 'street-level bureaucrats' (that is, public service workers engaging in face-to-face work with clients) adopted several coping strategies. Rationing or routinization of work helped to decrease the demands placed on them by their clients. Street-level bureaucrats also changed their own expectations of their work as well as altering their attitudes to their clients, often by resorting to a 'private assessment of the status quo' (Lipsky, 1980: xiii) within their employing organization. Midwives develop similar coping mechanisms (see Deery, 2005; Deery and Kirkham, 2006), which can be emotionally damaging rather than edifying. Over time these coping mechanisms become more and more difficult to sustain and eventually lead to emotional exhaustion and burnout (Sandall, 1997, 1998).

As was seen in Ruth Deery's clinical practice account, she was not able to engage emotionally with the women she was caring for:

> I had to be emotionally disciplined and keep a tight lid on my feelings. I was not able to engage with the women I was supporting and presented a detached demeanour, completing physical tasks and hoping that neither woman would make any requests that I did not have time to complete. This 'empty performance' (Bolton, 2005: 79) also helped me to control a situation that was becoming increasingly difficult to sustain. I made a choice to be 'absently present' (Berg *et al.*, 1996: 13) and withdraw emotionally from the situation in order to cope; to be a 'caring robot' (McCourt and Stevens, 2009); to be a 'faceless professional' (Edwards, 2009).

This is reminiscent of the classic psychoanalytic study of 1950s hospital nursing, in which Isabel Menzies Lyth provided an extraordinary picture of traditional task-oriented ways of working within hospitals (Menzies, 1970). She argued that the system functions as an organizational defence against stress and anxiety. Work that was task-oriented seemed to protect nurses from close contact with their patients, and depersonalization and categorization of patients meant that relationships were kept unemotional and distant. This happened within an organization that believed it was 'better to stick to dimensions of the work more subject to administrative manipulation' (Lipsky, 1980: 188) than to address the quality of relationships.

The strict routines and standard procedures that seemed to pervade the whole of nursing practice also minimized responsibility and decision making for nurses, thus protecting them from associated stresses (Menzies, 1960). Lipsky's street-level bureaucrats also saw detachment as a means of self-protection:

> Some bureaucracies so routinize their processing of clients that significant psychological interactions are minimal... [midwives] may adhere to interview formats that exclude personal elements and reduce the likelihood of decision making on the basis of inter-personal interactions. (Lipsky, 1980: 69, our addition of 'midwives')

Perhaps, on closer analysis, Ruth's self-criticism in her challenging clinical practice narrative appears overly harsh and simplistic. Insights from social science challenge us to look beneath the behaviour which is manifested, in order to access more nuanced interpretations. So the engagement and detachment in relationships may have multiple explanations. For example, in both of our research studies (Deery, 2003, 2005; Hunter, 2002, 2004), we found that midwives 'framed solutions' (Lipsky, 1980) by adapting their existing workloads in order to get through the working day. This entailed reducing the attention that midwives gave to some women and increasing the attention given to others. For example, community midwives in Deery's study described how they detached themselves from white, middle-class women, whom they perceived as demanding of emotional energy, stating that they 'got rid of them like hot bricks' when their 'usual' midwife was back on duty. As one of the midwives stated: '...the further you come up the social class... then the more demands they [the women] make on you... the demands they make are emotionally draining... they've got two sides of A4 paper of questions.' In contrast, Hunter (2002, 2006) observed that midwives spent more time with this group of women, who were culturally similar to the midwives in her study, rather than with those from differing social and ethnic backgrounds.

This accords with Lipsky's (1984) observation that overstretched public service workers differentiate between clients as a coping strategy, so that the ideal service is provided for at least a few: 'The street level bureaucrat salvages for a portion of the clientele a conception of his or her performance relatively consistent with ideal conceptions of the job' (Lipsky, 1980: 151). This entails 'creaming off' clients, so that those who are most likely to become successful 'cases' are selected. There were similar findings in the study by Kirkham *et al.* (2002). Midwives working under time and workload pressures were observed to spend a disproportionate amount of time giving antenatal advice to better-educated, middle-class women, rather than to working-class clients who were seeking advice and information. The result was an example of the 'inverse care law' (Tudor Hart, 1971), whereby those most in need of care are those least likely to receive it.

This 'creaming off' of clients may result in a lack of authenticity and flexibility. Midwives may find it difficult to calibrate their interactions; that is, to move and mediate in a sensitive and flexible manner between closeness and detachment. This ability to calibrate lies at the heart of midwives' skills in building relationships with women. The ability to move and mediate suggests that midwives can engage in constant rebalancing

(Carmack, 1997: 141), acknowledging that relationships can change. Other studies have indicated that midwives who are able to do this well have highly tuned levels of emotional awareness and that they know when it is important to engage emotionally and when it is not (Kennedy, 1995; Walsh, 2007). At the same time, the level of engagement will depend on the interpersonal emotion management (Francis, 1997; Thoits, 1996) and communication skills of the midwife. It will also depend on time and other organizational constraints, the amount of work to be got through, the woman, possible language and other communication barriers, and how all of the above are affecting the midwife. This balancing of engagement with detachment is important in midwifery because, as Carmack (1997: 142) states, 'one focuses on the here and now, recognizes limits, and does not attempt to over-control outcomes'.

> People who successfully balance engagement with detachment know what they can and cannot change or control. They are sensitive to their own emotional needs. They choose their level of engagement based on what they know they can handle at a particular time. People who successfully balance engagement and detachment understand the importance of self-care. (Carmack, 1997: 142)

Suggesting that midwives can rebalance within relationships implies that different levels of balance exist and, furthermore, that midwives can engage with women at different levels within the developing relationship. As Stapleton et al. (2002: 395) suggest:

> there appears to be a continuum of engagement between woman and health professionals. At one extreme the professional is entirely engaged with their own predetermined agenda and words addressed to the woman are largely instructional. Further along the continuum, the professional is still engaged with their agenda but shares with the woman, to a lesser or greater extent, the information gained during the consultation.'

However, the balance of the midwife–mother relationship can be disrupted if the midwife remains permanently anchored in either engagement or detachment. More importantly, engagement, detachment and rebalancing within relationships all assume that the woman and not the organization is the focus of the midwife's work.

Conclusion

In this chapter we have explored the emotion work created by the midwife–woman relationship. We have used a mixture of research data and personal reflection, underpinned by sociological interpretation, to consider how emotions stemming from this relationship may be experienced, and potentially managed, by midwives. It appears that the relationship between midwife and woman can be emotionally enhancing or, conversely, emotionally challenging.

We have attempted to explore why this disparity exists. Is it the result of individual characteristics of particular mothers and midwives? That is, some midwives and some mothers will have an instant rapport which leads to meaningful engagement, whilst others simply fail to 'click'? Or is it directly related to the workload of the midwife, so that an overstretched midwife will never have the emotional capacity to form mutually rewarding relationships with the woman she cares for? If midwifery services were fully staffed, would all relationships inevitably become emotionally rewarding ones? Or is the cause more subtle? Do midwives actually try to shape women to the organization? Perhaps it is the way in which midwifery work is organized and the model of care that is used which are most significant?

There is substantial evidence demonstrating that meaningful relationships are crucial to positive experiences for both women and midwives (Hunter *et al.*, 2008). However, despite this knowledge, we know that both women and midwives experience the maternity services as institutionalized and bureaucratic (Kirkham, 1999) and as 'cold, impersonal and clinical' (Wilkins, 2000: 46). The service is focused on meeting organizational demands rather than the needs of the woman or the midwife. But both women and midwives tell us that they need to feel seen, heard, acknowledged and supported – not to feel like they are 'just a thing' (Hunter, 2002).

What is missing in these cold and impersonal encounters is reciprocity. The potential for mutual 'give and take' (Hunter, 2006) is curtailed and thus the development of a mutually meaningful relationship for both the woman and the midwife is denied. So to return to our earlier questions: on the basis of the evidence to date, we would argue that it is the way in which midwifery care is organized that is most significant. Even if the delivery suite were fully staffed, it is likely that the focus on task completion and efficient 'throughput' of woman and babies would impede the development of mutually rewarding reciprocal relationships. A 'good midwife' in the eyes of the organization is the one who has successfully completed all tasks at the end of her shift, in compliance with relevant policies and protocols, and not the one who has disrupted the system by encouraging a new mother to talk through her birth experiences.

Drawing attention to these issues is crucial if midwives want to challenge the dominant industrialized model of childbirth and promote a smaller-scale approach to midwifery that will in turn help to develop reciprocal relationships with women.

References

Anderson, T. (2002) Feeling safe enough to let go: The relationship between a woman and her midwife during the second stage of labour, in Kirkham, M. (ed.), *The Midwife–Mother Relationship*, London: Macmillan Press.

Ball, L., Curtis, P. and Kirkham, M. (2002) *Why Do Midwives Leave?* Sheffield: Women's Informed Childbearing and Health Research Group, University of Sheffield.

Benner, P. and Wrubel, J. (1989) *The Primacy of Caring: Stress and Coping in Health and Illness*, Menlo Park, CA: Addison-Wesley Health Sciences Division.

Berg, M., Lundgren, I., Hermansson, E. and Wahlberg, V. (1996) Women's experience of the encounter with the midwife during childbirth, *Midwifery* 12: 11–15.

Bolton, S.C. (2000) Who cares? Offering emotion work as a 'gift' in the nursing labour process. *Journal of Advanced Nursing* 32(3): 580–86.

Bolton, S.C. (2005) *Emotion Management in the Workplace*, London: Palgrave Macmillan.

Bone, D. (2002) Dilemmas of emotion work in nursing under market-driven health care, *International Journal of Public Sector Management*, 15: 140–50.

Calhoun, C.C. (1992) Emotional work, in Cole, E.B. and Coultrap-McQuin, S. (eds) *Explorations in Feminist Ethics: Theory and Practice*, Bloomington, IN: Indiana University Press.

Carmack, B.J. (1997) Balancing engagement and detachment in caregiving, *Image: Journal of Nursing Scholarship*, 29(2): 139–43.

Deery, R. (2003) Engaging with clinical supervision in a community midwifery setting: an action research study, unpublished PhD thesis, University of Sheffield.

Deery, R. (2005) An action research study exploring midwives' support needs and the effect of group clinical supervision, *Midwifery*, 21: 161–76.

Deery, R. (2009) Community midwifery 'performances' and the presentation of self, in Hunter, B. and Deery, R. (eds), *Emotions in Midwifery and Reproduction*, London: Palgrave Macmillan.

Deery, R. and Kirkham, M. (2006) Supporting midwives to support women, in Page, L. and McCandlish, R. (eds), *The New Midwifery: Science and Sensitivity in Practice*, 2nd edn), London: Elsevier.

Deery, R. and Kirkham, M. (2007) Drained and dumped on: The generation and accumulation of emotional toxic waste in community midwifery, in Kirkham, M. (ed.), *Exploring the Dirty Side of Women's Health*, London: Routledge.

Dykes, F. (2005) A critical ethnographic study of encounters between midwives and breast-feeding women in postnatal wards in England, *Midwifery* 21(3): 241–52.

Edmondson, R. (2003) Social capital: A strategy for enhancing health? *Social Science and Medicine*, 57: 1723–33.

Edwards, N.P. (2005) *Birthing Autonomy: Women's Experiences of Planning Home Births*, London: Routledge.

Edwards, N.P. (2009) Women's emotion work in the context of current maternity services, in Hunter, B. and Deery, R. (eds), *Emotions in Midwifery and Reproduction*, London: Palgrave Macmillan.

Francis, L.E. (1997) Ideology and interpersonal emotion management: redefining identity in two support groups, *Social Psychology Quarterly*, 60(2): 153–71.

Halldorsdottir, S. and Karlsdottir, S.I. (1993) Caring and uncaring encounters during labour and delivery: from the perspective of women who have given birth, in *Midwives: Hear the Heartbeat of the Future: Proceedings of the International Confederation of Midwives 23rd International Congress*, Vancouver: Int. Confed. of Midwives 1993, 2: 967–71.

Halldorsdottir, S. and Karlsdottir, S.I. (1996) Journeying through labour and delivery: perceptions of women who have given birth, *Midwifery* 12: 48–61.

Healthcare Commission (2008) *Towards Better Births: A Review of Maternity Services in England*, London: Commission for Health Care Audit and Inspection.

Hollins Martin, C.J. and Bull, P. (2008) Obedience and conformity in clinical practice, *British Journal of Midwifery* 16(8): 504–9.

Hunter, B. (2002) Emotion Work in Midwifery, unpublished PhD thesis, University of Wales Swansea.

Hunter, B. (2004) Conflicting ideologies as a source of emotion work in midwifery, *Midwifery* 20: 261–72.

Hunter, B. (2006) The importance of reciprocity in relationships between community-based midwives and mothers, *Midwifery* 22(4): 308–22.

Hunter, B. and Deery, R. (2005) Building our knowledge about emotion work in midwifery: Combining and comparing findings from two different research studies, *Evidence Based Midwifery*, 3(1): 10–15.

Hunter, B. and Deery, R. (2009) *Emotions in Midwifery and Reproduction*, London: Palgrave Macmillan.

Hunter, B., Berg, M., Lundgren, I., Olafsdottir, O. and Kirkham, M. (2008) Relationships: The hidden threads in the tapestry of maternity care. Guest commentary, *Midwifery* 24: 132–7.

James, N. (1989) Emotional labour: Skill and work in the social regulation of feelings, *Sociological Review* 37: 15–42.

Kennedy, H.P. (1995) The essence of nurse-midwifery care: The woman's story, *Journal of Nurse-Midwifery* 40(5, Sept/Oct): 410–17.

Kirkham, M. (1999) The culture of midwifery in the National Health Service in England, *Journal of Advanced Nursing* 30(3): 732–9.

Kirkham, M. (2000) *The Midwife–Mother Relationship*, London: Macmillan Press.

Kirkham, M. (2003) *Birth Centres, A Social Model for Maternity Care*, Oxford: Elsevier Science.

Kirkham, M., Stapleton, H., Curtis, P. and Thomas, G. (2002) The inverse care law in antenatal midwifery, *British Journal of Midwifery* 10(8): 509–13.

Leap, N. and Hunter, B. (1993) *The Midwife's Tale*, London: Scarlet Press.

Lipsky, M. (1980) *Street-Level Bureaucracy: Dilemmas of the Individual in Public Services*, New York: Russell Sage Foundation.

McCourt, C. and Stevens, T. (2009) Relationship and reciprocity in caseload midwifery, in Hunter, B. and Deery, R. (eds), *Emotions in Midwifery and Reproduction*, London: Palgrave Macmillan.

Menzies, I.E.P. (1960) A case-study in the functioning of social systems as a defence against anxiety, *Human Relations*, 13: 95–121.

Menzies, I.E.P. (1970) *The Functioning of Social Systems as a Defence against Anxiety*, London: Tavistock Institute of Human Relations.

National Institute for Health and Clinical Excellence (NICE) (2007) *Intrapartum Care: Care of Healthy Women and Their Babies During Childbirth*, Clinical Guideline 55, www.nice.org.uk/nicemedia/pdf/IPCNICEGuidance.pdf, accessed March 2010.

Nilsson, C. and Lundgren, I. (2009) Women's lived experience of fear of childbirth, *Midwifery*, 25(2): 1–9.

Putnam, R. (1995) Bowling alone: America's declining social capital, *Journal of Democracy*, 6(1): 65–79.

Putnam, R.D. (2000) *Bowling Alone: The Collapse and Revival of American Community*, London: Simon and Schuster.

Redshaw, M., Rowe, R., Hockley, C. and Brocklehurst, P. (2007) *Recorded Delivery: A National Survey of Women's Experience of Maternity Care*, Oxford: National Perinatal Epidemiology Unit (NPEU).

Robinson, J. (2000) What are midwives turning nasty? *British Journal of Midwifery* 8(2): 143.

Rowe, R.E., Garcia, J., Macfarlane, A.J. and Davidson, L.L. (2002) Improving communication between health professionals and women in maternity care: A structured review, *Health Expectations* 5: 63–83.

Sandall, J. (1997) Midwives' burnout and continuity of care, *British Journal of Midwifery* 5(2): 106–11.

Sandall, J. (1998) Midwifery work, family life and wellbeing: A study of occupational change, unpublished PhD thesis, University of Surrey, Guildford.

Simkin, P. (1991) Just another day in a woman's life? Part 1: Women's long term-memories of their first birth experience, *Birth* 18: 203–10.

Stapleton, H., Kirkham, M., Curtis, P. and Thomas, G. (2002) Silence and time in antenatal care, *British Journal of Midwifery*, 10(6): 393–6.

Stevens, T. and McCourt, C. (2002) One-to-one midwifery practice part 3: Meaning for midwives, *British Journal of Midwifery* 10(2): 111–15.

Thoits, P.A. (1996) Managing the emotion of others, *Symbolic Interaction*, 19(2): 85–109, DOI 10.1525/si.1996.19.2.85.

Tudor Hart, J. (1971) The inverse care law, *Lancet*, 1: 405–12.

Twigg, J. (2006) *The Body in Health and Social Care*, London: Palgrave Macmillan.

Varcoe, C., Rodney, P. and McCormick J. (2003) Health care relationships in context: An analysis of three ethnographies, *Qualitative Health Research* 13(7): 957–73.

Walsh, D. (1999) An ethnographic study of women's experience of partnership caseload midwifery practice: The professional as friend, *Midwifery* 15: 165–76.

Walsh, D. (2006) 'Nesting' and 'matrescence' as distinctive features of a free-standing birth centre in the UK, *Midwifery*, 22: 228–39.

Walsh, D. (2007) A birth centre's encounters with discourses of childbirth: How resistance led to innovation, *Sociology of Health and Illness*, 29(2): 216–32, DOI: 10.1111/j.1467-9566.2007.00545.x.

Wilkins, R. (2000) Poor relations: The paucity of the professional paradigm, in Kirkham, M. (ed.), *The Midwife–Mother Relationship*, London: Macmillan.

CHAPTER 4

The Midwife: A Professional Servant?

MARY CRONK

As we go through life we continually make relationships. The mother-
-child relationship, formed after our birth, is arguably the most important
relationship of our lives (Raphael-Leff, 1991; Winnicott, 1987). As we
grow and mature we continue to form relationships with everybody we
meet and come in contact with. We constantly learn from the relationships we make.

Our family relationships teach us so much. The parent–child relationship is initially one of almost total dependence for our survival; whether
that relationship is good or bad, strong or weak, it is vital to our development (Niven, 1992; Rapheal-Leff, 1991; Richards, 1974; Winnicott,
1988). Siblings and other family members add their bit to the family
dynamic (Winnicott, 1965). During childhood links are formed with
others: perhaps child-carers, playgroup leaders, neighbours, teachers,
family friends, other children. We learn to negotiate our relationships as
we mature (Richards, 1974). As we grow older the base changes to a
more equal relationship with others.

We make acquaintances, friends and enemies, we identify our peer
group. The relationships have a form: equal relationships and others
where the power in the relationship is unequal. Relationships can be
loving, caring, formal, informal, welcome, unwelcome, constructive,
destructive, supportive, dependent, tentative, provisional.

As adults we make relationships with people from whom we purchase
goods or services. We choose the shops we use, the person who does our
hair. We choose the plumber, the window cleaner, the solicitor, the
dentist. With all these people we form a relationship. The power balance
with people we employ to provide us with services is different from those
of friendship or kinship.

So what factors are we looking at when we consider the optimum relationship between midwives and the people they serve? I was about to write 'women' instead of 'people', then I thought, 'It's not only women midwives care for, it's their babies and the babies' fathers and sometimes siblings as well', as hopefully we nurture the families we are involved with in providing maternity services as professional midwives.

A professional servant relationship?

The midwife is providing a service, either as an employee of a health service that has a contract to supply midwifery services or as an independent midwife directly employed by a woman to provide her with maternity services. Anyone providing a service is a servant. The midwife is a member of a profession. That means, surely, that she is providing professional services – she is a professional servant.

It may be difficult for many of us to think of ourselves as a woman's servant, albeit a professional one, but that is really what we are. I practise independently and therefore provide my professional services directly to people who employ me, and I do think of myself as their professional servant. Is that not the relationship all midwives should have to the people we serve? Nevertheless, it is not so, is it? Many of us presume we have a power over the people we serve, the people for whose benefit we practise, a power to 'allow'.

I am unclear how the power base between women and midwives changed, how it came about that we assumed a power that we do not have. How was it that we started 'allowing' women to eat, drink, walk, get out of bed, go to the loo and so on; 'letting' women have a companion in labour, feed their babies when they want to, even pick their babies up; 'giving' women permission to make a noise, or telling them not to make a noise? What happened to the employee–employer relationship between women and their midwives that enabled us to presume a power we had no right to presume, and use that power to control women?

I feel that perhaps the first Midwives Act – yes, our beloved 1902 Act in England and 1925 in Scotland – started the power shift. 'Ladies' became midwives. The bona fide unregistered, untrained midwife, who had previously cared for women who paid her, often in kind, was of the same social class as her clients; she was still around, and she hadn't really thought of herself as a professional, though she had been helping women in childbirth for a very long time. But she was not a 'lady'. The new 1902 professional registered midwife was very conscious of her status and her subservient role to the medical practitioners by whose grace and favour she practised (Heagerty, 1997). Remember, there was no requirement that a midwife sit on those first Midwives Boards, and the first batch of Midwives Rules has a great deal to say about the need for implicit obedience to the doctor's orders. If one has to obey orders about one's 'patients', one gives orders to one's 'patients'; if these patients were of a lower social order it wasn't difficult. The midwife employed and paid for by a Nursing Association or a Jubilee Midwife could and did give orders to the women for whom she was caring (Leap and Hunter, 1993). The bona fide midwife who had not been controlled by doctors, but by the people who employed her, was literally dying out.

The new registered midwife employed by a Nursing Association was required to wear a uniform. Uniforms are associated with military discipline, orders and hierarchy, and the registered midwife did have a relationship with her 'patients' that permitted her to give her orders. The private midwife was in a different position: she was directly employed and could be dismissed if she failed to give satisfaction. Ordering one's employer about rarely leads to a satisfactory relationship.

The arrival of the NHS in 1948 removed the remaining direct payment of the midwife from most midwife–woman relationships, and again our assumption of power grew. Midwives practising 'on the district', employed by the local authority and attending women in their own homes, gave their orders, but the woman in her own home often ignored orders that she didn't want to obey, or couldn't obey, or saw no need to obey. Then, in 1976, the reorganization of the NHS brought district midwives under the same employer as the hospital-based midwife. They were now expected to obey 'hospital policies'. Home births were phased out almost completely by the power of the employers of midwives, and the midwife obeying hospital policies relayed them to the woman as orders. The power dynamic of the midwife–woman relationship had changed almost completely, except for the few of us who practised independently and were employed by our clients.

The servant part of the professional servant status became almost forgotten. The various government reports *Changing Childbirth* in England (Department of Health, 1993) and *Maternity Care Matters* in Scotland (Scottish Programme for Clinical Effectiveness in Reproductive Health, 1998) did attempt to change the power base, although in practice not much has changed. Women still perceive themselves as being 'allowed' to go over their dates, 'allowed' to refuse routine interventions, 'given' choices.

So where do we go from here? Would it be a good thing if we remembered our professional servant status? I believe it would. I believe that for mothers and their partners in parenting to reclaim their rights will enhance their parenting. With rights go responsibilities. Parents are responsible for their children, aren't they?

For many years, and to a large extent still when a woman becomes pregnant, it is perceived that the midwife knows best; if she doesn't, well, the GP knows best, and the obstetrician certainly knows best how this pregnancy should be managed. After the birth (managed by those who know what is best), the midwife visits and knows what is the best way to feed, clean, hold, change and comfort the baby. After the midwife departs, along comes the health visitor. She knows best about lots of things: feeding, clothing, sleeping, potty training, immunizations; after all, she is a professional, of course she knows best. Then off to school. And who knows best there? Teacher knows best, and the local education authority certainly knows best, about what school little Darren or Ellie should attend.

Then all of a sudden it seems that the little darling is 16 or so and, as 16 year olds are prone to do, does something antisocial, if not downright diabolical. What does society say? Who is to blame? Why, parents of course. 'No sense of responsibility.' 'Parents must take responsibility for their offspring,' says society. 'Fine these irresponsible parents' scream the tabloids. It's a bit late, isn't it? I believe that our assumption of power over the women, for whose benefit we practise, at the beginning of their parenting can begin their disempowerment as parents and take from them the feeling of responsibility for their children on which good parenting depends. Our input in terms of nurturing, enhancing and respecting the development of feelings of parental responsibility will, I believe, benefit society.

If we want to do this, how can we set about encouraging the young mother to take and accept responsibility for herself and her offspring? How do we stop ourselves telling her what to do and taking responsibility? Would it be a good thing if we remembered our professional servant relationship with the people for whose benefit we practise? How could we start to do this? We would have to remember to give professional advice rather than orders. We would have to learn to cope with sometimes having our advice rejected. We would have almost to recondition women to feel more confident, more responsible, more in charge. I believe that changing the power basis in the relationship between midwives and women would enhance all the qualities that contribute to parents becoming competent, confident and responsible.

How can this power balance be changed? Perhaps one of the main ways for parents to feel that theirs is the responsibility would be if there were a change in the way maternity care was provided: to return the choice of midwife, continuity of care and control over their care to women. It is my hope that future maternity care will be a partnership model, with the woman choosing her professional attendants; more about this later. However, can we change within the structures we now have in the NHS, which do not by and large empower parents?

We would have to consider the words we use and our tones of voice. We would have to watch our language: no more 'allowing', no more 'giving' of choice, no more 'having' to do as we or Mr Highandmighty has ordered. It is difficult to remember to say 'I suggest we consider', or 'I advise', or 'I strongly advise', or 'it is recommended' or 'the evidence shows that', instead of 'you must', or 'you have to' or 'Mr Bloggs allows or doesn't allow'.

I have been practising independently for 15 years now, having been a district midwife and an NHS-employed midwife. I have worn a frilly nurse's hat and given my orders and thought I had authority to tell women what to do because I was a midwife and, of course, I knew what was best. I may have been a professional, but I had forgotten that my relationship with my clients was that of professional servant. Actually, when I think of all the things I knew best about over the years I cringe. A few to reflect on include mandatory shaving (in hospital, we didn't do it on the district), mandatory enemata, mandatory episiotomies (Mr Highandmighty liked them), telling all women how to push (they being too stupid to know how), forbidding women to get out of bed, ordering men to leave rooms (I knew the women didn't really want them there), forbidding women to eat or drink, taking their babies to nurseries, without even thinking to ask if that was what the woman wanted. I wonder if in ten years' time I will think the same about the things I think I know best about now?

If the woman is young, disadvantaged and/or unused to having her opinions sought, let alone valued, it needs to be remembered that she may find *not* being told what to do quite threatening, and it will require sensitivity on the part of her midwife to empower her gently, perhaps increasing her decision making as the pregnancy progresses.

In transactional analysis terms (Berne, 1961, 1964), personality encompasses three major aspects, which are defined as parent, adult and child and are reflected in the way we relate to one another. We want, surely, to have our clients relate to us as adults. Diagramatically this looks like Figure 4.1.

When the midwife says to the woman, 'You are 41 weeks now, so if you haven't had the baby before Monday you have to come in to be started

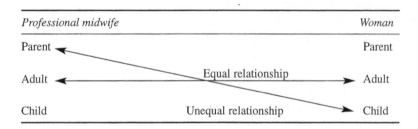

Figure 4.1   The midwife–mother relationship in transactional analysis terms

off', she is speaking in the parent-to-child mode. If the woman responds by saying, 'Thank you for your advice. I will think about it and let you know', she is converting the relationship to adult-to-adult and cutting across the relationship we have presumed we have with her. We should welcome this.

There are many other examples. One may, in the early antenatal period, have said something like, 'We do routine ultrasound scans here at X, Y and Z weeks, so that makes your first one on Wednesday week at 2.30 at the clinic on the first floor with a full bladder please.' If we are changing to professional servant or adult-to-adult mode, we might say something like, 'We offer ultrasound scanning checks here because it enables us to check that your baby is... How do you feel about this? Would you like to know more about ultrasound before you decide whether to have these scans?' Then, following discussion, we check that the woman has understood that we are advising and offering the service. 'Would you like to book your first appointment for next Wednesday? It is done in the antenatal assessment clinic on the first floor and we get a much better picture if your bladder is full.' Or, with something as ordinary, to us, as urinalysis: 'Have you brought a specimen? Well, dear, didn't you know you have to bring a specimen? You have to bring one every time you come; don't forget again, it's important.' The 'routine' blood tests, the abdominal palpation – there are all sorts of these scenarios in which reflection can help us see opportunities to empower the parents, to help them feel like responsible adults; these are times when it is all too easy to affirm them in the subservient child role they may feel it appropriate to assume.

The tone of voice we use should be similar to the tone of voice we would expect to be used to us by our solicitor, builder, hairdresser, optician, accountant – the people we engage to provide us with services. Are we likely to be addressed by them as 'dear', 'honey bunch', 'lovey' or 'duckey'?

Few of us would prick a baby's heel for the routine neonatal screening tests without informed consent by the mother, but it is also necessary to remember to ask, 'May I pick up, examine, check your baby? Is it all right if doctor has a look at baby?' All these phrases reinforce and affirm that this is *her* baby and we care for her with *her* permission because she is a responsible parent. Each time we pick up a baby without asking we are missing an opportunity for promoting responsible parenting. New mothers are so vulnerable, we have such power. Let's use it to empower.

Perhaps it would help if we thought to ourselves, 'Would this couple choose to have me as their midwife if they had the choice? If they could dismiss me and engage someone else, I wonder if they would do so? Would I speak to them as I have just done if they had that power?' It makes you think, doesn't it? We do not demean ourselves as professionals by fostering an adult-to-adult relationship between us and the people for whose benefit we practise and by whom we are paid, directly or indirectly, to give a professional service. The most powerful thing we can do as professionals is to empower the parents of the babies at whose births we assist.

Independent midwife–mother relationships

The relationship between midwives practising independently and the women who employ them has a different flavour to the relationship between an NHS midwife and her clients. These differences can be listed as follows. First, at the start, there is a consultation interview where both parties meet and basically see if they like each other. The woman decides if this is a person she wants to be her independent midwife (IM). The midwife, for her part, decides if she can meet this woman's needs. Secondly, the woman has chosen the midwife and is actually paying her directly. Thirdly, the midwife has agreed to be employed by the woman/couple. The woman may have interviewed several midwives before engaging this one's services and the midwife also has considered if she wants to be employed by this woman/couple before accepting the case. Many independent midwives have a written contract with their clients while, with others, there is an understanding of what each party expects of the other. This is detailed in the maternity notes which the woman holds during the pregnancy and of which she has a copy after the birth. Despite the commercial aspect, a relationship of friendship and mutual respect commonly forms and many independent midwives and their clients have built a relationship that will be there for years. With others, the midwife's services are engaged, the baby is born, the fees are paid and the relationship is terminated with mutual affection and respect.

The woman has the right to terminate the relationship and she can do this without giving any reason; while this is rarely done, it is the woman's right to do so. The woman exercising her right to dismiss the previously engaged midwife has no obligation to give any reason. Likewise, the midwife has the right to unbook a client, though she could be held to be behaving unprofessionally if she did this at the end of the pregnancy and without good reason. A midwife choosing to unbook a woman/client would be well advised to discuss the case with her supervisor of midwives and record this in her notes. Such breakdowns in the relationship are rare but are devastating for the midwife, and emphasize the importance of getting the relationship on the right lines at the consultation interview.

The relationship between the woman and her IM has many facets. The woman's decision to seek independent midwifery care outside the NHS has in most cases been considered carefully. Sometimes it is made early in the pregnancy, in many cases as a result of a previous unsatisfactory experience of care within NHS maternity services. The woman expecting her first baby and choosing to seek an IM is often influenced by local perception of the NHS care available. The common reason so often heard by IMs is the woman's desire to know the midwife who will attend her in labour; not only to know her, but to have chosen her and formed a relationship with her. The midwife taking on the case where the woman books early in the pregnancy has the opportunity to get to know her client and what 'makes her tick'. It is, in my opinion, a nonsense to treat all women the same; women are all individuals and pregnant women particularly need individual care. The IM, with her knowledge of the woman and her family circumstances, gained throughout the antenatal care, is particularly able to provide this individual care.

While it is beneficial to have had antenatal care provided by the IM, many clients will come to the IM late in pregnancy because relationships within the NHS have broken down. Many women in late pregnancy come to IMs because they have an unusual pregnancy which the NHS midwives do not, or cannot, cater for. Women with breech-presenting babies or twins, or who have had a previous caesarean section, may find that their care under the NHS does not meet their needs. Many describe the fragmented care and sometimes the withdrawal of midwifery care and the referral to unwanted medical care and management in such circumstances. The midwife who undertakes the care of the late-booking client has a difficult job to build up a trusting relationship with this client. In addition, she has to negotiate with the previous care provider and often make arrangements with local hospital staff. The woman may resent having to engage and pay for independent care.

There are many examples among IM clients of women with breech-presenting babies who book the midwife in the morning, relax that they have at last found a solution to their problem and go into labour that night! There has not been much time to form a relationship here and it is a skill that IMs have developed to gain the trust of a woman in one interview. Having said that, the late-booking woman does present relationship problems. In many cases she has feelings of resentment against her previous care provider; she can be apprehensive and fearful and wonder if she has done the right thing. While she is now employing the midwife, she has not had any time to establish a trusting relationship and such cases really challenge the IM to the full. If the labour needs help, and some do, the midwife may have to advise transfer to the very hospital that the woman has had difficulties with. The importance of documentation of all the aspects of care that were discussed at the booking and subsequently cannot be overemphasized, as well as the need to share with the woman the possibility of the labour needing help and transfer becoming advisable.

The relationship built between the late booker and the midwife is a challenge for the midwife who undertakes the case. She has to get to know a woman who is sometimes desperate and has perceived her care from the NHS to have been lacking. Her expectations of the IM may be unrealistic and it will take all the midwife's skill to meet her needs, but also to help the woman to move forward and leave behind her previous experiences. The woman/couple also have to find the professional fees for the midwife. This is something they have not budgeted for and for many it is a major problem. Most midwives have extended payment plans to assist clients in these circumstances, but the payment of fees can be a difficult area. The midwife needs to be direct and clear about her charges and how she expects to be paid. If there are requests for discounts that the midwife feels unable to agree to, she may decide not to take the case, as such disagreements about fees can interfere with and are damaging to the relationship. While it is hard to refuse a case, sometimes it does need to be done.

There are cases where an NHS Trust, finding itself unable to meet the woman's needs, has paid the fees for the independent midwife. These cases are rare, but if the aims of the One Mother, One Midwife/National Health Service Community Midwifery Model campaign succeed, women's need to have an IM and for a midwife to choose her clients could be met in this way (van der Kooy, 2009). In effect this is an NHS-based model, a scheme whereby any woman is enabled to have the option of choosing her midwife to supply one-to-one care throughout her pregnancy, her labour and the puerperium. Midwives choosing to join this model would be paid a set fee per case undertaken. This would be similar, in many ways, to how general practitioners practise, as contracted-in providers of care. This would enable the choice of midwife and the one-to-one care provided by the IM to be available to all women in Britain. While some Trusts do offer schemes to some women that provide one-to-one care, this is not with a midwife chosen by the woman and they usually have a geographical area in which a woman must reside in order to be included in the scheme. Further details of the One Mother, One Midwife campaign are available at www.onemotheronemidwife.org.uk.

The NHS Community Midwifery Model (van der Kooy, 2009) would allow all women to receive the model of care that is currently only available to those who choose, and can afford to employ, independent midwives. However, the government is proposing to make it compulsory for all health professionals, including independent midwives, to have professional indemnity insurance (against negligence claims). At present there is no such insurance available for independent midwives in the UK, and the government has refused to provide any. This proposal would effectively be proposing to make it illegal for midwives to work on a self-employed basis. This is an outrageous restriction on choice for women and midwives alike, particularly since there is no evidence that having insurance would improve outcomes for mothers or babies. If mothers and midwives value the relationships that are formed between them, they must make their feelings known to their MPs and the various organizations that represent the users of this service given by midwives as professional servants.

References

Berne, E. (1961) *Transactional Analysis in Psychotherapy*, New York: Grove Press.
Berne, E. (1964) *Games People Play*, New York: Grove Press.
Department of Health (1993) *Changing Childbirth: Report of the Expert Maternity Group*, London: HMSO.
Heagerty, B.V. (1997) Willing handmaidens of science: The struggle over the new midwifery in early twentieth-century England, in Kirkham, M.J. and Perkins, E.R. (eds), *Reflections on Midwifery*, London: Bailliere Tindall.
Leap, N. and Hunter, B. (1993) *The Midwife's Tale: An Oral History from Handywoman to Professional Midwife*, London: Scarlett Press.

Niven, C.A. (1992) *Psychological Care for Families, Before, During and After Birth,* Oxford: Butterworth Heinemann.

Raphael-Leff, R. (1991) *Psychological Processes of Childbearing,* London: Chapman and Hall.

Richards, M. (1974) *The Integration of a Child into a Social World,* Cambridge: Cambridge University Press.

Scottish Programme for Clinical Effectiveness in Reproductive Health (1998) *Maternity Care Matters,* Aberdeen: Dugald Baird Centre for Research on Women's Health.

van der Kooy, B. (2009) Choice for women and choice for midwives – making it happen, *British Journal of Midwifery* 17(9): 524–5.

Winnicott, D.W. (1965) *The Family and Individual Development,* London: Tavistock.

Winnicott, D.W. (1987) *Babies and Their Mothers,* New York: Addison-Wesley.

Winnicott, D.W. (1988) *Human Nature,* London: Free Association Press.

CHAPTER 5

Poor Relations: The Paucity of the Professional Paradigm

RUTH WILKINS

Why is one woman still aware of her community midwife's working hours a year after she last had need to know? Why does another claim to love her? Why did a third 'really mourn' the end of their relationship? Why does a fourth think her 'a saint', a fifth want her to be 'a friend'? Why is a sixth disappointed not to know her 'as a person', a seventh upset by her brusqueness, an eighth by her indifference? What on earth is going on?

I became interested in midwifery as one of the women referred to above. From my own experiences and discussions with other mothers, I became aware that the mother–community midwife relationship has a significance over and above its 'professional' functions. The mother–midwife relationship is often described as 'special' (Cronk and Flint, 1989; Flint, 1987; Page, 1988). I wanted to know what was 'special' and distinctive about it in the community setting.

I decided to research the mother–community midwife relationship from a sociological perspective for my PhD thesis. The research was a longitudinal study involving in-depth interviews with a group of 43 mothers and their principal community midwives about community midwifery in general and their relationship in particular. The study was preceded by a pilot study and supplemented by an observational study of community midwifery in the same district in the southeast of England, a substudy of some self-selected 'special' relationships (involving 7 of the 43 mothers) and a review of the relevant midwifery research literature (Wilkins, 1993).[1]

At an early stage in the research, I became aware of a profound lack of 'fit' between the viewpoint of the mothers and midwives I interviewed and the 'professional paradigm' that dominated the midwifery literature. The clash of perspectives was so fundamental that there seemed to be no way of incorporating what mothers told me was important or 'special' with prevailing conceptualizations of midwifery practice and the mother–midwife relationship. Consequently, I also become interested in the processes by which knowledge is constructed in academic and professional discourse.

In the first half of this chapter, I explore the paradox I had encountered and some reasons underlying it. I suggest that a 'professional' outlook is conceptually blind to the processes that make the relationship 'special' to mothers. It thereby overlooks important ways in which community midwives are (or can be) supportive of mothers. This, I shall suggest, is part of a wider incapacity to consider human relationships, emotions and biographical experiences as integral aspects of midwifery practice. This oversight is in turn explicable in terms of the assumptions concerning knowledge and meaning that support a professional perspective. A 'professional' outlook divorces mothers from midwives and midwives from themselves. For reasons I shall explore later, there was virtually no clue in the research literature to what mothers or midwives themselves hold to be special about the relationship, this despite the recognition that a 'special' relationship does, or can, exist.

In the second half of the chapter, I draw on findings from my research and suggest that the distinctive aspects of community midwifery practice lie in the '3 Rs': relationship, role and real social context:

- *Relationship*: The 'special relationship' of which so many women speak is a personal one in which they are emotionally engaged and each party becomes known to the other; placing the other within a personal and biographical, rather than a narrowly professional, context. This in turn requires continuity of carer.
- *Role*: The 'role' of the community midwife (compared with medical practitioners and health visitors) is woman centred and psychosocially oriented.
- *Real social context*: The 'real' social context of the community, and in particular the home, facilitates the development of relationship and role, making available those social, emotional and biographical aspects that underpin the distinctive role of the midwife as supporter, carer and clinician to childbearing women.

Outline of the professional paradigm

Although one can distinguish a profession, a professional, professional practice and the professional–client relationship, each is informed by the same underlying assumptions. A profession is:

A superior type of occupation… that requires advanced education and training. It thus has a specific and exclusively owned body of knowledge and expertise. A profession organises and, to some extent, controls itself by establishing standards of ethics, knowledge and skill for its licenced practitioners. (Oakley, 1984: 27)

Professional knowledge is exclusive, formal, discrete and cerebral. A professional is a person in possession of specialist abstract knowledge who thereby stands in privileged relation to his or her clients. Professional practice is the application of professional knowledge in an object-oriented relationship of domination and control, whether of a body, a mind or a situation.

In these ways, the professional paradigm (or worldview) enshrines and prefers concepts of rationality, objectivity, formal knowledge, culture and control (themselves associated with masculinity) in opposition to those of emotion, subjectivity, experience, nature and caring (which are in turn associated with femininity). These preferences are underwritten by ontological distinctions between object/subject, rational/emotional, knowledge/experience, mind/matter and culture/nature (Oakley, 1992; Wagner, 1986). Thus, the professional paradigm exemplifies 'normative dualism', a process in which:

Things that may be complementary or even inseparable [are conceptualised] in terms of exclusive disjunctions (either–or but not both)… They then value one disjunct more highly than the other. (Garry and Pearsall, 1989: xii)

In the professional paradigm, facts, reason, knowledge and science are actively pulled together, concertina fashion, along an epistemological drawstring called objectivity. The professional paradigm recognizes only one, 'professional' way of knowing. It prefers rational, formal knowledge, which it homogenizes and then monopolizes. It prioritizes professional practice (the active application of expert knowledge) and in so doing gives pre-eminence to the professional as the 'doer', overlooks the agency of the client and obscures other sources of knowledge. It also situates professional and client in wholly different 'planes of being' (or social dimensions), thus precluding any analysis of their relationship to each other and their similarities.

As Oakley (1984) notes, some sociologists, acknowledging the contradictions that this poses for a female professional, have labelled professions with a predominantly female workforce 'semi-professions' (Etzioni,

1969). Other sociologists, recognizing the masculinist normative prefer-ences inherent in 'professionalization', have questioned whether women should strive to become professionals at all. Addressing the nursing profession, Oakley (1984: 27) suggests:

> If a profession is by definition male dominated, then nurses might as well give up. Alternatively, nurses might ask the truly radical question as to what is so wonderful about being a professional anyway... the current crisis of confidence in medical care should tell us that profes-sionalisation is not the only answer.

The professional paradigm and midwifery research

The implications of this argument have not been fully articulated in rela-tion to the developments taking place in midwifery. Midwives are begin-ning to redefine the role, policy and practice of the midwife as distinct from that of medical practitioners. One aspect of this has been the assim-ilation of 'caring' as a professional objective. But this reversal of the 'care versus control' dichotomy in the medical professional model has led to neither a critique of related dichotomies nor, more radically, a critique of the normative dualisms on which the professional paradigm (and science) depend. Accordingly, midwifery continues to be articulated in a language appropriate to medicine rather than midwifery. For example:

> The midwife has a central place in the provision of care in pregnancy and childbirth, as it is in her role in particular that the main elements of maternity care – clinical assessment and monitoring and the provi-sion of advice and support – are combined. (Robinson, 1989a: 162)

The incorporation of the professional paradigm gives rise to a persist-ent tendency to conceptualize midwifery care in a conventional, object-oriented way in a manner that denies points of connection between professional and client and appropriates power and control to the 'expert'. There are three particular difficulties, as described below.

Location of mother and midwife in different planes of being

The professional paradigm situates mothers and midwives in different planes of being (or social dimensions). This gives rise to two particular shortcomings. First, it denies the validity and relevance of the midwife's biographical self to professional practice. That is, it alienates the midwife from herself, constructing her 'personal' and 'professional' selves as entirely separate. This is part of a larger failure to incorporate a subjective viewpoint. It denies the social self (and thus the possibility of sensitizing biographical experiences) and the psychological self, the midwife's culturally acquired 'ways of knowing' and 'conscious subjectivity' (Garry and Pearsall, 1989; Stanley, 1990).

Second, it denies points of connection between women. Mothers and midwives are conceptualized as if they inhabit mutually exclusive social spaces. The paradigm cannot accommodate the social and psychological identities that inscribe relationships between women in general, so cannot appreciate the gendered basis of the mother–community midwife relationship in particular. That is, it eclipses something of profound importance to women. It cannot explain many of the most emphatic statements they themselves have made, for example the importance of their community midwife being a woman and the desirability of her being a mother.

The paradigm is inadequate to the analysis of the mother–community midwife relationship. It is conceptually blind to the relationship as a dyad on the one hand and the points of connection within it on the other. It separates mothers from midwives and midwives from themselves.

Overemphasis on the professional

The professional paradigm prioritizes professional activity and professional knowledge and encourages an object-oriented perception of clients or patients. Emphasis is given to the activity and concerns of the professional. The professional paradigm invites practitioners to atomize the professional relationship and to fashion instead the entity 'professional practice', a discrete body of knowledge and expertise divorced from the social and relational context of its application. If the relationship is considered at all, as in some analyses of the 'midwifery process', it is instrumental to the professional objective, as for example with 'the provision of advice and support' (Robinson, 1989a), rather than being conceptualized in its own right.

The relationship is, however, often of value to mothers in and of itself, not instrumental to the provision of advice and support but an instance or expression of it. That is, it is the human relationship rather than merely the service or skill that is valued. It is not a package but a process, and the professional paradigm cannot see this. In order to understand the value of the relationship as it is lived, in order more fully to appreciate how midwifery is part of the social network, an aspect of social support, a real human relationship between two people, the professional paradigm has to be relinquished.

Alienation of women from their own experiences

The language of the professional does not articulate women's experiences. It is unable to accommodate what mothers value about their relationships with their community midwives and thus 'alienates them from their own experiences' (Smith, 1988: 86). It is the language of disinformation. It denies the need for a 'relationship' except for purely instrumental purposes and undermines women's own feelings. Women can be heard wanting a close personal relationship with their midwives:

> I'm hoping that a midwife will be almost like a friend's relationship with you. (Mother; Wilkins, 1993: 59)

yet recognizing these as 'outlaw emotions' (Jaggar, 1989: 145):

> But apparently that's unprofessional... you don't bring yourself, your own experiences, into that sort of thing... that's what I've heard... but I don't know whether I agree. (Mother; Wilkins, 1993: 59)

There are other, derivative difficulties. For example, the professional paradigm constructs and prefers 'knowledge' over 'experience', so that research, rationality and training are preferred over individual experience, whether professional or personal. The midwifery profession itself appears to be stratifying along these lines. Bodies and minds are also dichotomized, robbing mothers of their minds and midwives of their bodies. This approach also de-emphasizes and undervalues the practical basis of many professional skills.

In short, the professional paradigm is a way of constructing knowledge and human activity, one which relies on a series of dichotomies that polarize professionals and clients, midwives and mothers in turn. It is an ontology without a subjective viewpoint, ill disposed to relational analysis of any sort and capable of articulating relationships in only an instrumental and object-oriented manner. It is conceptually blind to subjective relationships, since there is no point of connection between expert and subject and therefore no way of understanding the emotionally connected and biographically grounded relationship that many women seek from their community midwife. It also prevents midwives perceiving that relationship in anything other than an object-oriented way.

This leaves midwifery conceptually impoverished. There is, for example, no way of differentiating the role of the midwife from that of the medical practitioner, except as a matter of emphasis. Furthermore, in failing to challenge professionalism's normative dualisms, the entire edifice remains intact. On this construction, 'care' will always remain less central to professional practice than 'clinical assessment', 'monitoring' and the 'provision of advice'.

Consequences of the professional paradigm in midwifery research

If we turn now to consider how the mother–community midwife relationship has been understood in the academic and practitioner-based literature reviewed, we find an almost total silence. The relationship between a childbearing woman and her midwife has been almost entirely neglected. This is an oversight that is all the more surprising when one considers that midwives are women's primary professional maternity care-givers, that midwifery is increasingly community oriented, that increased research attention is being paid to the psychosocial aspects of maternity care, and that midwives are re-establishing a distinctive professional role, practice and research tradition, a central tenet of which is the provision of care that is supportive of and 'sensitive' to the needs of the mother (Adams, 1987; Flint, 1987; Flint and Poulengeris, 1988; Kirkham, 1989; Methven, 1989).

If the relationship is recognized at all, it is characterized as an orthodox, if caring, professional–client relationship (Ball, 1989; Laryea, 1989; Methven, 1989; Robinson, 1989a, 1989b). It is recognized that the relationship is, or can be, 'special' (Cronk and Flint, 1989; Flint, 1987; Page, 1988), but there has been no attempt to specify how or why. This is part of a wider failing to incorporate the concept of human relationships into midwifery practice.

In addition, notwithstanding policy statements in favour of community-based midwifery care (Association of Radical Midwives, 1986; Royal College of Midwives, 1987), there has been no attempt to specify what is distinctive about the mother–midwife relationship in the community. With very few exceptions, the studies emphasize hospital rather than community midwifery and distinguish these for pragmatic or organizational rather than conceptual reasons (Wilkins, 1993).

It is in 'scientific' research that the contradictions implicit in midwifery research (those arising from the incorporation of the normative dualisms of science and professionalism such as object/subject, rational/emotional and knowledge/experience) are most acutely posed. In obstetric clinical research, the randomized controlled trial (RCT) has been vigorously advocated (Chalmers and Richards, 1977; Chalmers *et al.*, 1989; Enkin and Chalmers, 1982). A direct opposition is asserted between 'experience' and 'knowledge'. For example, Enkin and Chalmers refer to the 'shaky foundations of authority and clinical experience' and caution 'conscientious clinicians' to base their clinical practice on the results of scientific evaluation arising from the conduct of 'appropriately designed research' (Enkin and Chalmers, 1982: 278). Although they acknowledge that 'many things that really count cannot be counted' (*ibid.*: 285), there is no way of reconciling that sentiment with the putative superiority of scientific over other kinds of knowledge.

This approach has profoundly influenced the design and methodology of much midwifery research[1] and has three particular consequences. First, it undermines and deflects attention away from the midwife-researcher's biographical experiences as a source of professional knowledge, as well as from the skill and knowledge arising from that experience. Second, it denies the possibility of learning through identification with the client because it asserts an epistemic distinction between lay and professional knowledge corresponding to 'objective' and 'subjective' states (knowledge and experience respectively). In so doing, it implicitly (and erroneously) asserts the epistemic purity of scientific research through a sole reliance on 'objective' knowledge, methodologies and practice (Knorr-Cetina, 1981). Third, it seeks to confine 'subjectivity' to specific discrete and manipulable variables (and to research subjects), whereby subjectivity becomes divorced from other indices or outcome measures (for example, the degree of medical intervention during labour and delivery) and from the research process itself.

As noted earlier, this entirely fails to fit the central conclusions of my own research, which suggested that the importance of the mother–community midwife relationship lies precisely in those sources of 'knowledge' which the empirical scientist denies: the midwife's skill and experience on the one hand and her personal and cultural qualifications on the other. The personal, emotional and relational aspects of midwifery practice are crucial to both mother and midwife. Flint's *Sensitive Midwifery* (1987) abounds with examples of the importance of biographical experience and empathic identification to midwifery practice. Personal, emotional and biographical experiences are crucial aspects of the professional process, but this insight is denied by the perspectives of 'professionalism' and science. These perspectives denude the mother–midwife relationship and deny its richness and complexity. Moreover, since neither is able to appreciate the distinctive contribution of the midwife to maternity care, the midwife's contribution is indistinguishable from that of any other clinical provider.

Research findings: Distinctive aspects of the mother–midwife relationship

In the following section are presented findings from my own research, grounded in a viewpoint that relinquishes the normative dualisms of the professional paradigm, which reveals values and priorities that are not visible from a 'professional' perspective and that confirm the role of the midwife as distinct from that of other clinical carers of childbearing women.[1]

The best insights into what Cronk and Flint call 'that special relationship... on which so much depends' (1989: 9) come from direct experience rather than formal knowledge:

> Mothers and midwives are intertwined, whatever affects women affects midwives and vice versa – we are interrelated and interwoven... To be a midwife is to be with women (the meaning of the Anglo-Saxon word) – sharing their travail and their suffering, their joys and their delights. (Flint, 1987: viii, 1)

This implies two related aspects of the 'special' character of the relationship: a personal relationship between women and an emotional connectedness across the professional–client divide. This echoes the findings of my own research, which indicated in addition the rooting of the relationship in mothers' 'real', vital concerns. My research suggests that the community midwife's distinctive contribution lies in what I have termed the '3 Rs': the relationship, the role and the real social context respectively.

The relationship

The relationship was 'special' to the women interviewed to the extent that it was a *personal* relationship, akin but not identical to friendship. Mothers frequently expressed the wish to know, or the pleasure of knowing, their midwife 'as a person'. Moreover, for the women interviewed, it was indissolubly a relationship between women. They stressed the importance of a confiding, trusting, close relationship that held them, their emotions, experiences and concerns at its heart. Pregnancy and childbirth are in this sense a process of self-exploration shared with their community midwives. Such women want their midwife to be 'like a friend' to them. As the relationship deepens emotionally, so it expands socially; one mark of a developing relationship is the extent to which the social dimension extends into the 'clinical' encounter.

The role

The subjective, psychosocially oriented role of the community midwife concentrates on feelings and experiences. It also engages the midwife's culturally acquired 'ways of being' and 'ways of knowing'. This combination of professional role and cultural capability is a powerful and valued one. It is an important basis for the personal relationship referred to above. In addition, it places mothers and midwives in the same 'plane of being' and thus engages the midwife's personal as well as professional resources.

Many mothers valued the midwife's 'cultural qualifications'. Some valued the fact that she was a woman, others that she was a mother. If she was a mother, this was an important basis for sharing experiences and drawing the relationship closer. To many women, these cultural qualifications were important sources of professional expertise, encouraging empathy and social and emotional awareness. For these women, mother and midwife were drawn together through their mutual grounding in shared identities and experiences.

The role also enables mothers, through the medium of their midwives, to gain access to other women's experiences of childbirth. Here, midwives are valued for their rich and detailed knowledge of women's experiences of childbearing and the social and emotional transitions accompanying it, made possible by an empathic and supportive role and a sensitive and sentient attunement within it. It is an intensely subjective conceptualization of midwifery. Midwives are the embodiment of women's experiences of childbearing, an invaluable and unique resource.

The 'real' social context

The community context is the appropriate one for the role, rooting it within the psychosocial context it serves. In the community, midwifery is interwoven into the fabric of women's real, vital, immediate, practical and emotional concerns. Mothers usually feel more relaxed in their own homes and experience greater intimacy and personal connection in that setting. These visits also tend to be more leisurely. On this construction, the community context is both permissive (of the relationship) and a more appropriate venue to appreciate women's own concerns and priorities.

In the following pages, I explore each of these aspects (relationship, role and real social context) in more detail.

The mother–community midwife relationship

Midwives and mothers belong in the same 'plane of being', on the same 'side', in the context of an emotionally and practically important and supportive relationship. On this construction, what is 'special' is the *human relationship* within which midwives' skills and knowledge are embedded. What they value as 'special' and distinctive is an emotionally connected, supportive relationship that both draws on and expresses women's culturally acquired skills and experiences, one that is embedded in women's 'real' concerns and situations.

Bonds are formed from the sharing of intimate emotional experiences. So it is with childbirth. The deepest bonds are formed between mothers and community midwives who have shared an emotionally intense experience, be it the joy of birth or the trauma of bereavement. Birth, as one woman noted, is 'a very intimate experience to share with somebody'. Bonds may be formed unilaterally, but it is more usual for them to be mutual (although not symmetrical):

> I think if you're not prepared to reveal something of yourself you can't expect to get something back from somebody else. It's got to be a two way thing. You can't keep yourself aloof at the same time as expecting someone else to reveal their vulnerability. It's just not on. (Laura, midwife)

As this occurs, so the social dimension of the relationship is redefined. The emphasis switches from a role-based to a personally based relationship, with the consequent inclusion of social and biographical elements as the midwife is taken in by the mother from a personal perspective. These three elements – emotionality, mutuality and familiarity – are the core constituents of a close personal relationship:

> **Mother (Amanda):** I wanted a community midwife, yes, I did. Given the choice I had hoped it would be. Given the choice I had hoped it would be Anna as well.
> **Recorder:** And was it what you hoped it would be.

M: It was what I hoped it would be and an awful lot more. It was an amazing experience... totally because of Anna. Yes, it was totally different from Paula and it's what every woman's experience should be I think... but, yes, she just made it really.

R: What did she do; can you identify it?

M: Well first of all, I think it was just her reassuring manner, that everything was going as it should be and she helped me feel that I was in control of it, whereas when Paula was born it was very high tech – you know, she was monitored and forceps and epidural and everything. And it was just so totally different. I think just the reassurance that she gave that I was doing all right: even when I was sort of getting to the end and I remember hearing myself saying, 'No I can't do it any more, I can't.' And you know she said, 'Yes, you can and you've got to because that's the only way the baby's going to come.' And its the continual reassurance that the baby's doing all right; and yes it was just her whole professional manner really...

She was very good as far as Mike was concerned as well [involving him]. It was real sort of shared experience. There was no point that we felt she was sort of the medical person present; she was part of the whole situation, she was one of the active people involved in it all... We were both totally overwhelmed about what had happened and how she had made the experience for us. And she said it had been an experience for her as well, which was lovely.

And we were just given so much more time. I remember when Paula was born, we were very quickly whipped out of the delivery room and up to the ward. Here, we were left together for ages. And she brought a telephone into the room, it was all little things like that that just made it; and no rush to get out and into the system or anything... Absolutely marvellous, it really was...

R: Did that make it hard to say goodbye to her?

M: Very, yes it did, very very hard. Because in a funny way, it's almost like a sort of initial bonding when the baby's born, that then just bonds you with them. And you know the initial bonding you have when the baby's born, there's also that sort of feeling with the person who's delivered your baby. And yes, it was very very hard, very hard.

R: Did you have that feeling with the person who delivered Paula?

M: Um, no, not to the same extent, although she was lovely. But I was just one of a number. I mean I still am to all intents and purposes, but you were just made to feel very individual, I think that was the difference. I mean, yes, we were very grateful to the midwife who delivered Paula but it was a different... Right at the very end, that moment just before he was born, I was thinking, 'I really can't push any more, I've pushed all I can', and Anna suddenly said to me, 'Come on, say a prayer, you can do it.' And it really sort of brought me up and kept me going, and he was born within the next couple of minutes. It was amazing.

R: Did you get her a gift?

M: Well we did buy her something. We bought her a picture. It was one of those things where I knew what I wanted but couldn't go into a shop and say, 'I want this'; I knew it immediately I saw it. We both agreed that that's what we were going to do. But as you say, it was only a very, very small token of all that we'd had.

R: Have you got any plans to keep in touch with her?

M: Well yes, we have actually. She said to me before she went… she wants me to go up there… which would be lovely. She's such a lovely person. And it really did make the experience. That's not to say that Suzy [another midwife] is any lesser qualified because I'm sure the experience also would have been a wonderful one, but I think Anna was right for us… It's to be treasured really. It's not something you could write down; it's just something that I'll keep… It's what every community delivery should be. It's certainly what every woman should feel…

R: Did it make a difference as well when she came round afterwards; what difference did it make that she'd been there… did you talk it through or did it deepen the relationship?

M: Yes, it did… it was nice to have her reassurance, you know, the person that has actually delivered him and everything that he was going to be all right; I think it was just the reassurance of having Anna coming back every day, and not losing her, not letting go of her.

R: Did you talk over the birth?

M: I kept on saying what an experience it was, and I mean it was Anna who said that it was what every woman should experience and that was how they saw their role, but it was just a question really of man/womanpower and of the actual logistics of it all… A friend of mine who's expecting in June who I know is very apprehensive about it, she had a bad experience… I mean if I could sell it to her that it needn't be like that. Gosh, yes, if you could bottle it and sell it, you'd make a fortune. But I mean that is how it actually feels… It made me want to go and tell everybody, it really did.

The community midwife's role

Women seek an emotionally supportive personal relationship with their community midwife, one that is woman centred and pyschosocially oriented. This is the critical difference between the role of the midwife (particularly in the community) and that of other professional care-givers. The community midwife's role is empathically woman centred. Her role is to be 'with woman'. She therefore takes on the concerns of the woman, and it is this which gives her role its distinctive psychosocial orientation. The roles of GPs and health visitors, on the other hand, are not experienced by the mothers in such terms. The GP's role is seen as more objective and medically oriented, the health visitor's as more bureaucratic, advisory and interventionist. This places both GP and health visitor in a different plane of being from the mother and largely precludes an empathic, supportive, woman-centred role orientation.

This is not to deny that GPs and health visitors can be supportive, or that community midwives can be unsupportive; individuals may have a role orientation or personal disposition that departs from this, just as there is variability between midwives (Wilkins, 1993). It does, however, identify an important source of difference in mothers' experiences of their respective roles. These differences make it more difficult for a GP, for example, to be as socially supportive as a community midwife, whatever her or his personal outlook.

I was able to identify four distinguishing features of the midwife's role compared with that of the GP. First, the relationship is more personal and subjectively oriented. Women refer to the relationship with the community midwife as being more supportive, personal, intimate, friendly, informal, enjoyable and continuous.

Second, the role is psychosocially oriented. Her role involves greater intimacy between mother and midwife, in particular a more personal, caring, intimate and supportive orientation, more extensive and intimate contact with the mother's body and more contact with her in her own home. The lines of communication are more open between mothers and midwives. In particular, they feel more able to confide and to ask about 'little things' that they may feel are too trivial to mention to the doctor.

Third, the midwife is seen as the more appropriate professional, associated with childbearing in a way that medical practitioners are not. Midwives make more time, and there is greater continuity of care. The midwife 'sees you through' the whole experience, antenatally, intranatally and postnatally, in a way that the GP does not. These relational and role differences give rise to concrete differences of practice style. Women refer to midwives as better informed, as more thorough in the care they provide, and as providing better explanations. I observed that the style of consultation is more informal and the seating arrangements less confrontational with community midwives. Midwives and mothers are connected in a way that mothers and doctors are not.

An instrumental and clinical orientation defeats the expressive and psychosocial aspects that are such a crucial part of midwifery. In general, the relationship with the GP was described by the mothers as professional rather than personal. Essentially they felt the GP to be out of touch with women. Notwithstanding the need to foster a relationship for the purposes of subsequent contacts after the pregnancy, the GP was felt to be less interested in, and less sympathetic to, 'minor' or emotional aspects of care, and to have less understanding of women's needs and concerns. The mothers suggest there is less personal interest in the women themselves and, where interest is expressed, it is somehow less attuned to women's own feelings. The GPs resort to the notes, the computer or the midwives to avail themselves of details that community midwives grasp and retain informally.

Finally, women describe ways in which doctors are socially more remote than midwives. At one level this reflects class and status differences, but the distinctions they describe are sown into the fabric of the relationship in subtle ways that reinforce the dissociations inherent in the professional paradigm. The use of titles rather than first names reinforces social distance. Status distinctions underwrite social distance when women are called by their first name and doctors by their title. Doctors are very much 'that side of the desk' and women are summoned to consult them by a buzzer, in contrast to the practice of most midwives of going to greet and accompany the mother from the waiting room. There is less time, the GP is more busy (or mothers feel them to be), and they are conscious of the queues of people waiting behind them. The atmosphere is less relaxed and more formal. It is not an environment conducive to sharing and support.

There are superficial similarities between midwives and health visitors. Each is a health professional and almost invariably female. Each has contact with the mother in her own home. Each is concerned with facilitating the well-being of the family unit. Each is (usually) a trained nurse. Each has an advisory aspect to her role, and each is involved in a key life event.

The mothers' experiences and depictions, however, suggest the two roles are very different and mark something of a culture shock for the mothers. First, the health visitor has a more advisory role. Second, this lacks the supportive and intimate orientation of the community midwife. The relationship is less personal, less satisfying, less involved and less easy. Mothers often say that there is no sense of a relationship at all.

Third, the health visitor's remit is seen as the baby rather than the woman, and the woman may feel on trial as a mother. Fourth, it is a more dissociated, bureaucratized relationship marked by the mores of formal knowledge, including clinical measurement and textbook advice. Correspondingly, there is less emphasis, investment and immersion in experiential knowledge. Finally, mothers perceive a potential conflict of interest between themselves and the health visitor. The alliance between mother and community midwife is gone, replaced by the advisory, surveillance role of the health visitor.

With few exceptions, mothers painted a picture of mild antagonism towards the health visitor, who was variously perceived as unhelpful, out of touch or an inconvenience, there to instruct or test rather than support and befriend the mother. There were some positive comments, for example that she was involved, highly trained, gave good advice and was practical. Another woman whose child was physically challenged had major needs of the health visitor, was emotionally more invested and thus developed a stronger relationship. One health visitor in particular had a supportive orientation and was well integrated into the community. She tended to be appreciated in terms similar to those used for community midwives, but there was no suggestion of the 'special' relationship characteristic of community midwifery. Nonetheless, even some of these appreciative women still clearly distinguished the role of community midwife and health visitor along the lines indicated above:

M: Yeah, she played quite an important part. She was brilliant... She just knows everything. Yes, she was very good, very helpful, very positive person and I just think you need somebody like that...
R: Were there any differences from the midwife's role?
M: Well yeah, you know that the midwife is there to support you and help you through your labour, and there again it's attention on you; whereas the health visitor I used to think was just looking at the baby, she was just making sure that he was OK, nothing really about myself, whereas the midwife is as concerned for me as she is for my baby. (Lydia, mother)

In these ways, the roles of both GP and health visitor operate within the confines of the professional rather than the personal paradigm. In addition, the specific roles of the GP and the health visitor differ significantly from that of the community midwife, in a way that detracts from the supportive, intimate, woman-centred relationship that mothers themselves value.

The 'real' social context

I have suggested that the distinctive character of community midwifery rests on three key features: the relationship, the role and the real social context. The relationship is an intimate, personal one. The role is a psychosocial one, supportive of and centred on the mother. This leaves the third aspect, the real social context. The *context* of care fundamentally affects its character, creating some possibilities, precluding others. The community is the appropriate context for midwifery care, complementary to both role and relationship. It enables the personal and psychosocial aspects of midwifery care to be realized more fully. It does this by anchoring midwifery within the mother's social context, making visible and emphasizing her psychosocial needs and concerns.

This has four consequences for midwifery. First, it improves empathic understanding, which facilitates both role and relationship. The midwife has access at an experiential level to feelings, knowledge, relationships, environments and priorities that would not be apparent in the hospital. Second, it enhances the psychosocial dimension of midwifery care, which is central to the community midwife's role. Childbearing is as much a psychosocial as a biological event, and it is lived in the community. This is therefore the most appropriate site for the provision of psychosocial support. Mother and midwife experience the vivid realities of motherhood at the centre of the appropriate stage. Third, it enables the midwife to give more appropriate practical advice because, as noted, she has more direct access and exposure to the mother's environment. Conversely, the hospital setting is culturally discontinuous with the social and domestic context within which parenting occurs. This diminishes its practical utility. Finally, the community context facilitates the intimate and personal relationship. In the home context in particular, women typically feel more relaxed and more powerful, and this means that the relationship is more equal and open.

Both mothers and midwives indicate that it is easier to know and understand women in the community context as their circumstances and viewpoint become more visible. It is more the mother's domain, whereas the hospital is more the domain of professional experts. These are not absolute distinctions, but they are key distinctions for midwifery because the community setting provides information, experiences and understanding that would be unavailable to even the most sensitive midwife in the hospital setting. Compared to the hospital setting, women feel that they enjoy better care and better relationships in the community, and midwives feel that they gain a better understanding and appreciation of the women for whom they care. It is more personal, relaxed and humane, less clinical, medicalized, bureaucratic and rushed.

On the other hand, women experience the hospital as 'an institution': cold, impersonal and clinical. Mothers and midwives draw attention to three particular aspects of the hospital environment. First, it depersonalizes. Within such an environment, mothers and midwives are dissociated, care is stripped of its emotional aspect, and women become tongue-tied, anxious and angry. In hospital, you are 'just a number', anonymous, stripped of personal identity. You are redefined as a 'patient': sanitized, passive and helpless:

What do we do? We bring you in, we put you in a white gown and we put... a label on you. You're a patient, I'm a nurse. It's terrible... I feel it, every time I put a bracelet on a patient, on one of the women; now you're a patient. And they're not really. They're just in there because the facilities are there for them to have a baby. They're no different to me. (Joanna, midwife)

Second, the parties do not know each other, despite the existence of a team midwifery scheme. The interaction is more superficial, less grounded, less meaningful. In these circumstances:

I guess the answer you give is quite a stat answer. You just answer their question. It's not a meaningful one, it's not [like]... when they asked a question [in the community setting]. We did have some women that used to come up quite regularly and that was great: 'Oh a face I've seen before!' And they would latch on to you too. But yes, it is different [in the hospital]. You're just a midwife... there's not that personal contact... I was still myself but I just didn't feel I knew the person... I was desperately missing my women. (Joanna, midwife)

When Joanna returned to the community after an absence of three years, she had to re-establish the rebuilding of relationships with the women.

You just don't know any of the women... And I also feel it when they come in and say, 'Oh another face'... there's nothing I like nicer than walking out into the waiting room and spotting the woman who's next on the list, calling her by her Christian name and saying, 'Hi, how are you?' rather than going out there not knowing who's who, and just going out there and calling their name... And I missed the hands on...

And you're looking at the most non-maternal person. (Joanna, midwife)

The community midwife aspect of it, what makes it special has just got to be this continuity of care, and the fact that you do get to know the woman that you're looking after; and if you manage to stay in the same job for a while and they start coming back the second time around, that is lovely. (Elizabeth, midwife)

Third, the hospital is seen by many as an irrelevance, a waste of time. For them, impersonal care is impoverished care. With the exception of the scan, the clinical care offered in the hospital is seen as similar to that in the community, but the setting is less congenial and considerably more inconvenient:

You... go into a hospital and it's just so impersonal. As I say, although it's in my notes, I haven't even bothered to make an appointment to go up to the hospital because to me it's just a waste of time. I'm a number to them and they'll have my file but they won't know anything about me. Whereas I know at this stage if I've got a problem, I'll go down to see Anna or Suzy or Dr Peters and be dealt with in a much better, more humane way. And it won't take two and a half hours... That's something else, they will come back to you if there's a problem... I really don't see the point of [going to the hospital]. I mean, they look after you so well [in the community]; why go and sit up there and have exactly the same thing done to you that Anna can do? (Amanda, mother)

You don't know people. You go into a room cold. You've got minutes to get a rapport with that person... You can do it but it's not as satisfying. I can't remember their names, for instance. I can remember the incidents. It's not as satisfying as going into somebody's house that you know, is it? (Anna, midwife)

The second of these extracts tells its own story. In a hospital context, the midwife noted for her intimate orientation forgets the personal details, remembering simply the 'incidents', abstracted away from their contexts. She remembers incidents rather than people. Her recollection is fragmented, decontextualized and depersonalized.

It may be suggested that these distinctions reflect not the social setting *per se* but the organization of care, which in the hospital setting is typically more fragmented. According to this argument, if there were continuity in the hospital setting, the same relationships could be formed. But even if one could overcome the medicalized, bureaucratized and hierarchical culture of the hospital setting, and even if continuity, familiarity and sensitivity were fostered, the relationships would differ for the reasons indicated earlier: the woman's social context would be invisible, the relationship would be less personal and less psychosocially oriented, and the possibilities for realistic social support would be severely diminished because it would be enacted within an inappropriate environment, that of the expert rather than the client.

> Looking back on the time in hospital, when somebody comes in you put them in a nightie; that person's in a nightie. With the best will in the world, that person's still in a nightie. You've got no idea of their social background or their emotional needs. (Carol, midwife)

So the community provides a context within which midwives can most appropriately be 'with woman' and supportive, incorporated within a personal paradigm. The midwife becomes an aspect of the community, part of the social network and the family unit; not 'facilitating' or manipulating it but immersed in it, part of it, oriented to both in a way the hospital context prevents:

> I think you just feel that she's done this so many times before, and living round here she's delivered so many babies round here that she's sort of part of the whole – part of the area really. And you see all these people waving to her in the car. Everybody feels the same about community midwives I think; I mean, they're really part of their life really. They remember when their birthdays are and all that sort of thing... in a way I'd like to go and have these babies in a country where the midwife is really part of the village atmosphere, never far away... It's a very special job, very special... I don't know how emotionally they cope with being part of each little unit. Because I mean I almost cried when she left after 10 days... And I was thinking, 'I wish she could come every other day or something'; it would be nice if it almost was weaned off. I think it's quite sad... I remember feeling, 'It's like losing a member of your family really', as she was going... Do you know what I mean? She's gone... I'd have liked her to pop in... I really did feel very upset and bought her a present. (Virginia, mother)

I conclude this section by dealing briefly with the suggestion that what has been depicted as distinctive in community midwifery amounts in practice to 'being there' at a major emotional experience, that of child-birth. If this were true, mothers would feel similarly towards all principal care-givers present at the delivery. Certainly, when women describe their labours, it is not unusual for them to speak of strong feelings of affection and gratitude for their immediate care-givers, whether or not they had prior contact with them. Moreover, Klaus *et al.* (1986) refer to the socially supportive effects of *doulas*, or specialist lay attendants, who attend and support the mother during labour, with a statistically signifi-cant reduction in the number of perinatal complications in the general sample and a shorter labour in women requiring no intervention.

It is clear that 'just being there' is in itself not enough. Mothers often refer to the unimportance of GPs or students during labour. It is the prin-cipal care-giver who is likely to have a major impact, be it positive or negative. It is also well established that women do benefit from continu-ous emotional support during labour, although the nature of their requirements may vary.

Beyond this, two points can be noted. The first is that women's depic-tions of the delivery experience differ where the midwife is unknown, or relatively unknown, compared with the principal community midwife, even if the experience with hospital midwives has been emotionally intense and positive. Many women describe their hospital midwife as 'nice', 'friendly', 'lovely' and 'caring'. They may also describe social and biographical exchanges more typical of established relationships. But what is missing from their accounts is the relational element: the depth of relationship on the one hand and the sense of shared experience on the other. This manifests itself only in relation to community deliveries. Even if the most intense emotional attachment was with the unknown hospital midwife at delivery, the community midwife, as the one who 'knows you and has seen you through it', remains an enduring association.

In addition, the picture that emerges of *medical* care in hospital is the familiar one of a depersonalized, controlling service involving the elevation of the expert, and expert knowledge, within the professional paradigm. The 'patient' is overlooked, her insights are dismissed and her body is taken over. She becomes the object of professional practice: stripped of knowledge, emotional needs, social location and responsibilities, frag-mented, dislocated and objectified. This echoes the difficulties that women encountered in their dealings with GPs, but in the hospital context, anonymity, fragmentation and decontextualization compound these diffi-culties. The best endeavours of some medical practitioners cannot over-come structural obstacles to open and empathic communication.

Conclusion

For the past three centuries, midwives have increasingly had to compete with medical men for the privilege of delivering women's babies. To be a 'midwife' is to be 'with woman'. Until the sixteenth century, midwives had almost always been women. Symbolically, they were both feared and revered, representing women's powerful sexual and creative energies. The church took trouble to control them. For better or worse, midwives' skills were empirical, pragmatic and acquired through experience and apprenticeship. The rise of medicine and the invention of forceps, however, gave men both the power and the means to overcome this fearful female monopoly, to establish male supremacy and control (Donnison, 1988; Oakley, 1977). In essence, battle has been drawn along these lines ever since. On the one hand, there is woman, experience, intuition and allegiance. On the other, there is intervention, difference, medical/professional control and abstract knowledge.

However, battle wages not only between midwives and medical men, but also, more subtly, between mothers and midwives. On the platform of protests against medicalized childbirth, midwifery has begun to reassert itself and has gained in power and influence. As part of these developments, it has reclaimed its ideological heritage as comprising care-givers 'with woman', supportive of and allied with childbearing women. Midwives have taken their distance from the medical model of childbirth and begun to articulate a distinctive midwifery approach. Midwives, however, have rejected the medical model without relinquishing the conceptual apparatus, the professional paradigm, which supports it and which precludes an understanding of the important and unique contribution of the midwife.

During my research, I identified three broad tendencies in midwifery research. The first was a disaffection with and movement away from obstetric supremacy, reorienting the field of enquiry towards the nature and quality of the care provided by the principal care-giver, the midwife, and institutional/interprofessional impediments to appropriate and autonomous midwifery practice. The second, related tendency was an attempt to redefine the role, policy and practice of midwifery so oriented. This involved a critical reappraisal of medical procedures in midwifery practice, the ideological recognition of midwives as practitioners 'with woman' and a corresponding conceptualization of childbearing as 'an altered state of health', inextricably embedded in and influenced by psychosocial factors. The provision of continuity of care, and the development of team midwifery and the 'midwifery process', were central to this reorientation. Finally, as part of a broader tendency within obstetric and epidemiological research in the maternity services, there was a commitment to 'scientific' research practice. The dominant research orientation was evaluative, the dominant epistemology empiricist and the favoured method the RCT. There was an increased emphasis on the psychosocial aspects of care, but within an intellectual framework that located knowledge and control with the 'professional', whether a scientific researcher or a clinician. Consequently, midwifery ended up ideologically in conflict with itself, and the interests of both mother and midwife became articulated within a perspective that ultimately denied them.

The renaissance in midwifery therefore left it without a coherent paradigm on which to build a distinctive midwifery policy and practice. There remained a residual and unanalysed commitment to the professional perspective that underwrites medical practice on the one hand, and a related commitment to the research paradigms of epidemiologists on the other. In consequence, midwifery research developed on an uneven footing, its policies inclined in one direction and its paradigms in another. This tended to obliterate the insights and implications of the protests against medicalized childbirth and thus the possibility of recognizing the distinctive contribution of the midwife to childbearing women.

What implications does this have for future research, policy and practice? It suggests that mothers and midwifery research are facing in different directions. If midwives want to be 'with woman', they will have to do it without the professional paradigm. This does not mean that their outlooks have to be identical or wholly subjective. But the orientation of a 'caring professional' is not thoroughgoing enough.

As Methven's work (1989) indicates, language and concepts are among the most powerful definers of situations. If midwives really wish to challenge the medical model in their own practice, they have to address the professional paradigm that supports it. This is no small task, for ultimately it entails a critical re-evaluation of how we know what we know, who defines it for us, what goes on inside our own heads and hearts, and where we stand in relation to others. It restores mothers and midwives to the centre of the process, but in so doing it poses as many challenges as it meets. This is a challenge that other 'professionals' (among them sociologists, scientists and social workers) must also turn to face. Together we can find a voice.

Note

1. See Wilkins (1993) for a detailed discussion of the metatheory, methodology and research methods used in the research and the literature review undertaken in connection with it.

Acknowledgements

Three years is a long time to support somebody, and I would like to thank those who have supported me. I am grateful to the Economic and Social Research Council, without whom this research would not have been possible; to Ann Oakley and Jo Garcia for getting me started; and to Sara Arber and Sarah Nettleton, my PhD supervisors, whose insights and encouragement enabled me freely to develop my ideas. My gratitude to them is open ended, as it is to the research subjects (mothers and midwives) who generously allowed me to share such an important time in their lives. To my family and friends, a humble and sheepish thank-you, for 'taking it' when the tolls were high and the research absorbed me like a sponge, and for 'giving it' when you were so much needed. Without your love and support, I would have crumbled long ago. I hope it has been worth your efforts. Finally, my love and thanks to Rebecca and Rachel, my daughters, and Andrea, my midwife, for journeying with me through childbirth and teaching me so much about ways of knowing and growing in the world.

References

Adams, M. (1987) Deliveries: Mothers or midwives. A study of communication styles in midwifery, unpublished MSc thesis, University of Surrey.

Association of Radical Midwives (1986) *The Vision*, Ormskirk: Association of Radical Midwives.

Ball, J. (1989) Postnatal care and adjustment to motherhood, in Robinson, S. and Thomson, A. (eds), *Midwives, Research and Childbirth*, Vol. 1, London: Chapman and Hall.

Chalmers, I. and Richards, M. (1977) Intervention and causal inference in obstetric practice, in Chard, T. and Richards, M. (eds), *Benefits and Hazards of the New Obstetrics*, London: Spastics International Medical Publications.

Chalmers, I., Enkei, M. and Keirse, M. (eds) (1989) *Effective Care in Pregnancy and Childbirth*, Oxford: Oxford University Press.

Cronk, M. and Flint, C. (1989) *Community Midwifery*, Oxford: Heinemann.

Donnison, J. (1988) *Midwives and Medical Men*, 2nd edn, New Barnet: Historical Publications.

Enkin, M. and Chalmers, I. (1982) Effectiveness and satisfaction in antenatal care, in Enkin, M. and Chalmers, I. (eds), *Effectiveness and Satisfaction in Antenatal Care*, London: Heinemann.

Etzioni, A. (ed.) (1969) *The Semi-Professions and their Organisation*, London: Collier-Macmillan.

Flint, C. (1987) *Sensitive Midwifery*, London: Heinemann.

Flint, C. and Poulengeris, P. (1988) *The 'Know Your Midwife' Report*, available from 49 Peckarman's Wood, Sydenham Hill, London SE26 6RZ.

Garry, A. and Pearsall, M. (1989) 'Introduction' and 'Introduction' to Parts 1–7, in Garry, A. and Pearsall, M. (eds), *Women, Knowledge and Reality*, Boston: Unwin Hyman.

Jaggar, A. (1989) Love and knowledge: Emotion in feminist epistemology, in Garry, A. and Pearsall, M. (eds), *Women, Knowledge and Reality*, Boston: Unwin Hyman.

Kirkham, M. (1989) Midwives and information-giving during labour, in Robinson, S. and Thomson, A. (eds), *Midwives, Research and Childbirth*, Vol. 1, London: Chapman and Hall.

Klaus, M., Kennell, J., Robertson, S. and Sosa, R. (1986) Effects of social support during parturition on maternal and infant morbidity, *British Medical Journal* 293: 585–7.

Knorr-Cetina, K. (1981) *The Manufacture of Knowledge*, Oxford: Pergamon Press.

Laryea, M. (1989) Midwives' and mothers' perceptions of motherhood, in Robinson, S. and Thomson, A. (eds), *Midwives, Research and Childbirth*, Vol. 1, London: Chapman and Hall.

Methven, R. (1989) Recording an obstetric history or relating to a pregnant woman? A study of the antenatal booking interview, in Robinson, S. and Thomson, A. (eds), *Midwives, Research and Childbirth*, Vol. 1, London: Chapman and Hall.

Oakley, A. (1977) Wisewoman and medicine man: Changes in the management of childbirth, in Mitchell, J. and Oakley, A. (eds), *The Rights and Wrongs of Women*, Harmondsworth: Penguin.

Oakley, A. (1984) The importance of being a nurse, *Nursing Times* December: 24–7.

Oakley, A. (1992) *Social Support and Motherhood*, Oxford: Basil Blackwell.

Page, L. (1988) The midwife's role in modern health care, in Kitzinger, S. (ed.), *The Midwife Challenge*, London: Pandora.

Robinson, S. (1989a) The role of the midwife: Opportunities and constraints, in Chalmers, I., Enkei, M. and Keirse, M. (eds), *Effective Care in Pregnancy and Childbirth*, Vol. 1, Oxford: Oxford University Press.

Robinson, S. (1989b) Caring for childbearing women: The interrelationship between midwifery and medical responsibilities, in Robinson, S. and Thomson, A. (eds), *Midwives, Research and Childbirth*, Vol. 1, London: Chapman and Hall.

Royal College of Midwives (1987) *Towards a Healthy Nation: A Policy for the Maternity Services*, London: Royal College of Midwives.

Smith, D. (1988) *The Everyday World as Problematic*, Milton Keynes: Open University Press.

Stanley, L. (ed.) (1990) *Feminist Praxis*, London: Routledge.

Wagner, M. (1986) The medicalisation of birth, in Claxton, R. (ed.), *Birth Matters*, London: Unwin.

Wilkins, R. (1993) Sociological aspects of the mother–community midwife relationship, unpublished PhD thesis, University of Surrey.

CHAPTER 6

'There's so much potential... and for whatever reason it's not being realized'[1] – Women's Relationships with Midwives as a Negotiation of Ideology and Practice

NADINE EDWARDS

This chapter focuses on women's experiences of community team midwifery. It draws on lengthy interviews with 30 women who planned home births in Scotland, it is part of extensive work (Edwards 2001, 2005) to explore women's experiences of planning home births, and it takes account of women's ongoing reports at a busy Pregnancy and Parents Centre (formally known as BRC) in central Edinburgh (Armstrong *et al.*, 2006).

Until at least the beginning of the twentieth century, most women in Britain gave birth at home with women and midwives they knew. By 1980, almost all gave birth in hospital, often with strangers. Statistics suggest that home births are increasing slowly and, while research on complex issues cannot be definitive (Enkin *et al.*, 2006), it suggests that healthy women and babies attended by skilled midwives have excellent outcomes and enjoy important benefits (NICE, 2008).[2] The NHS still maintains a community midwifery service, government policies in England and Wales support an increase in home births, and overcrowding in maternity units might make this more likely (Morris, 2008). However, relationships between women and midwives are rarely focused on. In an area of southeast London where trusting relationships between women and midwives are deemed crucial, the Albany Practice midwives have a home birth rate of 47 per cent (Albany Midwifery Practice, 2009).

The need for supportive care for both women and midwives

Relationships are central to human experience, 'and these appear to be particularly influential during periods of emotional vulnerability, with new motherhood being a striking example' (Dykes, 2009: 99). The literature suggests that supportive care from and for midwives is key to women's experiences of childbearing and consistently provides excellent outcomes (Waldenstrom et al., 2004). Qualitative research suggests that caseloading midwifery and small birth centres, while not necessarily perfect, provide immeasurable benefits for women and midwives (Davis-Floyd et al., 2009; Kirkham, 2003; McCourt and Stevens, 2009; Sandall et al., 2001; Walsh 2007), but that team midwifery and care in large institutions are particularly problematic for both women and midwives and are associated with dissatisfaction, burn-out and 'long-term distress and emotional damage' (Ball et al., 2002; Hunter, 2009; McCourt et al., 2006: 154; Sandall, 1997). The paradox of 'Midwives... being asked to engage in meaningful support, when they themselves have impoverished support' (Deery and Kirkham, 2006: 126) denies women the support that supposedly protects them. The common thread running through research on relationships is the notion that a trusting relationship between woman and midwife is crucial for safe, supportive care during childbearing, that it provides similar benefits for women and midwives, and that these relationships are the key to its success and sustainability (Davis-Floyd et al., 2009; Huber and Sandall, 2006; Hunter, 2006; Kennedy et al., 2004; McCourt and Stevens, 2009). Yet continuity is almost completely lacking in maternity services in Britain, and continues to be contentious (Carolan and Hodnett, 2007).

The context

The ability of midwives and women to forge trusting relationships is usually beset with problems, because of the political context of birth and health care (Barclay, 2008; Deery and Kirkham, 2007; Dykes, 2009; Edwards, 2008, 2009; Hunter, 2003; Pollock, 2006). I found in my study with women (Edwards, 2005), as Ruth Deery (2003) also found in hers with midwives, that when community midwives are constrained by medical ideology, are unable to provide continuity of care and are stretched beyond their capacities, then relationships are fraught with tensions which drive deeply destructive wedges between women and midwives, and between midwives themselves. Social analysts indicate that this is because many of today's birth practices are rooted in an obstetric/technocratic ideology set in patriarchal, capitalist frameworks that maintain a particular social order (Davis-Floyd, 1992; Edwards, 2008; Murphy Lawless, 1998, 2006). These frameworks have led to truth being defined as a reified form of rationalism (science), in which bodily rhythms, women's knowledge, emotions and relationships are discounted and technology takes precedence. These frameworks have led to a particular form of market capitalism, where the pregnant woman is reduced to a consumer (Edwards, 2008; Murphy Lawless, 2006) in an increasingly privatized market. So while governments issue decrees about consumer-led health care based on greater choice, in reality overstretched services provide a more streamlined, centralized and standardized service than ever before, because where market forces are applied, throughput and profit become the driving forces. Within these frameworks midwives have no time or support to care for women (Deery and Kirkham, 2007; Dykes, 2009; Hunter and Deery, 2009). Of course, women and midwives continue to forge alternatives to the worst excesses of the market economy and engage across these difficulties, but successes are few and always under threat (AIMS, 2006). Here I present women's experiences of these complex, external factors through their relationships with team midwives.

In my study 27 of the 30 women booked with teams of six to eight community midwives; two of these women happened to have a midwife attend them during labour whom they had met on a number of occasions through their pregnancies. One woman received care throughout her pregnancy, birth and the postnatal period from an NHS midwife working in a semi-rural area, and two women received care from independent midwives later in their pregnancies, through birth and the postnatal period. All of the women expressed concern about the lack of relationships when attended by teams of six to eight midwives (a situation that has worsened in many areas as teams are now 10–20 midwives).

Team midwifery: Uneasy compromises

During pregnancy groups at the Pregnancy and Parents Centre, women frequently expressed unsolicited concerns about not being able to get to know the midwife who would attend them during birth. Young pregnant women attending one of the centre's outreach projects expressed the same concern. For those planning home births with community midwives, meeting a midwife for 15 minutes was not equated with forming a relationship, but was seen as better than hospital services, where 'there's a never-ending stream of trainees, students – anybody and everybody' and where six might be 'a lot, but it's better than just going up to the hospital and not knowing who you might get'. Women found it 'unnerving' that 'you don't know them very well', 'you've seen them once' but 'they're pretty much faceless'. This presented a conflict for the women:

> you see the problem is, if you see a different one every time you get to know them all, which is what you want, cos you don't know who's going to be at the birth – so you do want that – but you don't because you're not seeing the same person every time.

Rather than focusing on the woman's pregnancy, women might find 'a series of ladies rushing in to sort of present themselves' and have to decide whether or not there were any midwives who they did not want to attend them – but at the same time feeling unable to judge this, because 'I'm basing my assessment of people on little comments because, you know, I saw that women at the clinic for 15 minutes. I've no idea what she's like at all.' They did not wish to upset midwives – 'you know, I didn't want to be horrible' – and some women commented that a midwife they had been unsure about during pregnancy was extremely supportive during labour. They pointed out that some of us (women and midwives) take time to find ways of relating:

> the midwife who I've seen most often, I think I found it most difficult to start speaking to her but having met her several times, I think she's probably just like me. I'm quite hard to speak to when you first meet me as well and I think over that time, I've definitely built up to being able to speak with her.

Getting to know midwives, getting to know women

Like the women in Chris McCourt and Trudy Stevens' study, the women in my study agreed that getting to know a midwife is 'more complex than simply having met the person more than once, it was about the midwife knowing them' (McCourt and Stevens, 2009: 18). For example, as women in my study commented, 'I think it's very important to know what someone's fears are and what their strengths are, you know'. But midwives working within industrial models in busy hospitals focus on tasks (Deery, 2009). They simply do not have the time and wherewithal to allow questions or discussions to arise, especially about emotional issues (Deery and Kirkham, 2006: 136).

The following is what some of the women I interviewed experienced: 'what they did was checks, lots and lots of checks – which I didn't need... it was ignoring so much', and 'there is so much procedure and so many stock tests to be gotten through. By the time you've done that there's no slack in the appointments procedure for any chatting.' When I asked a woman if she had talked to her midwives about her thoughts about birth, she replied that she couldn't 'imagine that conversation. There's no way into that really. The times I've seen them, it's not been, you know, a natural progression of a conversation'; another commented: 'You know within that setting to try and bring up more emotional complex issues would feel quite wrong really, you would feel like you crossed the boundary.' Yet women need progressive conversations to be able to gather information and think through their decisions (Pairman, 2006: 86). This cannot happen when women are seeing a different midwife at each appointment, because as women pointed out, 'you chat about the same things with each of them that comes. You never really scratch the surface' and conversations remain 'superficial, I don't think I had a really proper conversation with any of them'. And:

> even if you manage to reach an understanding with one of them, you know, you don't know if they're going to be there and it's quite exhausting in fact to have to make that effort six times over, over the course of several months.

However, like the women in Chris McCourt and Trudy Stevens' study who valued care that included 'both their medical *and* their social and psychological needs' (McCourt and Stevens, 2009: 26), the same woman in my study quoted above, who felt that the 'checks' were unnecessary, even undermining, redefined this when she transferred from a team of eight midwives to one midwife who was able to provide more holistic care in the context of a relationship:

> the difference... is because I have time to get to know my midwife... we have a cup of tea, we have a chat... then... we do the check, so she will do all these things, but it seems relevant, it's like somebody you know who's caring for you, checking that you're okay, so it feels different

because you're not straight in the door and on the scales, or straight in the door lying on your back with your top up, you've actually engaged as an adult with somebody first.

Fom the women's perspective, concerns about not getting to know one or two midwives were exacerbated by a lack of commonality about birth ideology and practices. This made them feel vulnerable and uncertain:

I've found the relationship hasn't been able to develop for one reason or another, and yeah, I suppose you do feel a bit more vulnerable... I imagine they're going to be doing the best they can for you... but on the other hand, I just hear so many people planning home births and going in [to hospital] for what seem like very small reasons and I wonder you know, how can you sort of get round that.

Trust

A main issue to arise was that of trust in the face of vulnerability. Birth is a liminal rite of passage in which women's identities and bodies are changing and thus more vulnerable to external influences (Davis-Floyd, 1992; Kennedy and MacDonald, 2002; Shildrick, 1997). In order to feel safe, they need trustworthy others who will support their vulnerabilities, beliefs and values (Anderson, Chapter 7 in this volume; Pairman, 2006: 88). As women in my study said, 'I mean maybe it's not a bad thing to lose control, but you have to feel safe enough to be able to do that you know', and 'it's quite a big trusting thing to do'.

When midwives are constrained by obstetric policies, which include lack of time and continuity, trust cannot develop: 'I just don't know them well enough and some of them I've only met once for just a few minutes.' Mutual trust develops over time within a relationship and is based on mutual understandings about birth. A woman who received all her care from one community midwife observed:

you know, I really trust her and I trust her judgement you know, and I know when I go into labour and she'll come and she'll check every-thing and if she says everything's okay I'll believe her, you know, I'll trust her that it is okay.

Another woman stated that having a known, trusted midwife enabled her to approach birth with confidence:

the difference of just knowing I'd have someone more in line with my thinking, I didn't feel that I needed a birth plan any more. I don't need all these things because I trust her opinion and that way I don't have any fears. So I don't have to swot up so much and, you know, be so defensive.

When trust and confidence develop during the woman's pregnancy, the woman sustains this through her midwife even when birth is difficult:

obviously it was my decision as to how much I could take but in the end it was all fine... But I mean she [midwife] stayed as cool as a cucumber, which, you know, if she hadn't, if she'd at any point suggested that I wasn't going to make it then that would have had a huge influence on me, you know, cos I would have said, oh great you agree, okay, I can't do it.

Another woman who had a known, trusted midwife reported that it freed her to focus on her labour:

I knew that she would tell me if there was anything wrong and if she was ever really worried about the baby you know because it was a long labour.

Even when women in my study could see that midwives were constrained by hospital policies, they felt strongly that they could have dealt more constructively with ideological differences within the context of a relationship. As they said, 'you can't knock six of them into shape' but 'if I could get to know somebody. I could get round the little quirks or whatever' and 'engage'. This 'adjustment' (Kirkham, 2009) is crucial, especially when a midwife appears not to share the woman's beliefs about birth:

had it been somebody who I developed a rapport with, a lot of those difficulties could have been a lot less, just from knowing somebody and knowing where they're coming from and even just having longer to work out how it is that I can say things that otherwise would feel difficult because that's another way round, having to be bluntly assertive, is actually working out, well, how do you say this in a way that can be heard. You know, for me it can take quite a long time of negotiating around with somebody to find out what they can hear and what they respond well to and, you know, what I wouldn't be able to say or whatever.

This was confirmed by a story told by one of the women:

> However many they are [six], it's far too much. You can't really build
> up a rapport with your midwife which I think is the important thing
> really... And it should be one midwife or two you know, that one-to-one
> thing. Like my friend for example – that's the friend who did it [the
> one-to-one scheme]. She said, you know, initially she sort of like wasn't
> that keen on her midwife but in the end she just like thought she was
> absolutely fantastic and she was wonderful and she said she really sort
> of like got to know her.

Given the constraints of obstetric policies on team midwifery, lack of trust
is particularly acute around the issue of transferring to hospital, when
women are concerned about avoiding this unless absolutely necessary.
This can lead to fears on both sides that undermine safety:

> I don't trust her not to panic and send me off to hospital just because
> things are bit slow or something. And if there was a good reason for me
> going into hospital I still wouldn't trust that it was a good reason,
> because I wouldn't know that she wasn't just panicking or like plotting
> to get me away, you know.... And I don't think they trust me at all... I
> think [midwife] is very frightened that I'll stand there saying, I'm not
> going into hospital, and I'm staying here, you know, and just be really
> uncooperative and put her in a really difficult situation of not knowing
> what to do.

Yet care from a known midwife can have a positive impact on women's
experiences of tranferring to hospital (Kirkham, 2009: 230). Otherwise it
could seem like 'two worlds, not really living together terribly well, with
different rules for both' and women complained about seeing too many
practitioners, being given different opinions and repeatedly, 'having to
relate our story':

> I would have preferred for at least one of them [community midwives]
> to have been there, who knew me and could work with me.

Women are particularly vulnerable during a transfer to hospital, but
having a trusted midwife accompany them can enable women to continue
to focus on their labour and can lessen the need for them to focus on
negotiations with strangers. Known midwives can maintain a feeling of
security despite difficult changes in circumstances and environment.

When I asked if it made a difference, women said 'massively, yeah, yeah, yeah, totally' and 'definitely, definitely'. They appreciated midwives staying with them throughout, not automatically handing them over to hospital staff and routines, negotiating with doctors on their behalf, knowing what was important to them and supporting their wishes where they could.

Formulaic care

Without the potentially anchoring impact of relationships, women and midwives are pulled asunder by obstetric ideologies and are cast adrift by the structures arising from these ideologies that embed fragmented, standardized care as the norm. One woman commented above that there is no slack in the sytem for women, but there is no slack for midwives either (Hunter, 2009). They are obliged to disengage to protect themselves (Deery and Kirkham, 2007). When this happens, midwives feel like a 'cog in the wheel' (McCourt *et al.*, 2006: 158) and are less able to focus on women as individuals. Interactions become 'formulaic':

> They [midwives] were very helpful, but one thing I would say is that they seem to have been trained how to treat people [in general] and the sorts of anxieties people [in general] have, but, you know, you're an individual and... I didn't sometimes think that I was being heard. I think they had lots of answers, but some of them were to questions I hadn't posed and, do you know, I didn't feel there was a dialogue. I felt a little bit invisible... It was a bit smiley and a bit formulaic.

Care becomes insensitive to the individual woman's circumstances. For example, one woman said she was asked about antenatal tests when she was still bleeding heavily and unsure her baby would survive:

> do you want to get this spina bifida and Down's syndrome blood test, you know, which was just like too far down the line, you know, we were still, am I going to miscarry, and it was just like, oh, you're still bleeding, note it down and then on to something else that was on their agenda. Part of that was the lack of time that they'd got I suppose.

Without relationships and time, inappropriate blanket reassurance are likely to take the place of authentic engagement. Women understand that when midwives are overburdened they cannot respond otherwise, but:

I did find them quite quick to say, oh it'll be fine, you know which doesn't work in dispelling people's anxieties – at all. It doesn't matter how motherly you try to be, you know, you're not my mother... It wasn't what I wanted really... a kind of semi humorous, mothering type approach. I just didn't like that. I mean if people are scared, being humorous with them doesn't work, I don't think. And I really don't like that. I find that very minimising of my fear.

And yet within the context of a nurturing relationship, 'mothering' could be what women needed: 'what you want is a mother probably, to be mothered when you're just becoming a mother yourself'. This kind of mothering can increase self-esteem and provide an empowering role model. 'In this way the midwife acts more specifically as a 'mother' to the woman in order to facilitate her ability to nurture her baby: "mothering the mother to mother her baby"' (Mander, 2001: 82).

The battle over continuity symbolizes a conflict of philosophies about whether birth is defined as a social transition to motherhood in need of social support as well as physical care or a more medical event, mainly in need of monitoring. Thus, in the same way that obstetric safety cannot encompass women's complex meanings of safety (Edwards, 2008; Edwards and Murphy-Lawless, 2006), team midwifery cannot meet their needs for trusting relationships that will help them through the complex transition to motherhood.

Engaging with the social transition to motherhood

As I discuss above, when midwives feel overwhelmed they focus on getting through tasks as quickly as possible with minimal engagement (Deery and Kirkham, 2007; Dykes, 2009: 97; Hunter, 2009: 178). This is completely at odds with the enormity and potentially life-enhancing process of the real task – that of nurturing a mother to develop more of the resources she needs to nurture a new person into adulthood (Murphy-Lawless, 1998):

> my responsibility is to form a relationship. It's almost like that the birth is a rite of passage and by the end of it you've been through it together and you're in relationship to the baby, you know. It's sort of, the baby is what comes at the end of the process of giving birth, and I think the more connected I am with the birth, the more connected I am with the baby. And maybe my responsibility is to be open to having that connection with the baby.

Even if midwives align themselves with women ideologically, they cannot provide the kind of holistic care that can be provided by midwives who know about the woman's life context (Kennedy *et al.*, 2004: 19; Wilkins, Chapter 5 in this volume). This knowledge enables 'the midwife to orchestrate an environment of care to meet the woman's [physical and emotional] needs' (Kennedy *et al.*, 2004: 18) as she negotiates becoming a mother. Relationships form the basis from which to begin to understand women's needs as they become mothers:

> if they don't chat to you... they don't learn so much, you know, because you just walk out of there and you think, oh I forgot about, or you don't feel comfortable and you think, och, I won't bother... you know, I don't think they get so much and you don't get so much... But I suppose it's just getting to know somebody as well.

Mutual engagement and trust potentially increase growth in both women and midwives. As they negotiate decisions and come to mutual under-standings (Pairman, 2006: 86), they take more responsibility, see the consequences of their beliefs and actions and develop increased skills and self-trust (McCourt and Stevens, 2009: 26; Olafsdottir, 2009: 192; Pairman, 2006: 81). The potential for growth is largely lost when care is fragmented and midwives overworked (Deery and Kirkham, 2006: 136):

> I haven't really talked to her [midwife] at all. She just says things like, plenty of movements them? And I go, yeah. And then sort of afterwards I think, I wonder what plenty of movements means, you know, like, what is plenty, cos I don't know, and I've never really talked to her about anything.

This suggests that models that discount relationships undermine women's abilities to grow as mothers, and also midwives' abilities to hone their knowledge and skills. Midwives who caseload and women who receive care from them suggest that through the joint work of discovery within a relationship, women are more able to articulate their beliefs and values, and midwives are more able to provide care to women that is and feels safe – physically and emotionally. This 'shared knowl-edge and engagement may be key in understanding how midwives achieve positive outcomes. As many of the stories portray establishing a relationship with a woman and discovering her world and worries may alter a labour, create a lifelong memory, or help her find her inner strength' (Kennedy *et al.*, 2004: 21). This is unlikely in the context of team midwifery, where different midwives have different views and there is so little time to discuss even basic issues:

> it [talking about birth] never seemed appropriate. They always flew in. You offered them a cup of tea to try and make a little chat. Tried to communicate but, you know, sometimes it was me as much as them. You know I wanted them out of the house just as quickly as they wanted to get out of the house.

A woman needs time and trusting relationships to share her thoughts and concerns as she considers what becoming a mother means to her. She needs midwives who are able to listen and create space for her to talk about issues that are not always easy to discuss:

> if I were to think about the emotional or the spiritual parts of the birth it almost feels as if they're too tender and too soft to be talked about in that fast way and so I think that, you know, that sort of thing does narrow down what we would talk about.

This deeper sharing and openness (Kennedy *et al.*, 2004: 14; Pairman, 2006: 78–9) that women require to become mothers cannot occur in one-off meetings with overstretched, unsupported midwives. Women wanted to be able to raise their concerns (McCourt and Stevens, 2009; Pairman 2006: 80), but often felt unable to do so with team midwives, unless they happened to have got to know some of them over the course of several pregnancies and births, but: 'I would pick and choose who I spoke to. One or two of them, I would sit and think, na, I'll wait till next week.' Women need to trust before sharing information about themselves. Even with a known midwife, 'I was shocked the other day when a woman reached 34/40 pregnant before she was able to tell me that she had been sexually abused. It would never have come out in the conventional service' (McCourt and Stevens, 2009: 20). There are other examples of women sharing experiences of abuse and trauma that can form the basis of healing (Kennedy and MacDonald, 2002). Conversely, without trusting relationships women withhold (Edwards, 2005; Melender and Lauri, 1999).

This contrasts sharply with 'formulaic' care and tick-box birth plans which do not address women's unique concerns, or help them make important life decisions as they become mothers. Caseloading midwives find that they can best help women through the transitional process of pregnancy, birth and early motherhood by learning about the woman, and by helping her to work through her concerns and fears (Kennedy *et al.*, 2004: 21) so that she becomes more confident, and the midwife can 'focus on the watchful support that is so fundamental for normal birth' (McCourt *et al.*, 2006: 157). They find that having built up a trusting relationship, women 'are far more relaxed' (McCourt and Stevens, 2009: 21). In the context of a trusting relationship, women say the same:

> there was a kind of silence in the relationship, a stillness which was very important. And we'd done all the talking in the build up. So the talking was done. I felt confident that she [midwife] knew where I was coming from and vice versa. It was like we'd done all our dress rehearsal – what if... what if... And on the day there was nothing left to say really. So it just felt very calm, and I think that was the most important thing.

This deeper stillness is lost in industrialized models of birth. Yet 'tranquillity' helps women and midwives listen to their own inner knowledge: 'their own flow of thoughts, feelings and emotions', to ease the challenging journey through birth (Olafsdottir, 2009: 204). Consider the striking similarity between the observations of a woman in my study and those of an Icelandic midwife:

> it requires a certain amount of quiet round about you, and trust and respect really, and when that isn't given it's easy to doubt yourself or not to be able to hear what's actually going on [in your body].

> There has to be a certain calm, I need to be in a peaceful mind when instinct works with me. (Olafsdottir, 2009: 203)

In a social view of birth: 'Birth is not only about making babies. Birth is also about making mothers – strong, competent, capable mothers who trust themselves and know their inner strength' (Rothman, 1996). Thus part of the midwife's role is to nurture the woman's strength, by listening to her and helping her to 'find her strength and use her strength' (Kennedy *et al.*, 2004: 19). Becoming a mother and developing the resources needed to do this is ultimately about developing agency – a relational process that is best accomplished with supportive others.

Becoming 'strong, competent, capable mothers': Developing agency

Agency is described as valuing and developing self-knowledge, self-definition, self-trust, self-esteem and self-reflection and being able to make decisions and act on these. This confidence and trust in ourselves largely develops through relationships that are affirming of these characteristics (McLeod and Sherwin, 2000: 273).

Thus within the fraught political context of birth, in which women are vulnerable to the authority of obstetric ideology, they need trustworthy midwives who understand how they might become confident mothers. To do this, midwives need self-awareness, self-esteem, communication skills and 'emotional intelligence', which are usually difficult to acquire (Battersby, 2009; Deery and Kirkham, 2006: 125; Hunter, 2009). Indeed, the process of professionalization can lead to the very skills needed to support agency being lost in training and/or practice (Kirkham, 1999; Kirkham and Stapleton, 2001). Yet without this strong sense of agency, there is little possibility of helping women to develop theirs. Team midwifery, constrained by obstetric structures and policies and lacking in agency, leaves women isolated and having to assert their rights, which they find difficult. They struggle to remain true to themselves without causing 'waves', 'fuss' or 'alienation', but then feel self-critical for 'letting myself down' and being 'quite cowardly'. This is not a way to make 'strong, competent, capable mothers who trust themselves and know their inner strength' (Rothman, 1996).

It is distressing to observe that when relationships are not a priority, rather than growing in confidence women grow in anxiety, and instead of focusing on their pregnancies and becoming mothers, they are drawn into negotiating how to get to know midwives and their beliefs and practices: 'I wanted to be able to really experience it [pregnancy and birth] and think about it and dwell on it and not have to – or feel like I had to be running around sort of meeting expectations.' And when midwives comply with obstetric ideology and feel 'we have to do as we are told' (Deery, 2009: 82), this is passed on to women who then also feel that 'I should do as I was told' and that they are 'complying', to the extent that:

> your knowledge is totally overridden... I do find it totally unbelievable, and I don't think I appreciated that until I had a baby at home and realised that, you know, even although you're in your own home you still don't have great deal of control.

In other words, NHS community midwives working without support, constrained by obstetric ideology and providing fragmented care, might attenuate the immediate impact of medical ideology, but are less able to contribute to increased agency. To focus on becoming confident mothers, women need confident, self-aware midwives who provide them with opportunities to do this. As the women explained, without that support they were less able to make the decisions they wanted, and thus less able to assume responsibility for themselves and their families.

Thus, midwives, like women, need environments and situations in which to expand their own agency (Baker, 2009; Deery and Kirkham, 2006: 131; Dykes, 2009: 99). They appear to do this most easily in case-loading practices that facilitate relationships with each other, and with women. They develop skills to work through relationship difficulties with colleagues (McCourt and Stevens, 2009: 27; McCourt *et al.*, 2006) and a strong sense of self ('self actualization') that 'they had not found possible when working in the conventional services' (McCourt and Stevens, 2009: 24). Where midwives have to negotiate a 'tightrope' (Levy, 2004) between midwifery knowledge and obstetric practices in institutions, even the most committed, experienced midwives find that they have to compromise and worry about 'losing my clinical judgement in a space where standardised knowledge have priority over my sensual knowledge gained through years of experience' (Blaaka and Schauer, 2008: 348). For midwives to establish healthy relationships that encourage agency is not only ideal role modelling for women who are recipients of their care, but contributes to women becoming the 'strong, competent, capable' mothers they need to become. For example, a midwife observed that through listening to and acknowledging a woman over time, the woman learnt that 'not only was it her right, but she should demand to be listened to and was becoming a very strong woman' (Kennedy *et al.*, 2004: 20). Similarly, one woman in my study commented that 'in the beginning I didn't have the courage of my convictions', but:

> I think because of the way [midwife] answered questions you know, as though she was interested in your question and I think that made made me more and more confident... I think that did help me to grow because I thought that she trusted my ideas and she found them interesting so it made me follow through instead of just wishing. I got more and more confident about getting exactly what I wanted.

The work done between women and midwives can have positive, lasting impacts as women grow into motherhood: 'Women who feel empowered during childbirth will take that confidence with them as new mothers and this in turn will strengthen their families and society. The ripple effects of positive birthing experiences are far reaching and cannot be underestimated' (Pairman, 2006: 93). 'Story after story reflected women's sense of safety, accomplishment, power, and at times, transformation' (Kennedy *et al.*,, 2004: 20). My findings confirmed that confidence during birth 'ripples' out: 'I feel really proud of myself... so I think that just has ripple effects on the rest of your life, doesn't it', 'it knocked on into other areas of my life really, I just started to feel that my instincts were good', 'I still have the confidence of that whole period you know', 'it stays with me, and I think that will stay with me for the rest of my life, definitely a great sense of triumph really, it's incredible'. This growth potentially acts as a catalyst for new integrations: 'it's like I'm in the middle of a jig-saw that is my life and the pieces are starting to fit instead of which they used to be a wee bit all over the place'. This confidence and integration could be an anchor in times of stress:

> If I'm down about anything or I may have doubts about something I'm doing with [baby] you know. If I have a crisis of confidence, I think back to the birth and it's a very good anchor for me in that way. You know it makes me believe in my ability to make good choices and things like that and I think it's made a tremendous impact on how I can make decisions.

Understanding birth as a social transition to motherhood in which women need to develop knowledge, skills, strength and agency involves the midwife becoming an ally, a 'professional friend' (see Chapter 12, this volume) rather than a distant professional, for 'it is in the relationship between women and midwives as they go through the childbearing process together that the message of value and worth is given. It cannot be given by strangers mouthing words' (Pelvin cited in Pairman, 2006: 90).

Professional friendships: The building of trust, mutuality and authenticity

A professional friend is '*like* a family friend' or '*like* kin' (McCourt and Stevens, 2009: 19; Olafsdottir, 2009: 194). There is both closeness and distance. Reminiscent of Sigridur Hallsdorsdottir's work (1996), one woman in my study who got to know her midwife well explained the value and the complexities of the professional friendship, and the dance between closeness (that enabled her to feel engaged and comfortable) and distance (that prevented her midwife's issues from encroaching on her own):

Another thing that I've found important is that she's a warm person, but she's also quite a private person and I quite like that. She's not private in a way that, you know, some people can be private in a way that would make you feel awkward... because they're so closed or something. She'd be warm and friendly, but her life's her life and she has a kind of demarcation and I like that... I feel much more comfortable than I would have imagined possible, but the funny thing is, you build up a relationship that is in some way – it has a lot of trust, implicit trust in it. But at the same time you both know that it's built around a professional thing. It is built up quite quickly. So that you know in a way, I'm asking her to behave like a very close friend on one level – and she's isn't. And I know that, and she knows that and that's okay.

This professional friendship enables the midwife to support the woman in the best way: 'I'm definitely more in tune with the women I look after and I certainly respect [the] women – because I know them and I'll do the best to help them make the choices they want...' (McCourt and Stevens, 2009: 20). This can happen where mutual respect and adjustment occur, and where women and midwives value each other's contributions and knowledge (Kirkham, 2009: 230; Pairman, 2006: 79). This kind of 'mutuality emerged as foundational for the midwife's relationship with the woman' (Kennedy *et al.*, 2004: 16) and requires time and mutual trust, especially when women's trust and confidence in themselves and others has been undermined.

The mutual confidence, trust and respect enable midwives and women to create appropriate boundaries (McCourt and Stevens, 2009; McCourt *et al.*, 2006: 155–6). In the context of supportive relationships, women tend not to 'disturb their midwife unless it was urgent' (McCourt and Stevens, 2009: 31). This is different from not 'bothering' people because they have no capacity to respond: 'I mean, you don't like bothering people because I know they are SO SO busy...' (Dykes, 2009: 95; see also McCourt and Stevens, 2009). Women in my study made similar comments: 'I'm always aware that [the midwives] are pushed for time and I don't want to blether... I feel I need to get on and out of their hair sort of thing.' But this is indicative of enforced disengagement, not of confidence.

A professional friend is very different from a friendly professional:

For the childbearing woman, there is a world of difference between having a known and trusted midwife who is with her through the whole of pregnancy, birth and the early weeks of the newborn life, and being in the care of strangers, no matter how kind. (McCourt et al., 2006: 141)

Without relationships midwives are 'kind and concerned... and try their best to provide... good care. But they don't know the women and the women don't know them' (Pairman, 2006: 92). As women in my study frequently said, midwives are 'well-intentioned', 'friendly', 'lovely', 'but they're still, you know, quite a lot of strangers'. While ongoing, support-ive relationships are potentially transformative, continuity of care rather than carer provides basic care, which cannot easily contribute to this potential.

Power: The underside of relationships

If decisions are more easily made and acted on in relationship with others (Mackenzie and Stoljar, 2000), and if women need to be listened to, respected (McLeod and Sherwin, 2000) and trusted, in order to make decisions for themselves (Mackenzie, 2000), then relationships exert a great deal of power. As Susan Brison suggests, dialogic exchanges are influential:

> If we are 'second persons' – not just in the sense of having been formed by others in childhood, but also in that we continue to be shaped and sustained by others – then other's speech to and about us and ours to and about them are crucially important in the development and endurance of our autonomous selves. (Brison, 2000: 287)

So if we are distrusted and prevented from acting on our decisions, our identities are undermined. And even though self-worth is complex, and (fortunately) women are resilient, Brison remarks that 'one assailant can undo a lifetime of self-esteem' (in Mackenzie, 2000: 141), as birth accounts sometimes demonstrate. While there is potential for the devel-opment of agency and even healing, the woman's concerns can be tram-pled on 'beyond your wildest dreams' (remark made by a woman at the Pregnancy and Parents Centre) and her integrity is therefore open to abuse during a vulnerable process (Fleming, 1994; Kennedy and MacDonald, 2002; Smythe, 1998; Wilkins, Chapter 5 in this volume). In other words, 'only if principles and fairness are in place and processes within a social structure are ethical, can trust contribute to well-being' (Thiede quoted in Huber and Sandall, 2006: 449). Partnership must be within a context of high levels of self-awareness on how one influences another (Pairman, 2006). It also goes without saying that practitioners are responsible for maintaining their own good practice skills, as 'liking or trusting their care provider might well be precisely what makes women feel their care is of high quality even when it is not' (McCourt *et al.*, 2006: 144).

It is easy to forget just how socially constructed and prescriptive the relationships between mother and midwife are. Since legislation and regulation in England and Wales in 1902 and in Scotland in 1915, the midwife has had to work within a series of restrictions and expectations. This can be more clearly seen in the recent legislation and regulation in North America (Davis-Floyd and Johnson, 2006; MacDonald, 2007). While not comparable to changes in Britain in the nineteenth and twentieth century, they remind us about both the inclusionary and exclusionary aspects of the regulation and professionalization of midwifery, how that affects pregnant women, and the altogether uneasy foundations on which the midwifery/woman relationship is built (Davis-Floyd and Johnson, 2006; Heagarty, 1997; MacDonald, 2007). The high profile given to the small but increasing number of women having births without midwives provides important opportunities to look at power imbalances and the role of the midwife 'with institution' (Kirkham, 1999). More recently, the relationship has been further defined and constructed through emphasis on the duty of midwives to report any concerns about babies to Social Services. We know little of the impact of meeting women's diverse needs for empathic engagement through a framework of rationed-out, standardized surveillance, but reports to AIMS from women who have been reported to Social Services suggests that this can happen when they question obstetric policies. This has devastating consequences on families (Beech, 2003) and indicates that the tensions between personal agency, professional agency and state support and surveillance have not been considered carefully enough in relation to the role of the midwife and other practitioners.

Concluding thoughts

'Birth remakes us and makes us revalue our way of being in the world' (Murphy-Lawless, 2006: 444). As Jo Murphy-Lawless explains, how birth is done in ever larger, centralized, technological obstetric units largely reflects our dominant beliefs about the importance of individual wealth, competitiveness and consumerism. But when birth is done differently, it can help us develop an ethical stance that questions this unsustainable, exclusive and inhumane model and starts to revalue connection – connection between mind and body, mother and baby, within families, between woman and midwife, between family and community and between disparate communities sharing similar struggles to make life more humane.

Increasingly, research suggests that midwives have an important role to play within this broader context of improving the lives of communities, and that it is working in this broader context that sustains both midwives and midwifery (McCourt and Stevens, 2009). In other words, continuity of carer provides very similar benefits to midwives as it does to women. Both report positive growth, increased knowledge and self-esteem, and increased agency.

Not all midwives want to work in caseloading practises, but in New Zealand where midwives can do this within the health-care system, by 2002, 40 per cent had chosen to (Pairman, 2006: 76). And when a midwifery/social ideology is shared, it becomes a haven for women and midwives: 'It's like going to heaven being with midwives that work the same way... I felt this big cloud had lifted' (McCourt and Stevens, 2009: 25). Similarly, a woman who booked with a midwife she trusted found 'a weight going off my shoulders... the confidence came surging back. It was like, no, this wasn't a figment of my imagination. It is possible to have a home birth.' Of course, relationships alone cannot improve birth outcomes; this depends not only on how we do birth, but how we do public health and social welfare. Within maternity care, however, three main ingredients for positive outcomes are cited again and again:

> a close personal and trusting relationship with a midwife in a one-to-one caseload model; a strong belief in childbirth as normal physiology; a familiar environment for birth that enhances and supports the normalcy of childbirth. (Pairman, 2006: 85)

Despite the often unbearable circumstances in which women give birth and midwives practise, there is still the will to do the best they can: women tenaciously repeat their stories, attempt to engage and explain their beliefs and values. There are shining examples of midwives working with women to dismantle ways of working and practices which alienate women and over-medicalize birth. They thwart the system in myriad ways to get a measure of the women they care for, give more personal care and convey trust and confidence in the little time they have together. But the costs are high, and the achievements, particularly of midwives working within the NHS, are against the odds. It would be far more beneficial if relationships were part of the 'warp' (Hunter et al., 2008) of maternity care, so that the efforts of women and midwives could be less fraught and bear more fruit. Given what we know about the important benefits of relationships between women and midwives, it seems particularly perverse to prevent those midwives who wish to provide this. As one or two women commented in my study, even if the midwife wanted to provide more continuity and attend her during labour, she appeared to be lacking the support and flexibility to do this within team midwifery. It seems equally perverse to maintain systems of fragmented 'care' that traumatize and alienate many women and midwives when there are examples of midwifery models based on relationships that provide excellent outcomes, promote growth and agency in all those involved, and are good for families and society (Albany Midwifery Practice, 2009; Birthinangus, 2009; Davis-Floyd *et al.*, 2009; Kirkham, 2003; Walsh, 2007).

To work towards relationships being central to midwifery care, women and midwives need to form relationships beyond the childbearing one, in order to work together to find locally acceptable, sustainable ways of working within midwifery that develop agency for both and that are mutually beneficial (Bourgeault *et al.*, 2006; Davis-Floyd *et al.*, 2009). In other words, women and midwives need to work together for changes within society that will sustain their work together, changes that include better working and payment conditions for midwives, more resources for maternity services to provide more midwives, more care in the community, and more public welfare for families.

Notes

1. All unreferenced quotations throughout this chapter are from the interviews I carried out in Scotland, with 30 women planning home births. These are reported in my book, Edwards, N.P. (2005) *Birthing Autonomy: Women's Experiences of Planning Home Births*, London: Routledge.
2. For example, recent figures show that the home birth rate for the UK is 2.55 per cent: 1.36 per cent in Scotland, 2.69 per cent in England and 3.53 per cent in Wales. These national figures hide regional differences. In Orkney in Scotland, for example, there were no home births recorded in the latest statistics, while in East Lothian where a dedicated team of midwives have long supported home birth, the figure is 4.8 per cent. In England, numbers of regions have home birth rates of over 10 per cent, and in Wales, Powys has a home birth rate of 10.7 per cent (see BirthchoiceUK).

Acknowledgements

I would like to thank Peter Edwards, Mavis Kirkham, Jo Murphy Lawless and Irene Walton for their support and comments on previous drafts.

References

AIMS (2006) Birth Centres Journal: Still standing and proud, *AIMS Journal* 18(3).

Albany Midwifery Practice, www.albanymidwives.org.uk/albanymidwivesfactsand figures.php, accessed August 2009.

Armstrong, F., Clayton, L., Crewe, J., Edwards, N., St Clair, A., Seekings-Norman, L. and Wickham, S. (2006) The Birth Resource Centre: A community of women, in Wickham, S. (ed.), *Midwifery: Best Practice*, Vol. 4, London: Books for Midwives.

Baker, K. (2009) Peeling onions: Using drama to explore emotion, in Hunter, B. and Deery, R. (eds), *Emotions in Midwifery and Reproduction*, Basingstoke: Palgrave Macmillan.

Ball, L., Curtis, P. and Kirkham, M. (2002) *Why do Midwives Leave?* London: Royal College of Midwives. Available from www.rcm.org.uk/info/docs/Why%20 midwives%20leave%20full%20report.pdf, accessed March 2010.

Barclay, L. (2008) Woman and midwives: Position, problems and potential, *Midwifery* 24: 13–21.

Battersby, S. (2009) Midwives, infant feeding and emotional turmoil, in Hunter, B. and Deery, R. (eds), *Emotions in Midwifery and Reproduction*, Basingstoke: Palgrave Macmillan.

Beech, B. (2003) The effects of child-protection investigations on maternity care, *AIMS* 15(1): 8–9.

Birth Choice UK, www.birthchoiceuk.com/BirthChoiceUKFrame.htm?http://www. birthchoiceuk.com/HomeBirth.htm, accessed August 2009.

Birthinangus, www.birthinangus.org.uk/, accessed September 2009.

Blaaka, G. and Schauer, T. (2008) Doing midwifery between different belief systems, *Midwifery* 24: 344–52.

Bourgeault, I.L., Luce, J. and MacDonald, M. (2006) The caring dilemma: Balancing the needs of midwives and clients in a continuity of care model of practice, *Community, Work and Family* 9(4): 389–406.

Brison, S.J. (2000) Relational autonomy and freedom of expression, in Mackenzie, C. and Stoljar, N. (eds), *Relational Autonomy: Feminist Perspectives on Autonomy, Agency, and the Social Self*, New York: Oxford University Press.

Carolan, M. and Hodnett, E. (2007) 'With woman' philosophy: Examining the evidence, answering the question, *Nursing Inquiry* 14(2): 140–52.

Davis-Floyd, R.E. (1992) *Birth as an American Rite of Passage*, Berkeley: University of California Press.

Davis-Floyd, R.E. and Johnson, C.B. (eds) (2006) *Mainstreaming Midwives: The Politics of Change*, London: Routledge.

Davis-Floyd, R.E., Barclay, L., Daviss, B.-A. and Tritten, J. (eds) (2009) *Birth Models That Work*, Berkeley, CA: University of California Press.

Deery, R. (2003) Engaging with clinical supervision in a community midwifery setting: an action research study, unpublished PhD thesis, University of Sheffield.

Deery, R. (2009) Community midwifery: 'Performances' and the presentation of self, in Hunter, B. and Deery, R. (eds), *Emotions in Midwifery and Reproduction*, Basingstoke: Palgrave Macmillan.

Deery, R. and Kirkham, M. (2006) Supporting midwives to support women, in Page, L.A. and McCandlish, R. (eds), *The New Midwifery: Science and Sensitivity in Practice*, 2nd edn, Oxford: Churchill Livingstone/Elsevier.

Deery, R. and Kirkham, M. (2007) Drained and dumped on: The generation and accumulation of emotional toxic waste in community midwifery, in Kirkham, M. (ed.), *Exploring the Dirty Side of Women's Health*, London: Routledge.

Dykes, F. (2009) 'No time to care': Midwifery work on postnatal wards in England, in Hunter, B. and Deery, R. (eds), *Emotions in Midwifery and Reproduction*, Basingstoke: Palgrave Macmillan.

Edwards, N.P. (2001) Women's experiences of planning home births in Scotland: Birthing autonomy, unpublished PhD thesis, University of Sheffield.

Edwards, N.P. (2005) *Birthing Autonomy: Women's Experiences of Planning Home Births*, London: Routledge.

Edwards, N.P. (2008) Safety in birth: The contextual conundrums faced by women in a 'risk society', driven by neoliberal policies, *MIDIRS*, 18(4): 463–70.

Edwards, N.P. (2009) Women's emotion work in the context of current maternity services, in Hunter, B. and Deery, R. (eds), *Emotions in Midwifery and Reproduction*, Basingstoke: Palgrave Macmillan.

Edwards, N.P. and Murphy-Lawless, J. (2006) The instability of risk: Women's perspectives on risk and safety in birth, in Symon, A. (ed.), *Risk and Choice in Maternity Care: An International Perspective*, Edinburgh: Churchill Livingstone.

Enkin, M.W., Glouberman, S., Groff, P., Jadad, A.R. and Stern, A. (2006) Beyond evidence: The complexity of maternity care, *Birth*, 33(4): 265–9.

Fleming, V.E.M. (1994) Partnership, power and politics: Feminist perceptions of midwifery practice, unpublished PhD thesis, Massey University, New Zealand.

Halldorsdottir, S. (1996) *Caring and Uncaring Encounters in Nursing and Health Care: Developing a Theory*, Linkoping: Department of Caring Sciences, Faculty of Health Sciences, Linkoping University.

Heagarty, B.V. (1997) Willing handmaidens of science? The struggle over the new midwife in early 20th century England, in Kirkham, M.J. and Perkins, E.R. (eds), *Reflections on Midwifery*, London: Balliere Tindall.

Huber, U. and Sandall, J. (2006) Continuity of carer, trust and breastfeeding, *MIDIRS* 16(4): 445–9.

Hunter, B. (2003) Conflicting ideologies as a source of emotion work in midwifery, *Midwifery*, 20(3): 261–72.

Hunter, B. (2006) The importance of reciprocity in relationships between community-based midwives and mothers, *Midwifery*, 22(4): 308–22.

Hunter, B. (2009) 'Mixed messages': Midwives' experiences of managing emotion, in Hunter, B. and Deery, R. (eds), *Emotions in Midwifery and Reproduction*, Basingstoke: Palgrave Macmillan.

Hunter, B. and Deery, R. (eds) (2009) *Emotions in Midwifery and Reproduction*, Basingstoke: Palgrave Macmillan.

Hunter, B., Berg, M., Lundgren, I., Olafsdottir, O.A. and Kirkham, M. (2008) Relationships: The hidden thread in the tapestry of maternity care, *Midwifery* 24(2): 132–7.

Kennedy, H.P. and MacDonald, E.L. (2002) 'Altered consciousness' during childbirth: Potential clues to post traumatic stress disorder, *Journal of Midwifery and Women's Health* 47(6): 380–82.

Kennedy, H.P., Shannon, M.T., Chuahorm, U. and Kravetz, M.K. (2004) The landscape of caring for women: A narrative study of midwifery practice, *Journal of Midwifery and Women's Health* 49(1): 14–23.

Kirkham, M. (1999) The culture of midwifery in the National Health Service in England, *Journal of Advanced Nursing* 30(3): 732–9.

Kirkham, M. (ed.) (2003) *Birth Centres: A Social Model for Maternity Care*, London: Books for Midwives.

Kirkham, M. (2009) Emotion work around reproduction: Supportive or constraining? In Hunter, B. and Deery, R. (eds), *Emotions in Midwifery and Reproduction*, Basingstoke: Palgrave Macmillan.

Kirkham, M. and Stapleton, H. (2001) *Informed Choice in Maternity Care: An Evaluation of Evidence Based Leaflets*, Sheffield: Women's Informed Childbearing and Health Research Group, School of Nursing and Midwifery, University of Sheffield; NHS Centre for Reviews and Dissemination, University of York.

Levy, V. (2004) How midwives used protective steering to facilitate informed choice in pregnancy, in Kirkham, M. (ed.), *Informed Choice in Maternity Care*, Basingstoke: Palgrave Macmillan.

MacDonald, M. (2007) *At Work in the Field of Birth: Midwifery Narratives of Nature, Tradition, and Home*, Nashville, TX: Vanderbilt University Press.

Mackenzie, C. (2000) Imagining oneself otherwise, in Mackenzie, C. and Stoljar, N. (eds), *Relational Autonomy: Feminist Perspectives on Autonomy, Agency, and the Social Self*, New York: Oxford University Press.

Mackenzie, C. and Stoljar, N. (eds) (2000) *Relational Autonomy: Feminist Perspectives on Autonomy, and the Social Self*, New York: Oxford University Press.

Mander, R. (2001) *Supportive Care and Midwifery*, Oxford: Blackwell Science.

McCourt, C. and Stevens, T. (2009) Relationship and reciprocity in caseload midwifery, in Hunter, B. and Deery, R. (eds), *Emotions in Midwifery and Reproduction*, Basingstoke: Palgrave Macmillan.

McCourt, C., Stevens, T., Sandall, J. and Brodie, P. (2006) Working with women: Developing continuity of care in practice, in Page, L.A. and McCandlish, R. (eds), *The New Midwifery: Science and Sensitivity in Practice*, 2nd edn, Oxford: Churchill Livingstone/Elsevier.

McLeod, C. and Sherwin, S. (2000) Relational autonomy, self-trust, and health care for patients who are oppressed, in Mackenzie, C. and Stoljar, N. (eds), *Relational Autonomy: Feminist Perspective on Autonomy, Agency, and the Social Self*, New York: Oxford University Press.

Melender, H.-L. and Lauri, S. (1999) Fears associated with pregnancy and childbirth – experiences of women who have recently given birth, *Midwifery* 15: 177–82.

Morris, A. (2008) Pregnant women are urged to give birth in their own homes, 8 December, http://edinburghnews.scotsman.com/health/Pregnant-women-are-urged-to.4770315.jp, accessed December 2008.

Murphy-Lawless, J. (1998) *Reading Birth and Death: A History of Obstetric Thinking*, Cork: Cork University Press.

Murphy-Lawless, J. (2006) Birth and mothering in today's social order: the challenge of new knowledges, *MIDIRS Midwifery Digest*, 16(4): 439–44.

National Institute for Health and Clinical Excellence (2008) *Intrapartum Care of Healthy Women and Their Babies during Childbirth*, CG55 corrected June 2008, www.nice.org.uk/guidance/index.jsp?action=download&o=36275, accessed January 2009.

Olafsdottir, O.A. (2009) Inner knowing and emotions in the midwife–woman relationship, in Hunter, B. and Deery, R. (eds), *Emotions in Midwifery and Reproduction*, Basingstoke: Palgrave Macmillan.

Pairman, S. (2006) Midwifery partnerships: Working 'with' women, in Page, L.A. and McCandlish, R. (eds), *The New Midwifery: Science and Sensitivity in Practice*, 2nd edn, Oxford: Churchill Livingstone/Elsevier.

Pollock, A.M. (2006) *NHS plc: The Privatisation of Our Health Care*, London: Verso.

Rothman, B.K. (1996) Women, providers, and control, *Journal of Obstetric, Gynecologic, and Neonatal Nursing* 25(3): 254.

Sandall, J. (1997) Midwives' burnout and continuity of care, *British Journal of Midwifery* 5(2): 106–11.

Sandall, J., Davies, J. and Warwick, C. (2001) *Evaluation of the Albany Midwifery Practice*, London: King's College Hospital.

Shildrick, M. (1997) *Leaky Bodies and Boundaries: Feminism, Postmodernism and (Bio)Ethics*, London: Routledge.

Smythe, E. (1998) 'Being safe' in childbirth: A hermeneutic interpretation of the narratives of women and practitioners, unpublished PhD thesis, Massey University, New Zealand.

Waldenstrom, U., Hildingsson, I. and Christie, R.I. (2004) A negative birth experience: Prevalence and risk factors in a national sample, *Birth* 31(1): 17–27.

Walsh, D. (2007) *Improving Maternity Services: Small is Beautiful – Lessons From a Birth Centre*, Oxford: Radcliffe Publishing.

CHAPTER 7

Feeling Safe Enough to Let Go: The Relationship Between a Woman and her Midwife During the Second Stage of Labour

TRICIA ANDERSON

Very little is known about women's experience of the second stage of labour and what aspects of midwifery care help or hinder them in the process of giving birth. As Kirkham and Perkins write, 'the voices of women are muted by the experts, although only women experience birth' (1997: 185). The increasingly technological aspects and professionalization of childbirth mean that women's experiences are too often neglected, yet unless we know what they are going through, how can we provide appropriate and sensitive care? This chapter is based on a study that tried to redress that balance by recording women's experiences of the second stage of labour and their perceptions of midwifery care during this crucial time (Anderson, 1997). The impetus behind the study was this simple question: 'What can I do, as your midwife, to help you during the second stage of labour?'

Sixteen women, given pseudonyms in this chapter, who had given birth normally without epidural analgesia, were interviewed in depth using the grounded theory approach. Full details of the methodology can be found in Anderson (1997). The women were asked about their experience of the second stage, which for them incorporated elements of the transitional phase of labour as well as the 'pushing' phase. Eight had given birth at home and eight in hospital; five were primiparous, eleven multiparous, and all gave birth normally with minimal intervention. These women are not representative of other women in their area, let alone all women giving birth in England. These findings cannot therefore be generalized to groups from other cultures or to women who experience, for example, augmentation, epidural analgesia or instrumental birth. These are, however, women who have achieved a normal birth with minimal intervention and analgesia within a Western cultural context; listening and analysing their stories may help midwives caring for women who want to give birth normally.

The intense physical sensations of the second stage

The second stage of labour is associated with the onset of new and frightening physical sensations, which appear to follow a predictable pattern. Women describe sensations such as bulging, cracking, splitting, opening and breaking, as the uterine cavity is fully open and the baby begins its internal descent:

> I remember the sensation of my pelvis coming apart – unzipping. I suddenly thought 'Christ, my pelvis is cracking open'! I was really scared, because it was a bit like wild horses tied to either side of your pelvis, running in opposite directions... I didn't want to push, because I thought if my pelvis unzips any more, I'm going to come apart. (Anna)

On feeling these overwhelming sensations, women have to overcome a barrier of fear that initially prevents them pushing wholeheartedly. As Flint writes:

> I feel that when nature asks us women to push a baby out, it is probably the bravest thing we ever have to do. The feeling that trauma must ensue is so strong; in a way, a woman has to abandon her own comfort and safety in order for her child to emerge. (Flint, 1997: 186)

Women describe an initial sensation of holding back – for fear of opening their bowels, for fear of their backs cracking in half or their pelvis splitting open, for fear of nobody being there ready to catch the baby, for fear of losing control or for fear of simply more never-ending and worsening pain:

> You go through a sort of mental barrier, definitely. Before I stood up,

it was like 'oh my god, this is so painful' and like just going with the pain. But when I stood up and started pushing, you suddenly just think 'well, I've got to do it. No matter how painful it is, I've got to get this baby out, and I've got to push and just forget about the pain.' You become a lot stronger all of a sudden. (Julie)

Price (1993) talks of the importance of body image and how this is constructed of, among other things, a concept of body boundaries – a perception of where one's body ends and the outside world begins. Any change in this body image can be profoundly traumatic, possibly no more so than during the process of giving birth, in which a woman's body literally opens up, the boundaries being breached and no longer clear and intact:

When I felt her first really descend, that was when I got a bit frightened... it was like a huge powerful thing that was happening to me... a fear that she was coming out beyond my control, there was a fear of the pain, and the fear that my body couldn't possibly open any more. (Anna)

In this process there is an inevitable loss of control. This is the 'regressive boundary-permeable phase'. One coping strategy is to seek external boundary control by grasping out for physical contact with something – with anything. If this need is not met, then, Price theorizes, a woman will enter the third, aberrant phase, known as 'desperate-body boundary-diffuse phase', which may lead her to believe that her body is going to break up and she is going to die. Natalie, a primigravida, explains it thus:

I was convinced, absolutely convinced there was no way I could survive this kind of pain... I kept saying 'I can't survive another contraction.' I was desperate to die – I thought that would get rid of the pain. (Natalie)

Fear of losing control

Perhaps surprisingly, however, the predominant fear seems to be that of losing control, which for many women is the main hurdle that needs to be overcome in order to give birth normally. Rhiannon talked of how women need to 'let go' in order to give birth, yet women report the greatest satisfaction in childbirth when they feel 'in control' (Green, 1993). Are these two states incompatible? As Bluff and Holloway (1994: 161) point out, the issue of control is 'ambiguous, with women wanting to be in control of events even though they acknowledged that maybe they were not':

> It's quite nice to have the contractions stopping and a different thing happening, but it's scary at the time. It's almost like you're losing your control over the whole process and that's the scary bit. (Rhiannon)

Waldenstrom *et al.* (1996) explain how being in control seems to be associated with birth satisfaction, and, indeed, the women kept returning to this idea. The concept of control is complex and can mean different things for different women. Waldenstrom *et al.* suggest that it might be linked to a sense of being an active subject rather than the passive object of the event.

Brewin and Bradley (1982) also looked at women's perceived control and the experience of childbirth. Interestingly, they found that women who either perceived themselves to have control over labour or perceived the staff to have control over labour reported less pain. It would seem that the worst option of all is for no one to have control over labour; that is, for the labour to be 'out of control'. Neither the midwife nor the woman is in control and, importantly, neither does the woman's body feel as if it knows what it is doing. This resonates with Daniella's experience: when the second stage of her labour seemed to be prolonged, she lost all sense of both internal and external control, and her saviour was a midwife, 'an angel', who came in and took charge of the situation:

> It was like at last somebody's here now who's in control and who's going to do something. (Daniella)

Altered states of consciousness

The severity and intensity of physical sensations lead women to a instinctive primal survival technique, that of entering an altered state of consciousness. This equates with Rhiannon's suggested need to 'let go' or Isobel's 'just disconnect'. This was one of the strongest findings in this study; all but one of the women talked of a sense of separation of mind from body, which was not a frightening experience and paradoxically enabled them to retain control:

> I was aware of having a kind of out of body experience... It was a suddenly kind of floating feeling like I wasn't really there and then the contraction would come again and wake me up. I was just floating

away, really comfortable, no pain, it was really quiet, really peaceful. There was nothing around me. I could have been totally on my own, just not aware of anybody. (Natalie)

The women did not equate entering an altered state of consciousness with being out of control; on the contrary, it was a powerful coping strategy that increased their sense of being *in* control. This corresponds with Davis's (1989) paradoxical notion that, to gain control, one has first to go through a process of losing it. She talks of how the key to gaining control is often to lose it, to surrender ideas, desires and fears in order to merge with and then master the experience:

> I didn't feel in control. But I didn't feel like the midwife was in control, either. I just felt like my body was in control. But not my mind at all. (Emma)

Letting go

The women talked a lot about their bodies being in control. It seems that there is a sense of 'letting go' on a psychological level that allows the physical body to take control. Thus, the woman still retains her sense of control and physically embodies Waldenstrom's idea of being the active subject. The woman is the body that is in control. In this sense, there is no loss of control:

> At that point you're not in control, society's not in control, no one's in control apart from your body and what your body has learnt to do by itself over generations and thousands of generations. (Rhiannon)

This psychological state is similar to that described by Cosmi (1995) as a hypnotic trance. It is characterized by a perceptual shift of awareness in an atmosphere of trust and security. Subjects describe a 'distancing' that they later describe as a feeling of being outside themselves, peripherally 'watching' what is happening to them. Cosmi points out that severe pain and stress seem to enhance the ability of an individual to enter this state. Machin and Scamell (1997: 82) described their participants as experiencing 'a trance-like state of consciousness, indicative of the transitional state of a rite of passage'. Odent (1991) suggests that this might be similar to a 'near -death' experience, in which there is a sudden, massive release of endorphins, which might explain the women's feelings of floating – a calm and peaceful euphoria.

Davis (1989) explores the concepts of different types of brain wave, the alpha, beta, theta and delta waves demonstrated on an electro-encephalogram. She suggests that women in labour are in the theta state, the same state that is induced by deep hypnosis or near-death experiences, which would explain their euphoria, sense of oneness and lack of temporal or physical awareness. Isobel put this concept in her own words:

> What she [the midwife] said did get through to me though, even though I was on another level... it's like a different level of the brain picks it up, and that bit of the brain reassures the rest of the brain that's doing it that it's all right, even though it's not a big part of it. (Isobel)

The level of endorphins, the body's naturally produced, powerful opiate-like substances, is at its highest during transition and the second stage, producing a sense of well-being and peace, altering the perception of place and time, yet curiously co-existing with the feelings of extreme pain (Odent, 1994). To be able to 'just disconnect', as Isobel described, minimizes the negative effect of the stress hormones (adrenaline and noradrenaline) on the strong oxytocic response needed to facilitate the contractions of the uterus and thus the birth.

Cathy was intrigued by this notion, and commented that 'it's not the kind of thing I've ever heard people talk about'. She pointed out that 'if you're talking to someone in labour, don't expect an answer straight away. Wait for something to happen, and then you'll get an answer.'

Entering this altered state appeared to be unconnected to use of analgesia (only three of the women being given pethidine) or the length or duress of the labour; even Rhiannon, whose entire labour was less than two hours in total, experienced a sense of separation. She gave birth at home without any intervention, any vaginal examination or any physical contact from the midwife, and was able to take this one step further:

> For me, it was not so much a separation but more a kind of 'oneness'. It was a separation from the intellectual side of life... when you're there and you're giving birth and your body is in total control. It's a trust and it's an animal thing. It's a separation from thinking. You couldn't intellectualise it. You have to separate your emotional thinking side of you to cope with it. (Rhiannon)

A sense of timelessness

All the women experienced temporal and locality distortion, and a sense

of timelessness. Beck (1994) studied this phenomenon of temporal awareness and found that labouring women's sense of time fluctuates throughout the process. This has implications for midwifery practice: telling a
woman that the anaesthetist will be here in 20 minutes or that the baby
will be born within half an hour may not be helpful or relevant to her
(although it may be of benefit to an anxious partner!). The woman may be
experiencing time at a completely different pace, one in which half an hour
may seem like a day or like a few minutes. This is similar to the temporal
distortion undergone by those experiencing altered states of consciousness
in other ways, through meditation, for example, or through hallucinogenic
drugs (*Scientific American*, 1972). It may well be that, for the labouring
women, losing track of time is a very helpful coping strategy.

Andrea's story: The exception to the rule

Not all women may feel that the sense of going into an altered state
applies to them, as seen, for example, with one woman in the study.
Rather than being an anomaly to be ignored, Andrea's experience is
worthy of special mention as it throws up an important point. She
explains that, even while pushing, she was worrying about her housework:

> I wasn't able to do that [go into another world]. I was worried about
> my husband. And you've got a lot of things going on in your head…
> Everything's got to be just right in this house. Housework, dusting and
> all the rest of it. Making sure my eldest was all right at school, making
> sure the other one was going to be in bed at the right time and just
> thinking 'oh dear, I haven't cleaned this and I haven't cleaned that and
> what are people going to think'. Thinking about the washing, thinking
> 'I hope this isn't going to make a mess cos I've got to wash more
> sheets!' I think it helped take my mind off things.

Rather than floating off into a private world, Andrea used her domestic worries as a distraction from the pain of the contractions. More than
that, however, Andrea lived in an abusive relationship, her husband
having a record of violent behaviour, towards both her and health professionals. Andrea's prime concern was to ensure the birth went smoothly so
that her husband did not become violent. Thus, she had an overwhelming primacy of fear: in her rank of competing concerns, her fear of her
husband and of her husband's abuse held sway over any fear of labour,
pain or even death itself. This necessitated Andrea keeping herself very

much 'together' and alert during the process of giving birth; any sense of separation or disconnection might have had disastrous consequences for her and her family. Had her husband's violence surfaced during the birth, Andrea knew that she risked having her children taken away.

Note how she quickly glosses over the fact that she is worried about her husband and moves on to a long description about housework. Women's lives are multifaceted and ongoing, and giving birth takes place in a complex context that has been long in its weaving. Midwives need to be aware of the whole picture, or at least be aware that the picture they see is not necessarily complete.

Supporting or undermining: The power of the midwife

The women were unanimous in their belief that the contribution of the midwife was critical, having the power to make or break the woman's birth experience, and this centred on the issue of control. They agreed how vulnerable and susceptible to suggestion they were during the second stage of labour, which corresponds to the idea of an altered state of consciousness, and just how much power the midwife had to influence and direct them. Women in labour are in a vulnerable state of separation, a dangerous state in which the power of the surrounding people and their messages can be irresistible.

> I felt completely in the midwife's hands, and would have obeyed anything she told me to do! (Tracy)

> The midwife told me to stand up when I was laying down, and I did not want to stand up, but I just got up because she had told me to. I was told to get up, I got up. I was told not to push and pant, I panted. It's like being back at school... I remember looking at my husband and the GP, thinking 'she said pant, guys. Pant! The midwife says pant.' The midwife is more in control than you think. (Cathy)

Midwife as safe anchor: Feeling safe enough to let go

The women talked about having to trust the midwife; a failure to do what the midwife tells them could put their baby's life at risk (Beaton, 1990; Bluff and Holloway, 1994; Kirke, 1980). Those women who gave birth at home had the opportunity to get to know their midwife, and without exception they rated this opportunity to build up a relationship of trust before the birth as being very important. Andrea talked about how the midwife was able to treat her as an individual as she had come to know the family and Andrea's own wishes regarding how she wanted to give birth, and then respected them. The trust was based on some foundation. Rhiannon agreed:

> The most important thing for me is to have somebody there who I trusted, who I knew beforehand, who was familiar with my family and was familiar with what I wanted, who I trusted and liked, and someone that I could feel completely at ease with and know that I could just get on with what I needed to do and give birth. (Rhiannon)

Isobel talked of how it was important that she knew and trusted her midwife 'not to laugh at me, or something'. Feeling safe enough to enter an altered state of consciousness was much easier in front of someone you knew, she thought. But even the women who gave birth in hospital and who had never met their midwife before labour talked of how they automatically trusted her and assumed that she knew what she was doing: 'You have to, don't you?' (Julie). Their trust was based on blind faith rather than any solid foundation. As they were in such a vulnerable state, they had no choice but to trust the unknown midwife. Tracy, a young woman having her first baby in hospital, goes one step further and talks of how the midwife takes on a mothering role to the mother-to-be, a firm-handed mother figure who has to be obeyed:

> You have to obey and listen to what the midwife's telling you. You know that she does it all day, every day. She's the expert. It's just automatic. There isn't time to rationalise it. You're in pain, the contractions are coming fast. You really want your mum, don't you? The midwife is the surrogate mum. (Tracy)

The midwife is in an extraordinarily powerful position. In her care, she has a woman who is vulnerable and in extreme pain, hypersuggestible and experiencing perceptual distortions and loss of control:

> You're at the most vulnerable point, because you can't do anything. If someone starts telling you to do something, you just do it. When the midwife told me that I wasn't to push or to do something – like turn over – I felt like a little schoolgirl: 'Oh, all right then – if I have to.' So midwives are in a real position of power which they mustn't abuse. (Rhiannon)

This power on the part of the midwife can be used sensitively and wisely or, as Rhiannon points out, can be abused. Lukes (1986) explored how power affects behaviour. *A* has power over *B* to the extent to which *A* can get *B* to do something that *B* would not otherwise do. *A* (the midwife) may not exercise her power, but *B*'s (the client's) knowledge of this power gains her willing compliance. Emma talked of how the midwife made her lie on her side, which Emma intuitively felt was wrong and subsequently proved to be so. On being asked whether she told the midwife this, Emma answered:

No, I didn't say anything to her about not lying on my side. It was like 'OK, I'll lie here. Whatever you say.' The schoolgirl syndrome. If she'd said, can you just swing on this rafter, you'd go 'OK.' You haven't got time to think about it, have you? Everything is happening so quickly, you just don't have the time. You just do as you're told. (Emma)

Trust sustained

When this power is appropriately channelled, a skilled midwife can provide a sense of security that enables women safely to enter the disconnected state and thus facilitate the birth process:

It's the midwife's job to keep everything safe. She's the anchor that helps you go off into that altered state... I also felt really assured that they were competent. That was very reassuring, that they know what they were doing. It was all alright, it was all normal. They anchored me and allowed me to feel safe going through all that. (Isobel)

For this to happen, women need a midwife to be present yet unobtrusive. Berg *et al.* (1996) found that the midwife's 'presence' was key. If trust is lacking, if women feel undermined and unsupported and do not feel that the midwife sees them as individuals, they perceive the midwife to be 'absently present':

She [the midwife] didn't spend much time with me, coming in and out... she seemed quite distracted, like her mind wasn't really in the room. (Judith)

Calm and quiet

Quietness and calm are attributes that women frequently mention they

value in a midwife. Yet paradoxically, when women are off in a disconnected state, the midwife's role is for many of them surprisingly peripheral, which may illustrate how well she can perform her task as guide,
safe-keeper and anchor:

> I wasn't even aware of anything, even of which side she [the midwife]
> was standing. I don't remember much of what she was saying, I really
> don't. I'm sure it was all really good stuff... I'm sure probably if she
> hadn't been saying anything I would have noticed. (Natalie)

This idea of a midwife who sits, watches and is quiet is mentioned by
Odent in his discussion of the role of the birth attendant (Odent, 1987).
He proposed that the foetus ejection reflex can only happen when the
attendants are conscious that the process of parturition is an involuntary
one, and that one cannot help an involuntary process but simply not
disturb it. If labour is going well, a woman needs little input from the
midwife other than her simple presence:

> The perfect midwife for me would be someone who would be able to
> understand when she was needed... But if everything's going well, just
> to be left by yourself, knowing that she's there, knowing that there's a
> woman there to deliver the baby, catch the baby, hold the baby. She's
> there if anything goes wrong. But it must be difficult – only experience
> can probably give a midwife that kind of knowing – when to step in and
> when not to step in. But I think that's the most important thing – not
> to spoil the whole flow of the birth process. That continuity of peace
> and tranquillity and privacy. (Rhiannon)

> Just a guiding through, yes. Just to reassure you you're doing the right
> thing. But I would say that it's good for the midwife and everybody else
> just to stand back, really. You don't really want to listen to anybody. (Anna)

Yet for some women, the midwife, and in particular her voice, can be
acutely important, the only thing that keeps them safe and holds them
anchored in this world:

> I was very much tuned into her voice. If my husband had said
> anything, I probably wouldn't have heard it, but my ears were focusing
> back towards where the midwife was and very tuned in to what she was
> saying. It was very dark, and all I could hear was the midwife's voice,
> saying 'keep breathing'. (Joanna)

As well as quietness and calm, the women valued praise, positivity, simplicity, reassurance and gentle encouragement in their midwives to help them get through the second stage. They talked of how important it was that the midwife gave them confidence, confidence in both the midwife's skills and their own ability to give birth. The midwife needs to believe that the woman can do it and convey that belief to her.

Jones (1989) talks about the importance of care-givers having insight into the mind–body process of labour, which will result in them giving support that is far more appropriate to the mother's lived experience than if they only know the anatomical and physiological aspects of labour. 'As far as I'm concerned, teaching about the mother's altered state of mind is far more important than teaching about cervical dilatation', he writes (Jones, 1989: 19).

> The midwife said, 'you can do it..., you can do it'. She didn't tell me to push or anything. I didn't need telling to push this time. I felt really confident that I was in safe hands. (Isobel)

> No, what the midwife said, and the encouragement was just right. It wasn't too over the top. I think if she'd said more, I probably would have wanted her to shut up. You don't want to be bombarded with instructions. You just want it very simple, clear, consistent... You almost want to hear the same thing again and again... to reassure you that that's all you have to do. (Joanna)

Unobtrusive

It is important that midwives know when to stand back and not intrude or distract women from focusing on the intense natural process of pushing. This important distinction was very well summarised by Berg *et al.* (1996), who described a woman's need to be supported and guided by the midwife *but on her own terms*. Supporting and encouraging women to listen to their own feelings and instincts are very different from imposing a pre-learnt, arbitrary set of instructions. When guidance is given, women still need to be able to retain their sense of control. This idea was beautifully summed up by one of their respondents, who said: 'Even if I received expert help... it wasn't the intention of someone else that dominated, but my own desire' (Berg *et al.*, 1996: 13). The women themselves wanted to be the authorities at their own births, even though they all recognized and valued the need for professional assistance and guidance. Women – both multiparous and primiparous – acknowledged the expertise of the midwives but wanted to retain control and give birth actively:

> I was very much in control of the whole thing. And the midwife helped that. She could have easily cluttered the whole process. I liked the way that she was very, very easy, and didn't say 'right' and roll her sleeves up and say 'now, let's do this.. and let's examine you... and... I'll break your waters... and...' It just all happened and felt so natural. (Joanna)

Importantly, women value how the midwife does not take control of everything but facilitates their own ability and confidence to be in control. This leads to overwhelmingly positive feelings about the experience:

> After you've given birth, you can do anything. You could move a mountain... And the midwife helps you do that, doesn't she, as long as she doesn't interfere too much. (Cathy)

Back to the school room: The naughty schoolgirl

Difficulties arise when midwives abuse their position, undermining the woman's sense of being in control rather than reinforcing it. Six women in the study talked unprompted of feeling like a naughty little schoolgirl, with the midwife that well-known authority figure, the harsh and unkind schoolmistress:

> You go back to being a schoolgirl and do as you're told. You feel vulnerable, and you think that somebody in authority, which the midwives are – they're the people that know about what's going on – you listen to them and do what you're told. (Julie)

Several women were called 'a good girl' when they did well. More often, though, they talked of a sense of 'not doing it right' or 'not doing it very well'. They were sure that there was a 'right' way to do it and that they were inadequate or deficient in some way:

> Everybody kept saying to me 'I've got to try and push harder' and I really felt inadequate that I wasn't doing it right at all. (Tracy)

Women were praised by the midwife if they got it 'right' – 'she kept saying I was doing it just right' – and berated if they were not doing it 'right' – 'she shouted at me to stop shouting and start pushing'. All the women talked of times, either in this birth or from a previous birth experience, when the midwife had been at best intrusive, and at worst overbearing and rude. They cited examples of care by the midwives that had distressed them and, in the case of the multiparous women who had chosen to give birth at home, it was their memories of poor treatment during previous births that had been one of the motivating factors in opting for a home birth.

Two women mentioned how intrusive they found the midwife's constant note taking during the second stage:

> I can remember the midwife was scribbling notes all the time. That's about all I can remember of what was going on around me. That's all she seemed to do. (Emma)

> Midwives should spend less time doing paperwork and give more attention to the women they're going to deliver! (Rhiannon)

The timing of a midwife's questions can sometimes be inappropriate and insensitive:

> Every time one of the midwives went to say something to me, I couldn't answer because it was at a time when a contraction was coming and you're trying to say something but you can't. It was irritating. (Sonia)

Sadly, some midwives can be rough, hard and insensitive:

> A lot of the midwives seemed very butch, very manly. Maybe that's the way they've got to be. They're all rough. (Judith)

Maybe 'doing things' helps the midwives to feel useful, rather than being of help to the woman:

> It would just be an invasion of space if they leant in and said 'come on, dear...' Unless the woman is saying 'I can't do this', which I don't think happens at that stage. Maybe it would help the midwives, to think that they were helping, but I don't think you need to hear it. (Anna)

Some of the other women remembered being shouted at, which was never appreciated:

With my second daughter… by the end of it I was legs strapped up, big set of pliers and the midwife shouting 'you will fucking push this baby out!' like some headmistress! (Isobel)

Andrea recalled the second stage of her first birth, which she remembers as a terrible experience. While she was giving birth, a cleaner came in and carried on cleaning the room as if nothing was happening:

When I had my first baby, I had a cleaner walk in when I was pushing! She just walked in, had a dust round and off she went again. She picked me knickers up off the side to dust round them… I was pissed off about the whole thing. I had a husband who was sat there drunk asleep at the time. Great! And just people walking in and out all the time. It's not much fun. And then when you're in the stirrups, it's just… There is a lot of people there. I had forceps and so you end up with a paediatrician, doctors, junior doctor. It's like a side show. (Andrea)

Feelings of anger

The imagery of the circus was used by several different women: they described the medical staff as the circus and themselves as the freak or side show. It was fairly clear from some of the women's accounts exactly who was in control:

I was very angry because she'd taken him away. The midwife wanted to get him dressed instantly – instantly he came out! Quick, get his clothes on! Oh my god! They wanted to take him away and give me a cup of tea and it was like 'I don't want a cup of tea actually – go away! I want my baby in here with me and everyone else can go away… I was so angry. I was so angry. I was really angry. I felt that, after going through this whole empowering thing of giving birth where you've got so much strength, then all of a sudden in come the circus and you're totally disempowered. (Rhiannon)

So I screamed at L that I wanted to push, and she said 'No, don't push, don't push…' and then with every contraction then it seemed just more and more strongly that I wanted to push. And that's when she made me get out of the bath… I would have happily stayed in there – no problem at all, because it was really comforting actually being in the water. In the bath, she was saying 'we'll get you out of the bath and then I'll examine you to see how we're getting on'. (Natalie)

Note the use of the first person plural in the last sentence: exactly whose labour is this? Brook (1996) uses the term 'maternalism' to describe the way in which midwives may act towards a labouring woman more like the authoritarian mother of a small child rather than someone in a professional adult relationship:

> The midwife [who] delivered my first baby was quite old fashioned. I didn't feel relaxed... I felt very stressed actually, because she was very kind of sergeant majorish – 'come on then, up you get, into the bath with you'... It was like 'what's this woman doing in my house!' She broke my waters and stuff. But now I think about it, she did want to control my pushing. I did listen to her. I did do what she said. I did, yes, I did. And at the time she said it, I found it incredibly irritating and I was quite angry because it was going against what my body was telling me to do. I didn't like it, and I just wanted to tell her to bugger off – just shut up! (Rhiannon)

Julie's comments are thought provoking:

> It's not the midwife that forces you to be like that, is it? Like a school-girl? It's you. I suppose it's just going back to childhood really. The last time you felt so out of control, so helpless. I think it's just a natural thing. I don't think you can help it. (Julie)

As is obvious from some of the other women's stories, when a midwife uses her presence wisely, the adult labouring woman need not feel like a schoolgirl; it is not necessarily a 'natural' thing. Women do not equate entering the altered state with a return to childhood. Yet Julie believes that regression to childhood during labour is inevitable, as a midwife has taken the schoolmistress role at both her births. Julie's belief in her ability to give birth as an adult woman is undermined by the midwife taking the power and exerting her influence as the adult, relegating Julie to the position of child. As Julie is on the brink of becoming a mother, this seems wholly inappropriate.

Intrusive directions

> Giving birth is a completely free-willed thing and it doesn't listen. I think if it had to listen to something, that's when things start going wrong. (Rhiannon)

Interventions in the natural process of giving birth may be intended by the midwife to confirm normality, and she may believe it to be reassuring for the client. However, the very act carries with it the message that things might very possibly *not* be going well, for otherwise, why intervene at all? Professional surveillance brings doubt and anxiety into the process, and because of the supposed greater power, education and (assumed) gender status of health professionals, women are socialized into believing that the professionals' version of reality must be more accurate than their own.

That intervention in labour, such as monitoring the foetal heart, is of value is not in question, but, as an intervention, its proponents must be aware of its costs and benefits. If, by a simple procedure or examination, women are made to doubt their own bodies' ability to give birth ('I worried about it after that'), midwives must develop their communication skills of reassurance to try to root out the seeds of uncertainty that they have sown. This process also undermines a woman's sense of control and self-awareness: 'I feel *X*, but the midwife says *Y*; therefore I must be wrong':

> At one point I thought I felt a bit pushy and she was examining me at the time, and she said 'oh no, you don't feel like pushing yet'. And I thought 'Oh. No, OK then.' That made me feel a bit stupid, I suppose. Well no, not stupid, but just a bit like 'oh, I must be wrong. I'm not doing it right. I was just a bit confused, really. I didn't feel angry – just confused, and like I was wrong and she was right, because she's the midwife and she must know. So I must have been mistaken in what I felt, which is stupid really. (Julie)

Being undermined

Many women quoted instances when the midwife had completely under-mined and disregarded what they were feeling, which made them feel angry and sapped their confidence in their own bodies. If the midwife's instruc-tions were at odds with their physical sensations, this resulted in feelings of uncertainty and confusion. As already noted, women are so sure that the midwife must be right, and therefore their own body must be wrong:

> I thought I wanted to push, but she [the midwife] said I couldn't possi-bly. (Sonia)

Thomson, in her review of the management of the second stage of labour, writes:

There appears to be an impression among the midwifery and obstetric profession that control has to be exerted over the labouring woman as soon as the second stage begins... the delivery room can resemble a rugby scrum with everyone present peering at the woman's vulva while urging her to exert greater effort. (Thomson, 1988: 77)

Midwives have traditionally exhorted women to 'take a deep breath in, hold it, and push.........sh' (McKay *et al.*, 1990: 192), responding more often than not to their own overwhelming urge to push (Sargady, 1995). McKay *et al.* (1990) showed how the instructions that women received were more often than not completely at odds with their body's sensations, and Evans and Jeffrey (1995) found that pushing directions were the most frequently mentioned areas of conflict in information needs between midwives and clients.

Trust betrayed

The women explained how important it is that the information given is accurate: 'white lies' are not appreciated, even when meant to encourage. For, if they are found out, the trust that the woman has placed in the midwife is instantly betrayed and any sense of control that the women has maintained is lost. None of the women appreciated being kept in the dark or being given inaccurate information or false hope. Dianne experienced this in her first birth: she had an epidural, the midwives were telling her how well she was pushing, yet in fact there was no progress whatsoever:

You're not quite sure that when she says 'oh, you're doing really well' whether you really are doing really well, and you're thinking 'well, am I?' I obviously wasn't doing very well. Why didn't they tell me I wasn't doing very well? You're just lying there, thinking 'oh this is easy' with a big smile on your face, and then you find out that you're not doing it right at all. Nothing's happening. You just assume that everything's going all right, because they've just told me it is. (Dianne)

Wrong assumptions

Many of the women incorrectly anticipated events, based on either past birth experiences or what they had learnt in antenatal classes. The multiparous women expected events to unfold in the same way in which they had previously, and kept waiting for the midwives to do or say certain things. Nowhere was this more evident than when to begin pushing:

I was actually waiting for them to tell me what to do. That was a problem, in that I was waiting for them to tell me what to do, and of course they're letting you do what you want. I was waiting for permission to push, because that's what we'd been told in the classes… But then I didn't say anything to them anyway, so it was my fault as much as anything, because I assumed it would be the same thing as last time. (Julie)

Rose Driscoll has collected birth stories from 50 women of different generations and from differing cultures – England, Ireland and Italy:

Something else many women agreed on was that once labour had begun there seemed to be great disagreement over the subject of when to push. When you're thrashing around in agony and wanting to push, it's not much fun to be told you can't. Unless you have the confidence of a gladiator you do as you're told. You wait for them, you don't make a fuss, you submit to their demands. They know best. (Driscoll, 1997: xvi)

But midwives are changing the way in which they practise towards more evidence-based care. One such significant change is the move away from the intervention of directed pushing to free women to follow their own body's instincts. This has a solid foundation in research evidence (Nikodem, 1995). However, it is important to realize that this change has implications for women. First, all midwives do not change their practice at the same pace in the same way and at the same time. It is a piecemeal affair, with midwives even in one labour ward working the same shift using very different styles. Second, women clearly have a received knowledge of what they expect from the midwife, which is that she will tell them when to push. This is implied even in a guide issued by the NCT (Nolan, 1996), and Dianne mentioned how she learnt her birthing behaviour from what she had 'seen on the telly':

I didn't go to any antenatal classes… so luckily, you've seen it all on the telly so you know more or less what you've got to do. (Dianne)

This illustrates nicely just how pervasive the notion of enforced pushing has become within Western society. It is possible that this received knowledge can be changed over a period of many years by consistency in childbirth classes, literature and other media, but in the meantime childbearing women are left in a very confusing situation. This was apparent from many of the discussions. The confusion over whether or not to push was widespread. All of the women had attended antenatal classes, for either this baby or a previous baby, and had clear expectations that the midwife would tell them when they could push. If this did not happen, they were left in limbo and not in control, not knowing whether or not to push:

> A lot of it, I was holding back for, because when I went to antenatal classes with the twins we were told 'don't push; if you want to push, then say so and we'll tell you when you can push'… because they check that there's no membrane across or something. So of course, I'm saying that I want to push, and I'm not being told 'no, don't' but I'm not being told 'yes, do!' And I'm thinking that they will tell me when I can. In the end I was saying 'if I want to push, can I push?' (Dianne)

For many women, there appears to be a conflict between their own and their care-giver's readiness to have them push. This can occur in one of two ways: the woman wanting to push and being told not to, or her not wanting to push yet being told she should. The most undermining and confusing of all would be when both things happen, as it did with Daniella.

Daniella's experience

> I was too exhausted to take her in. I was crying tears, but I wasn't even crying. I was crying from inside.

Thus spoke Daniella about the birth of her baby. For her, the second stage was a repeating nightmare that was out of control: Daniella was the one woman in this study for whom the second stage of labour was an extremely negative experience. As we have seen with Andrea, the exception sometimes provides some interesting food for thought.

Daniella's first birth had ended in a long two-hour second stage and a bad perineal tear, which she remembers two doctors taking two hours or more to suture. She recalls not being able to walk for three weeks, and she could not resume sexual intercourse for a year and half. She felt brutalized, with her sexual identity in tatters. Daniella felt so traumatized by the memory of that second stage that she considered opting for an elective caesarean section for this birth, but decided in the end to have a vaginal delivery. The first stage went easily and quickly, and she needed no analgesia; then the second stage began, she panicked and it all started to go horribly wrong:

I thought I was pushing as much as I could. You can be pushing because you're told to push, or there's that point where I got these natural urges, they were real, and then I did really push for all I had. But the rest of the time I was having to force myself to push because they weren't sort of natural and the midwife was saying not to force it, so I thought well I won't push then, because I'll be forcing it. I was just so confused. Should I be waiting for the natural urges to push and then give it all I've got, all the welly, or should I just be pushing? The midwife was saying that I was using my breathing too much and I thought well, I've got to do something for this pain. (Daniella)

The midwife told Daniella to 'go with her body', which left Daniella confused over whether or not she should push. Yet when she did get an urge to push and tried, the midwife told her not to, which undermined what little confidence she had. Midwives were coming in and out of the room, and Daniella very quickly felt that everything was slipping out of control. The midwife was not taking charge, Daniella did not feel in control and, importantly, her body was obviously not to be trusted. Daniella did not know what to do, whether to push or to breathe, and then there was the continuing, excruciating pain. But then came her 'angel'. A second midwife came in after this had been going on for an hour and a half, 'took charge' and assisted Daniella to give birth vaginally by giving clear, precise directions:

This midwife came in and took charge, almost with military precision, and you just felt confident with her. She said 'Right, Mrs X', and she just looked at me and she took my arm and she was an angel sent from heaven. I suddenly had a surge of energy. It brings tears to my eyes, because she really did. (Daniella)

There are two points to be made here. First, the lack of continuity of care is painfully obvious. The midwives did not know Daniella's history: she had asked for it to be documented, but when she arrived in labour they could not find her notes. So they were unaware of her fears of the second stage of labour and Daniella's trust in them was shaken. Second, the time for midwives to sit in the background is when all is going well, but all the women agreed that it was to the midwives that they expected to turn when things started to go awry. Daniella felt that the first midwife let her down for failing to initiate what Simkin (1989) has termed the 'take charge routine'. As previously mentioned, the worse scenario of all is if the woman feels things are 'out of control'; Daniella trusted the midwife to restore control, and felt betrayed when this did not happen.

Two key studies point to a significant discrepancy between a woman's perceptions of her own pain during labour and the midwives' perceptions of the pain that a woman is experiencing (Bradley *et al.,* 1983), which indicates a lack of connection. Rajan (1993) suggests that this phenomenon is self-perpetuating because it remains unspoken: neither women nor professionals fully understand the reality of each others' feelings and beliefs. They seldom truly listen to each other:

> They've got this way of saying to you 'that's not a very big one [contraction]!' I was in the hospital, and some woman was strapped up and she was having some quite nice peaks on there, and she was in a lot of pain, and they were going 'you're not in labour, don't be so silly'. She was only 28 weeks, and she had the baby that afternoon. I mean, for goodness sake! It makes you feel like slapping them sometimes. (Andrea)

This echoes Kirkham's plea for the recognition of the value of story telling (Kirkham and Perkins, 1997) in the hope that women's voices may be heard, which will facilitate a sense of what Belenky *et al.* (1986) call 'connected knowing': through a process of collaboration, they can begin to measure personal knowledge against the authority of others and develop a constructed (or reconstructed) knowledge of childbirth based in lived experience. In an age when women-centred care is held up as the new ethos, this is surely essential.

Anxiety-provoking interventions

The phenomenon of interventions bringing doubt and uncertainty was confirmed by many of the women. It prevented them from 'letting go'. They talked of how they were not at all worried about the baby's well-being until the moment when the midwife went to listen for the foetal heart or rupture the membranes. Then they worried:

> She listened to it about every ten minutes or so, and every time she said it was fine. But it is a worry when she starts doing it because you think 'oh-oh is it going to be all right? Is there something wrong with the baby?' (Julie)

I can remember the midwife wanting to break my waters. I said, 'why do you want to do that – is the baby OK?' 'Yes, yes, everything's fine – I just want to break your waters.' When she was talking about it I thought, 'oh my goodness, is something wrong? Maybe the baby's not OK.' (Rhiannon)

I always remember this nurse asking me continually if I wanted the gas. Me saying 'no, I'm fine. Why, am I not fine? Is there something I don't know? Is there something wrong with me?' (Cathy)

Anna highlighted how important it is for the midwife to give feedback quickly after every intervention. Having made the decision to intervene, silence is the worst possible outcome, implying that something is most definitely wrong:

I was worried for the baby's safety. Yes. When the midwife listened. I was really relieved when the midwife said 'that's fine'. So would it almost be better if the midwife didn't listen to the baby's heartbeat at all. And it would have been awful if the midwife hadn't said anything – if she hadn't said 'that's fine'. That's very important. Had she not said anything, I would have assumed that there would have been something wrong. (Anna)

Andrea took this concept one step further when she talked of how technology comes between the midwife and the woman in labour and plays a disempowering role. At home, without access to cardiotocography, the midwife has to trust the woman far more:

I don't think you need to be strapped up the whole time, because then you spend the whole time staring at the monitor, watching the heart going up and down and thinking 'ohhhh'. And watching your contractions, and they say that they're a bit pathetic, not good enough – all this sort of stuff, whereas as home, the midwife couldn't tell me that my contractions were worth having or not. So without the monitors, the midwife has to trust us much more, and if I say I'm having a contraction, then I am! (Andrea)

Some of the women were pleased not to have any vaginal examinations whatsoever, which they felt allowed labour to progress very spontaneously:

She didn't do any. Even when she first arrived. That amazed me, because I thought she'd want to know how dilated I was. But because she didn't, it felt incredibly natural. (Joanna)

Andrea specifically did not want any vaginal examinations. She equated them with the midwife taking control away from her and asserting her professional power and authority over Andrea's labour. This is exactly the implicit function of vaginal examinations demonstrated in Bergstrom *et al.*'s study (1992) – a ritual to communicate the care-giver's control and the woman's corresponding passivity:

That was another thing. I didn't want any internals... I just felt that I would know. I know my body well enough now to know when it was all ready. I really wanted to trust myself. It would have been the midwife saying 'right, now it's time to push or no, you can't push'. I just wanted it to happen and be very natural. So I'm in control, I'm doing it. I mean, I know you can feel you want to start pushing before it's ready to push, but I just trusted my body to do it the right way. (Andrea)

Several multiparous women talked unbidden of how they were aware of a direct connection between them and the foetus they were carrying. They were very much conscious of how the baby was, and 'knew' that he or she was all right even though the professionals were thinking otherwise. They seemed surprised when asked to explain themselves more – to them it seemed self-evident:

She did say that I'd been fully dilated for an hour and it's policy that we tell somebody, which I immediately thought sounded a bit suspicious! There's obviously something wrong. But I didn't *feel* that there was something wrong. In my body I didn't feel anything was wrong. (Julie)

I wasn't worried about the baby at any point. I knew she was fine. When I had my second baby... I remember being on my knees and thinking, no, this is not right. The baby was not happy. It was wrong. It was just not right. At no time with this baby did I feel anything like that. When the waters broke, the midwife said 'they're lovely and clear' and I remember thinking 'that's all right, because I know she's all right'. I wasn't worried. I know if they're fine. (Cathy)

Several women quite disingenuously and intuitively suggested that there was a clear link between fear and distress – the mother being afraid and the baby becoming distressed:

Not afraid. I don't think you're allowed to be afraid. I think if you're afraid, your baby is in distress. My sister was afraid, and her baby was in distress. Because she was afraid, because she did have distress. I think the afraid comes with it. I think if I was afraid, I wouldn't be so sure of myself that the baby was all right. I would say that you being afraid helps the baby get distressed. I think they definitely go together, fear and distress. (Cathy)

This intuitive idea is identical to the findings of Levinson and Shnider (1979), who looked at the role of maternal catecholamines, maternal fear and foetal distress. They found that the raised level of catecholamines in anxious labouring women resulted in a lowered uterine blood flow, thus reducing the amount of oxygen available to the foetus. A robust foetus will be able to compensate for this drop, but a previously compromised foetus is less able to do so and will show signs of distress. But how did Rhiannon, Cathy and the others know that?

Davis (1989: 5) talks of women's intuition being the 'apprehension of reality exactly as it is'. The participants 'knew' something on an internal, subjective level that has only been recently confirmed by scientific method (and is not yet widely accepted). Belenky et al.'s (1986) work on women's ways of knowing shows how women pass through five stages of 'knowing'. The third stage (in which most of the women in their study were to be found) is a dualistic state of connecting with an inner voice that is contradicted by those on the 'outside'. The women 'knew' that maternal fear and foetal distress are connected, a notion that would be derided by many contemporary 'experts'.

The existence of intuition or 'gut feeling' is controversial. Baron (1988: 26) defines it as an 'unanalyzed and unjustified belief', yet Orme and Maggs (1993: 273) define it as 'a state of heightened perceptual aware-ness which emanates from subconscious thought'. By constant profes-sional intervention and monitoring, a woman's own intimate knowledge of her own body and the foetus within is undermined and devalued. As Gilligan (1982: 88) puts it, 'All knowledge is constructed, and the knower is an intimate part of the known.' In this instance, the 'knowers' – for example Cathy and Rhiannon – are most certainly an intimate part of that which they know, for nowhere is there a greater, more tangible exam-ple of connectedness and intimacy than between a woman and her foetus. By not even recognizing this knowledge, midwives undermine a woman's belief and confidence in her own body, which in turn makes her unable to feel in control of her labour.

Conclusion

Midwives are called the experts of normal childbirth, yet so little work has been done exploring what normal childbirth is that it is hard to know how they can deserve this accolade. This study set out intentionally to study the normal second stage of labour. The women themselves described how, in order to cope with the enormity of the sensation that they experienced during a normal second stage of labour, they entered an altered state of consciousness, in which the mind 'let go' and allowed the body to be in control. The part played by the midwife is crucial to the success or failure of this strategy. A skilled and sensitive midwife can create a unobtrusive atmosphere of safety and calm, which allows a woman to feel secure enough to 'just disconnect' mind from body. An insensitive and intrusive midwife can just as easily block a woman's being able to do this, undermine her confidence in her own body and turn her experience of giving birth into a nightmare.

Midwives are extraordinarily powerful when a woman is in labour; these findings may help them to use that power wisely to the best advantage of the women in their care. By examining the components that go towards creating a normal second stage, listening to women's stories and establishing what they find helpful and what hinders them, midwives may create and use their own body of midwifery knowledge to help more women achieve the very thing that so many of them desire – to give birth normally.

References

Anderson, T. (1997) Women's experiences of the second stage of labour, unpublished MSc dissertation, University of Surrey.

Baron, J. (1988) *Thinking and Deciding*, Cambridge: Cambridge University Press.

Beaton, J.I. (1990) Dimensions of nurse and patient roles in labour, *Health Care for Women International* 11(4): 393–408.

Beck, C.T. (1994) Women's temporal experiences during the delivery process: A phenomenological study, *International Journal of Nursing Studies* 31(3): 245–52.

Belenky, M.F., Clinchy, B.M., Goldberg, N.R. and Tarule, J.M. (1986) *Women's Ways of Knowing*, New York: Basic Books.

Berg, M., Lundgren, I., Hermansson, E. and Wahlberg, V. (1996) Women's experience of the encounter with the midwife during childbirth, *Midwifery* 12: 11–15.

Bersgtrom, L., Roberts, J., Skillman, L. and Seidel, J. (1992) 'You'll feel me touching you, sweetie': Vaginal examinations during the second stage of labour, *Birth* 19(1): 10–18.

Bluff, R. and Holloway, I. (1994) They know best: Women's perspective of midwifery care during labour and childbirth, *Midwifery* 10: 157–64.

Bradley, C., Brewin, C.R. and Duncan, S.L.B. (1983) Perceptions of labour: Discrepancies between midwives' and patients' ratings, *British Journal of Obstetrics and Gynaecology* 90: 1176–9.

Brewin, C. and Bradley, C. (1982) Perceived control and the experience of childbirth, *British Journal of Clinical Psychology* 21: 263–9.

Brook, C. (1996) Supportive interactions between midwives and childbearing women, *Birth Issues* 5(2): 15–19.

Cosmi, E.V. (1995) Hypnosis and birth, *Prenatal and Perinatal Psychology* 7(4): 461–3.

Davis, E. (1989) *Women's Intuition*, Berkeley, CA: Celestial Arts.

Driscoll, R. (1997) *Plain Tales from the Labour Ward*, London: Minerva Press.

Evans, S. and Jeffrey, J. (1995) Maternal learning needs during labor and delivery, *Journal of Obstetric, Gynecologic and Neonatal Nursing* 24(3): 235–40.

Flint, C. (1997) Using the stairs, *MIDIRS Midwifery Digest* 7(2): 186.

Gilligan, C. (1982) *In a Different Voice: Psychological Theory and Women's Development*, Boston: Harvard University Press.

Green, J.M. (1993) Expectations and experiences of pain in labour: Findings from a large prospective study, *Birth* 20(2): 65–72.

Jones, C. (1989) The laboring mind response, *Texas Midwifery* VI(2): 19–21.

Kirke, J. (1980) Mothers' views of obstetric care, *British Journal of Obstetrics and Gynaecology* 87: 1029–33.

Kirkham, M.J. and Perkins, E.R. (1997) *Reflections on Midwifery*, London: Baillière Tindall.

Levinson, G. and Shnider, S.M. (1989) Catecholamines: The effects of maternal fear and its treatment on uterine function and circulation, *Birth and the Family Journal* 6(3): 167–74.

Lukes, S. (ed.) (1986) *Power*, Oxford: Basil Blackwell.

Machin, D. and Scamell, M. (1997) The experience of labour: Using ethnography to explore the irresistable nature of the bio-medical metaphor during labour, *Midwifery* 13: 78–84.

McKay, S., Barrows, T. and Roberts, J. (1990) Women's views of second stage labor as assessed by interviews and videotapes, *Birth* 17(4): 192–8.

Nikodem, V.C. (1995) Sustained (Valsalva) vs exhalatory bearing down in the second stage of labour, in Enkin, M.W., Keirse, M.J.N.C., Renfrew, M.J. and Neilson, J.P. (eds), *Pregnancy and Childbirth Module of the Cochrane Database of Systematic Reviews, 1995* (updated 24 Feb 1995), London: BMJ Publishing Group.

Nolan, M. (1996) *Being Pregnant, Giving Birth: A National Childbirth Trust Guide*, London: HMSO.

Odent, M. (1987) The fetus ejection reflex, *Birth* 14(2): 104–5.

Odent, M.R. (1991) Fear of death during labour, *Journal of Reproduction and Infant Psychology* 9(1): 43–7.

Odent, M. (1994) The love hormones, *Primal Health Research* 2(3): 3–7.

Orme, L. and Maggs, C. (1993) Decision-making in clinical practice: How do expert nurses, midwives and health visitors make decisions? *Nurse Education Today* 13(4): 270–6.

Price, B. (1993) Women in labour: Body image, loss of control and coping behaviour, *Professional Care of Mother and Child* November–December: 280–2.

Rajan, L. (1993) Perceptions of pain and pain relief in labour: The gulf between experience and observation, *Midwifery* 9: 136–45.

Sargady, M. (1995) Renewing our faith in second stage, *Midwifery Today* 33: 29–31, 41–3.

Scientific American (1972) *Altered States of Awareness: Readings from* Scientific American, San Francisco: WH Freeman.

Simkin, P. (1989) *The Birth Partner*, Boston: Harvard Common Press.

Thomson, A.M. (1988) Management of the woman in normal second stage of labour: A review, *Midwifery* 4: 77–85.

Waldenstrom, U., Borg, I., Olsson, B., Skold, M. and Wall, S. (1996) The childbirth experience: A study of 295 new mothers, *Birth* 23(3): 144–53.

CHAPTER 8

The Midwife–Mother Relationship Where There is Poverty and Disadvantage

Anna Gaudion and Claire Homeyard

> The ideological opposition between motherhood and consumption both casts individualising blame upon and renders invisible the lived realities of many people whose life situation make it especially difficult to cherish the illusion that mothering can somehow remain free and pure of issues and commodification. (Taylor, 2004:4)

Unpacking this statement reveals the very women that the Department of Health policy (Department of Health, 2004, 2007a, 2007b) and *The Confidential Enquiry into Maternal and Child Health* (Lewis, 2007) define as hard to reach, vulnerable and marginalized. Every woman and her situation is individual, but the women who do not access and engage fully with maternity services are frequently those who are financially strained, including asylum seekers and refugees, teenagers, migrant women, routine and manual workers and women within chaotic or restricted social set-ups because of problematic addiction, mental ill-health or domestic abuse.

Even when these women do access care, a number of issues can hinder helpful provision of midwifery services, including lack of trust of professionals, language barriers and perceptions of care. This can result in unsatisfactory and discriminatory treatment by health service providers, uninformed consent, and misunderstood health advice and information (Homeyard and Gaudion, 2008).

This chapter will share the learning from five projects undertaken between 2004 and 2008 that shed some light on the everyday realities for these women. The projects include the making of a documentary film, *Florence: The Experience of Becoming a Mother in Exile* (Gaudion *et al.*,

2005); the development of an access and advocacy pack (Gaudion, 2005, 2007); a maternity services needs assessment (Gaudion and Allotey, 2008); a health equity audit of access to maternity services in SE London (Gaudion, 2008); and the work undertaken by the Polyanna Project around access and engagement (Gaudion *et al.*, 2007, 2008). The work bears witness to the perceptions of midwives working with economically disadvantaged women and in turn gives evidence and space for the women themselves to speak back.

If as professionals the imperative of partnership with women is to be more than rhetoric (Department of Health, 2004, 2007a), listening to these women's voices, although uncomfortable, provides the insight and learning to improve. Overwhelmingly during the projects women reiterated that where the midwives had some understanding of their lived experience and respected them, the relationship was positive; where they did not, the women felt shunned. Areas of importance to the women included access to services and information, the difficulty of eating a healthy diet, lack of choice in their lives, being self-conscious about appearing as 'lesser mothers' because they did not have slippers or lovely new things for the baby, but most importantly the attitude of the midwife towards them. The chapter will conclude with some markers learnt in conducting the projects about how this relationship can be crucial in influencing outcomes and empowering these women.

Exploring what is meant by 'economically without'

Every day the newspapers report that the financial crisis has affected many people, but even prior to the credit crunch the disparity in income between the rich and poor was already a gulf (Toynbee, 2004, 2008). Consumption of commodities is a means by which people seek to define themselves in the world, not just for basic needs but to achieve self-respect and social identity (Miller, 1997, 2004; Taylor, 2004). Thus, for example, brands, goods and gadgets associated with babies offer a type of public currency that is instantly recognizable (Clarke, 2004). For the women under consideration here, the question is 'what must and what can I buy?' (Taylor, 2004). Respectability, Jean Davis notes in the foreword to *Poverty, Pregnancy and the Healthcare Professional* (Hunt, 2004), is an important concept, but one that is more difficult to achieve where there is inadequate income.

In 1999 the then Prime Minister made a commitment to end child poverty. Some eight years later in 2007 the government reaffirmed this commitment, describing it as a 'goal for this generation'. However, when the three-year Comprehensive Spending Review (2008 to 2011) was published it revealed the promises to be modest: an extra £1 a week (in addition to the previously announced £3 a week) on Child Tax Credit by 2010; the national roll-out of the In-Work Credit for lone parents returning to work; an increase in the amount of child maintenance a parent can receive before starting to lose Income Support; and an increase in the benefit rates for 16 and 17 year olds to bring them into line with those for 18–24 year olds. Though welcome in themselves, these measures are nowhere near enough to create an approach commensurate with the scale of the challenge. The stereotypical image of a lone parent in poverty as a young teenage mum is unfounded, as lone parents under the age of 25 account for just one in eight of all young adults in poverty and only a fifth of all the lone parents in poverty. Most of the lone parents in poverty are aged 25 or over (Palmer *et al.*, 2007).

Approximately 40 per cent of people from ethnic minority groups live in income poverty, double that for white people. A household is defined as being in income poverty if its income is less than 60 per cent of the contemporary median household income in Great Britain. In 2004/05, this was £183 a week for lone parents with two dependent children and £268 a week for a couple with two dependent children. Almost half of all ethnic minority children live in income poverty (Kenway and Palmer, 2007).

Poverty can exclude people, it affects dignity and self-esteem and the ability people have to make choices. Not being able to afford a newspaper, a drink or a bus fare is beyond the comprehension of people who are not poor (Toynbee, 2008). The poor are the anthropological 'other'; for women and their children who are poor social exclusion is bound up with the stigma of state support:

> the support of poor women and their children tends to be decried and resented as an illegitimate use of other people's money. (Taylor, 2004: 6)

Women who have no recourse to public funds are particularly vulnerable, not just in terms of health care but in the whole remit of social provision for themselves and their children. Public funds include a range of income-related benefits together with housing and homelessness support. No recourse to these funds applies to people who are from a country that is not part of the European Economic Area; people with limited leave to enter, for example those on a work permit, student or marriage visa; people at the end of the asylum process who have not been successful in their application; migrant workers without a permit; and trafficked women.

In 2004 the journalist Polly Toynbee recorded her experience of living on a council estate and taking whatever was on offer at the job centre. This included cleaning, working as a dinner lady and work in a nursery. Living on the minimum wage, her understanding of exclusion was made apparent:

> It is a large 'No Entry' sign on every ordinary pleasure... a harsh apartheid. (Toynbee, 2004: 239)

Accessing maternity services

The most recent confidential enquiry into maternal and child health (Lewis, 2007) and the Department of Health Direction to reduce infant mortality (Department of Health, 2007b) illustrate too well that for poor and therefore disadvantaged women the outcomes for mother and baby are worse. The rate of infant death among social classes 1 to 4 is around 4 per 1000 live births, compared to 5.5 for those in social classes 5 to 8 (Palmer *et al.*, 2007).

In the white paper *Building on the Best, Choice, Responsiveness and Equity in the NHS* (Department of Health, 2003), the lived experience of negotiating health services for more vulnerable populations was recognized:

> All of us – not just some among the affluent middle classes – want the opportunity to share in decisions about our health and health care, and to make choices about that care where appropriate; we want the right information, at the right time, as well suited to our personal needs as possible... our health needs are personal, and we would like services to be shaped around our needs, instead of being expected to fit the system. (Department of Health, 2003: 7)

Project London, which operates a free clinic in East London for people who have difficulty in accessing care, is registering increasing numbers of pregnant women who have not accessed care from all over London. In 2006 there were 39 women and in 2007 a total of 118 women:

> Mrs S came to us during her 38th week, having had no prior antenatal care. She had been refused maternity access at her local GP surgery and had been informed that she would not be able to deliver at her local hospital. (Project London, 2008: 18)

more than 25% of the women were more than 18 weeks pregnant and had had no antenatal care. (Project London, 2008: 18)

Confusion over the 2004 regulations regarding entitlement to NHS care has affected access to care for some women (Kelly and Stevenson, 2006). The guidelines for entitlement to health care are under review, but the current Department of Health guidelines state that maternity care is termed as immediately necessary care and should always be given. All antenatal, birth and postnatal care should be provided irrespective of ability to pay (Department of Health, 2004).

Within maternity services, some women are expected to fit the system, but are sadly disadvantaged by attitudes and reactions from health-care professionals; other women experience individualized care, care here being the operating word.

Although class is spoken of less in British society today (Toynbee, 2008), listening to women in four of the projects highlighted that financially poor and therefore disadvantaged women describe themselves as 'other'. For many this was accompanied by loss of self-esteem, for others anger and frustration. Certainly, negotiating maternity services was difficult. Women were amazed at the notion of choice, that interpreting services could be arranged and that maternity services were interested in how they felt. Although the Department of Health champions choice (Department of Health, 2003, 2004, 2007a) and partnership working, most of the women reacted by saying that this would not apply to them:

> For people like us it is different, you help yourself or fall by the wayside, people don't give you help. I would not ring. (White woman with problematic addiction)

Unsurprisingly, one of the issues highlighted in listening to women is that encounters with health professionals, where they were told what they should do, were negatively received. Information was wanted, but so was discussion and time to make a decision. Irish travellers at a health fair noted that some of the health professionals: 'Just gave out to us and don't have a clue what it's like or what our way of life is.' Women were very receptive to being asked for their perspective:

> It is better to do the consultations than making assumptions because professionals can pressurise and tell people what they should and would need. (Advocate)

Although women recognized that it would be good to have the luxury of a consultation with a midwife early in their pregnancy and to have regular contact, the reality of their lives meant that this was not always possible. Other issues such as housing, hate crime, domestic abuse, transport and day-to-day living took priority over a pregnancy. If they had other children, lack of social relationships with people who could look after the children or collect them from school while the mother attended a hospital appointment presented difficulties. Consultations where everything was done at the same appointment were appreciated; if phlebotomy or ultrasound departments were in a different location it made it more difficult for women to accommodate them. Appointments with housing, immigration or citizens advice were more pressing, and there was a general consensus that as long as the baby was moving the pregnancy could wait.

Cost of access and engaging with services

Lacking access to those services that it is normal for most people to have is an important part of the experience of poverty and social exclusion. This dichotomy does not only exist in access to ordinary pleasures – an ice cream, a daily newspaper or a bubble bath – but to access to and engagement with health services. Households without a car are much more likely to report difficulties accessing local services than households with a car. In 2006, 20 per cent of women lived in households that did not have a car. Two-fifths of women either lacked a car in their household or did not have a driving license (Palmer *et al.*, 2007).

Many women felt that cost was a barrier to access and engagement: the cost of transport or ringing for appointments or needing to change appointments. The cost of phone calls to the midwives' number and being put on hold while listening to classical music and being put through to different people before you could eventually talk to a midwife was prohibitive and exasperating; time is money.

Midwives providing enhanced midwifery care for asylum seekers, refugees, women with problematic addiction, homeless women, women experiencing domestic abuse or poor mental health and those working with teenagers under the teenage pregnancy strategy (Department of Health, 2001, 2004, 2007a) were able to divert some of the cost of engagement to the service provider by facilitating access by text messaging, actively ringing the women, home visits and local drop-in clinics.

Midwives working within the main structure of maternity services, in the hospital and community setting, articulated frustrations at the lack of social provision for women who 'were a financial burden on the service', either because they did not attend appointments and therefore midwives had to waste time trying to follow them up or because they occupied a bed for longer than 'the norm':

Asylum seekers present a particular challenge because they have nowhere to live or clothes for the baby and they effectively block a bed which is costly and a poor use of services. (Midwife)

Bed occupancy is an issue... longer stays in hospital. In a recent case... woman with a new baby was not allowed to remain in accommodation with her baby and returned to hospital... homeless, baby admitted... cannot justify readmitting mother... irresponsible of her, we have the image of being a soft touch... there are no boundaries... people think they can just come here... I am concerned about the babies, they are vulnerable... it is just a strain on the service. (Midwife)

Ideally would like a mother and baby unit, information and a system of ongoing support, not necessarily midwifery support. Hospital does have constraints... migrants come because it is better in this country... opportunistic. (Midwife)

There is lots of abuse of the NHS... women know how to use it, if they book late it is because they want to, English people do that too. Use of ambulances just to get a couple of paracetamol, they know if you ring 999 it has to be answered... they should be charged... come to the UK with the idea that it is Utopia, may be late bookers because they have just arrived or choice, like English people and travellers. (Midwife)

In a focus group of midwives, no one challenged the following statement:

Plus they have different values... whatever Allah wills... they don't have the same concerns as us, they are more used to hardship, although I do see some precious ones... who have money and leave and have high expectations when they get here when they could have paid for private care in their own country. (Midwife)]

Unfortunately such perceptions were not lost on the women:

The word for it is rejection, no one is interested. (Woman from Irish traveller community)

She said now bath your baby and I bathed my baby and it was a test, she said there was not enough beds in the hospital and if you can bath your baby you can go home... your husband I know will not help you, no one will help you but there is no room here. In that time I was having antibiotics and medicine. (Woman from Iraq)

Communication

Communication is not just the spoken or written word but a spectrum of non-verbal information which may enhance or damage relationships, a smile or a look of anger for example. Women talked often of how 'stretched' maternity services were and how they therefore did not want to 'bother' the midwife or take up too much time:

In Poland there are less pregnant women, midwives and doctors have more time for you, here it is more busy. You feel lonely, and wonder why they do not want to talk to you but I know they are busy. (Polish woman)

The midwives are always so busy, always in a rush, very friendly but always in a rush.

Lots of midwives helped me, my care was excellent, I was in hospital before my baby was born, they were really friendly, but they showed me everything and were very helpful. (White British woman on benefits)

Communication is key in any relationship. Where, because of lack of interpreting services, some women either did not understand what was being said to them or were unable to express their particular needs and circumstances, the partnership relationship favoured by the Department of Health in the National Service Framework for Children, Young People and Maternity Services, Standard 11 (2004) and *Maternity Matters* (2007a) was severely compromised:

You have to get by with pointing and mime... sometimes you have your husband there... no one ever asked about how we were feeling or domestic violence. We have to sign if we want water or if we have pain... feel safe though, it is good care because they care about us and send an appointment. (Woman from Afghanistan)

The way they treat you and look at you sometimes is not right. Last time I went with my friend and the people, the 'nurses' just ignore you, don't ask what is your name or ask if you are OK... they took no notice at reception. They do not see it as important did not speak to [us], not even in English. Just ignored... no communication. (Chinese woman)

The value of being listened to by a midwife was expressed many times and echoed relationships of respect and trust:

After the baby was born it was so nice because the midwife came to the house and check me and the baby... midwife was nice... the midwife asked me how are you? How are you feeling? Are you happy? When I feel sad I can talk to the midwife or my friends or my daughter. (Chinese woman)

Don't see the midwife enough... I would like to see her more because it feels better after I have talked to her. (Bangladeshi woman)

I learnt from my midwife Claire how to have a baby, she was lovely, I trusted her. (Moroccan woman)

This sentiment was repeated many times in slightly different guises:

My midwife was a Sure Start midwife, she was lovely. If I am negative she makes me feel positive and that really helps, this is what should happen. (Bangladeshi woman)

My midwife made me feel comfortable, she listened to me and I felt supported and less vulnerable... you are so scared about feeling like an outcast. (White woman with problematic addiction)

Information

Access to advice and information, awareness of what to expect and what was expected, especially for women who lacked confidence and self-assurance and were not adept at negotiating services, often came through as a topic for discussion. In awe and somewhat distrustful of organizational powers, women wanted information to be available before they encountered particular services.

Where a midwife was visible and appeared friendly or was recommended by a relative or friend, for example a midwife working with young people in a children's centre, the women perceived the midwife to be:

> More like us... and you can ask her anything. (Teenager from the Caribbean)

Parent education sessions were warmly welcomed, either individually or in groups that were aimed at young people, people in language or faith groups, especially where advocates were part of the provision, as was peer support facilitated by a midwifery team, for example breastfeeding support.

The breastfeeding DVD from the Department of Health is to be given to all pregnant women, but what of the women who do not have a DVD player to watch and gain from this resource? Overheard conversation and 'statemented facts' reflect an inability by some midwives to think laterally, to distribute information within the community or to provide facilities within children's centres:

> I have been in some dreadful flats, they don't have much but they always have a huge television, its what they want to spend their money on... they always have that. (Midwife)

Reduced income, reduced choices

Awareness of the restriction that lack of money can place on choice, be it clothes, food or housing, is instrumental in the pivotal relationship between mother and midwife.

In the making of the film *Florence: The Experience of Becoming a Mother in Exile* (Gaudion, 2005), a young woman described the difficulties she had buying healthy food to eat during her pregnancy. Off camera she talked about the difficulty of shopping in a foreign country where she did not recognize the food available, the facilities she had for cooking, the cost and her inability to buy cheaper items in bulk because of having to carry them home and a lack of storage facilities. The film records her heating rice, which was all she had in the house to eat. She reports that she had been lucky, her midwife was fantastic, she cared for all of her not just her pregnancy, and she had invited her to a group where she had met other young people, learnt where to buy things locally and gained cooking tips. Her midwife, Maggie, had given her self-esteem, had always listened to her and had given her time to signpost her towards appropriate help.

In Hillingdon, young pregnant women who had arrived in the UK as unaccompanied asylum-seeking children (UASC) were accommodated in housing away from good shopping facilities or markets and were therefore forced to purchase food from more expensive local stores. Many of the teenagers were originally from China and shared that they lived mainly on a diet of 'takeaway rice'. This food, they argued (through an interpreter), could be obtained without having to say very much. Their accommodation facilities often included a microwave but no cooker:

> it is not possible to stir fry food in a microwave. (Young Chinese woman)

Everyday kindness and respect collectively meant much to the women. Midwives who were interviewed talked of ransacking bounty bags, bringing in the second bottle of conditioner or soap from home when there had been a special offer of 'buy one get one free' and setting up systems for women who were 'without' to collect used baby clothes and equipment from the hospital or children's centre. There was evidence that kindness of this sort built relationships between the women and professionals:

> I was [in London] with the first child until I was 5 months then I was moved to [Scotland] my blue book stayed in [Scotland]... just temporary, I was not there for a long time and then I moved back to London. It was difficult moving whilst I was pregnant but [the hospital in Scotland] very nice hospital, very nice team. I have no idea about hospitals in the UK but they gave me confidence, they were very nice to me, they gave me clothes for the baby and sheets and nappies and soap and shampoo, they were very kind as I had nothing. (Woman from Iraq)

Poverty undoubtedly restricts choices, even about where you live. Asylum seekers are moved, dispersed within the National Asylum model; people fleeing domestic abuse may 'camp' on friends' floors for periods of time and then move on; the homeless live in temporary shelters and at temporary addresses, often for only a couple of nights at a time, and do not develop support and friendship structures or know about local organizations that could help them:

> I have just one room, there are five rooms here, all different people... all similar situations, shared kitchen. When I was 7–8 months pregnant they moved me here... they don't move you till the end... I need more

support. Money is the biggest worry and I do not know the other girls, one did not clean up after herself. (Chinese teenager with a 10-month-old baby and pregnant)

The ward scared the hell out of me, I did not know what I was supposed to do... I didn't have the right stuff, you know, pretty dressing gown, slippers. (Black British woman with problematic addiction)

Negative encounters

During the course of the projects women were often cautious about what they said, later saying that they feared that if they spoke out women like them would have an even worse time. What mattered most to them was to be cared for by someone kind. They talked to each other, often telling negative stories about their maternity experience. Such stories spread through social capital could have the adverse effect of putting other women off accessing maternity care. They talked of attitudes that excluded them:

The midwife was really nice, but some of them are useless, they just ignore you. (Woman from Egypt)

I put it off, going I mean till I was 8 months gone, it was their attitude, therefore I put it off... it makes you afraid... they did not want to know... I mean the organic women, you know those ladies with partners and flowers and a bag packed, they get treated differently, they get asked not told. (Woman with problematic addiction)

Every mother is supposed to be equal and needs care because every child is supposed to matter and be equal, but some matter less. (Eritrean woman)

The other one when she said go to your own country, I felt really bad but she surely has to do her job, I felt so helpless, I wished I was not pregnant so that I would not have met such a person. (Woman from Afganistan)

Some midwives treat you differently, you need to be warned that this might happen... not everyone is nice. (Somali woman)

I think their attitude should be a higher standard. When I see the kind woman I think of her as my mum and it is nice, when I see the other one who was cruel I feel suicidal, I want to die, some people think we are not human beings because we come from another country and that we know nothing... it is very important we need interpreters and some people just do not care. (Woman from Afganistan)

It is not just prejudice against Black and Asians it is white people too, but the poor ones. (Somali woman)

If women living in poverty perceive that midwives do not have a good understanding of the context of their lives, then they are less likely to act on health advice and more likely to perceive the interaction as negative.

Enhancing relationships, the midwife's role and conclusion

Midwives can feel overwhelmed when confronted by the many issues related to poverty and disadvantage in pregnancy. For many of these women, the liminality of their lives results in a complex variety of interconnected issues and concerns. Part of the midwife's role is to try to minimize the impact of poverty.

In researching her book *Hard Work*, Toynbee (2004) spent a few months living in social housing on minimum wage, but she admits that she went home occasionally and had meals with family and friends. The midwife too enters for short periods the estates of the poor, bears witness to chaotic lives ruled by drug or alcohol addiction or mental health, but leaves and goes home paid on a Band 6 or 7 salary. The women living these lives are the unrecognized experts in the reality of living in poverty. Most importantly, recognizing and respecting this helps:

Communities are wise, if you give us a choice and include and embrace our voices, allow us to bring forward our experiences and visions, we can become doorways rather than divisions. (Woman from Uganda)

People just make assumptions about us. We get worse care than the white British. Need to involve the community to change strategy... not always leave us as the outsiders... we are not illiterate, we are not given an opportunity to be involved... it is about recognition and respect. (Somali advocate)

It is essential to begin with the woman's view of the world, not the professionals':

> As part of the booking process, a midwife should carry out an early needs assessment on the expectant mother, with the resulting needs profile informing their subsequent antenatal care. Women with high medical needs, for example, would need additional obstetric antenatal care. Women with high social needs (for example women with mental health problems or misusing alcohol or other substances) would need active help to engage them with relevant services and co-ordinate care across multiple agencies. (Darzi, 2007: 45)

Although some of the midwives interviewed had excellent creative partnerships in outreach services and within children's centres, the central issue of support was a common one. Midwives expressed feeling alone and overburdened, often coined the 'emotional labour' of midwifery. What was missing was the central element of true partnership working, of engaging with other services to provide for individual need; it is not about the midwife 'doing it all' or being all things to all people. Listening to women talk about being asked about domestic abuse routinely in the antenatal period was welcome; what was also liked was the fact that this also involved being given a helpline number. Midwives can be signposters, supporters and facilitators of choice. Working in this way enhances the relationship; it admits that the midwife does not have to be expert or knowledgeable about everything. The needs, risk and choice assessment is about finding out what the woman's individual needs are and working with her to make a holistic plan.

A prerequisite for providing care in partnership with a woman is to avoid stereotyping, to listen to the woman and to gain an understanding of her individual needs. In the Equity Audit conducted in Southeast London, a large percentage of the maternity population lived in areas of deprivation (Gaudion, 2008). Policy direction recommends enhanced care for these women, but they represent a majority, therefore it is up to each individual midwife to listen, signpost to sources of support and above all respect these women. Negative attitudes are brick walls to reducing inequity and inequality. Senior midwives, supervisors' of midwives and lecturers have an important task in acting as role models in their attitude, not just in the clinical area but in the changing rooms and coffee areas of their workplaces. The Midwives Rules (2004) and Code (2008) make it clear what the midwife's duty is and professionally make everyone responsible.

References

Clarke, A.J. (2004) Maternity and materiality: Becoming a mother in consumer culture in Taylor, J.S., Layne, L.L. and Wozniak, D.F. (eds), *Consuming Motherhood*, New Brunswick, NJ: University Press. .

Darzi, A. (2007) *A Framework for Action*, London: Healthcare for London, www.healthcareforlondon.nhs.uk, accessed March 2010.

Department of Health (2001) *Better Prevention, Better Services and Better Sexual Health: The National Strategy for Sexual Health*, London: Department of Health, www.dh.gov.uk/en/Publicationsandstatistics/Publications/PublicationsPolicyAndGuidance/DH_4003133, accessed March 2010.

Department of Health (2003) *Building on the Best: Choice, Responsiveness and Equity in the NHS*, London: HMSO.

Department of Health (2004) *National Service Framework for Children, Young People and Maternity Services, Standard 11*, London: HMSO.

Department of Health (2007a) *Maternity Matters: Choice, Access and Continuity of Care in a Safe Service*, HMSO: London.

Department of Health (2007b) *Review of the Health Inequalities Infant Mortality PSA Targets*, London: HMSO.

Gaudion, A. (2006) *The Reaching Out Project: Report on the Preliminary Consultations, May–July 2005*, www.medact.org/content/reaching_out/report%20preliminary%20consultations.doc, accessed March 2010.

Gaudion, A. (2007) *The Development of the Maternity Access and Advocacy Pack (MAAP)*, London: The Polyanna Project, www.thepolyannaproject.org.uk/what-we-do.html, accessed March 2010.

Gaudion, A. (2008) *Health Equity Audit of Access to Maternity Services in SE London: Maternity Matters Early Adopter Site Report*, London: Guys and St Thomas' NHS Hospitals Trust and Kings College Hospital Trust (internal report).

Gaudion, A. and Allotey, P. (2008) *Maternity Care for Refugees and Asylum Seekers in Hillingdon: A Needs Assessment*, Uxbridge: Centre for Public Health Research, Brunel University (internal report).

Gaudion, A., Homeyard, C., Murshali, H. and Field, V. (2005) The experience of becoming a mother in exile, *RCM Midwives* 8(9): 387–9.

Gaudion, A., Godfrey, C., Homeyard, C. and Cutts, H. (2007) *The Hackney Women's Wheel Visual Diary*, London: The Polyanna Project, www.thepolyannaproject.org.uk/resources/wheel_visual_diary.pdf, accessed March 2010.

Gaudion, A., Godfrey, C., Homeyard, C. and Cutts, H. (2008) *The Barking and Dagenham Women's Wheel Visual Diary*, London: The Polyanna Project.

Homeyard, C. and Gaudion, A. (2008) Safety in maternity services: Women's perspectives, *The Practicing Midwife* 11(7): 20–23.

Hunt, S.C. (2004) *Poverty, Pregnancy and the Healthcare Professional*, London: Books for Midwives.

Kelly, N. and Stevenson, J. (2006) *First Do No Harm: Denying Healthcare to People Whose Asylum Claims Have Failed*, London: London Refugee Council.

Kenway, P. and Palmer, G. (2007) *Poverty among Ethnic Groups: How and Why Does It Differ?* London: New Policy Institute, Joseph Rowntree Foundation.

Lewis, G. (ed.) (2007) *The Confidential Enquiry into Maternal and Child Health (CEMACH). Saving Mothers' Lives: Reviewing Maternal Deaths to Make Motherhood*

Safer 2003–2005. The Seventh Report on Confidential Enquiries into Maternal Deaths in the United Kingdom, London: CEMACH.

Miller, D. (1997) *Capitalism: An Ethnographic Approach*, Oxford: Berg.

Miller, D. (2004) How infants grow mothers in North London, in Taylor, J.S., Layne, L.L. and Wozniak, D.F. (eds), *Consuming Motherhood*, New Brunswick, NJ: Rutgers University Press.

Nursing and Midwifery Council (2004) *Midwives' Rules and Standards*, London: NMC, www.nmc-uk.org.

Nursing and Midwifery Council (2008) *The Code: Standards of Conduct, Performance and Ethics for Nurses and Midwives*, London: NMC, www.nmc-uk.org.

Palmer, G. MacInnes, T. and Kenway, P. (2007) *Monitoring Poverty and Social Exclusion*, London: New Policy Institute, Joseph Rowntree Foundation.

Project London (2008) *Report and Recommendations: Improving Access to Healthcare for the Communities most Vulnerable*, London: Project London, www.medecinsdumonde.org.uk/doclib/155511-plartwork.pdf, accessed March 2010.

Taylor, J.S. (2004) Introduction in Taylor, J.S., Layne, L.L. and Wizniak, D.F. (eds), *Consuming Motherhood*, New Brunswick, NJ: Rutgers University Press.

Taylor, J.S., Layne, L.L. and Wozniak, D.F. (2004) *Consuming Motherhood*, New Brunswick, NJ: Rutgers University Press.

Toynbee, P. (2004) *Hard Work, Life in Low-Pay Britain*, London: Bloomsbury.

Toynbee, P. and Walker, D. (2008) *Unjust Rewards*, London: Granta.

CHAPTER 9

Pakistani Muslim Women– Midwives Relationships: What are the Essential Attributes?

KULDIP BHARJ AND MARGARET CHESNEY

To be 'with woman' is more than giving physical and technical care. It involves providing social, emotional and psychological support for women and their families. There are a number of concepts which enable midwives to be 'with women', for example giving women information, enabling them to participate in the planning and delivering of care, facilitating women to have control over the care they receive, believing women, listening to women and developing trusting relationships with them.

This chapter sets out to highlight the attributes that contribute to development of a meaningful relationship between Pakistani Muslim women and midwives. It draws on data from an interpretive ethnographic study conducted in the north of England to examine Pakistani Muslim women's experiences of labour and maternity services (Bharj, 2007) as well as from an empirical study that examined the experiences of women who had given birth to their babies in Pakistan (Chesney, 2004).

Pakistani women in Kuldip Bharj's study (2007) perceived the 'woman and midwife' relationship to be central to their childbirth experiences and described the impact this had on their encounters. Similar findings are echoed in a number of worldwide studies drawing attention to the woman–midwife relationship (Anderson, 2000; Berg *et al.*, 1996; Davies, 2000; Edwards, 2005; Halldorsdottir and Karsldottir, 1996; Kirkham, 2000; Lundgren and Berg, 2007; McCrea and Crute, 1991; Walsh, 1999). This evidence highlights that midwives play an essential role in the life of women during their most significant period: they are the orchestrators of their labours, having the power either to augment or ti mar women's experiences of childbirth.

Pakistani women's narratives (Bharj, 2007) provided insights into the midwives' attitudes and behaviours that were instrumental in shaping relationships between them and the midwives. The majority of women in this study asserted that they were unable to develop deep and meaningful relationships with their midwives during labour, indentifying ingredients of interpersonal interactions which either assisted or hindered the development of their relationships with their midwives and other healthcare professionals. For many women the quality of their relationship with their midwife affected their childbirth experiences, positively and negatively. The data from the midwives in Kuldip Bharj's (2007) and Margret Chesney's (2004) studies provide an insight into the challenges of communicating with Pakistani women who are not fluent in English.

Relationship development: Facilitators and hindrances

Pakistani women in Kuldip Bharj's study (2007) gave insights into their *emic* worldview of their relationships with midwives. They spoke of their relationship with the midwives being either close or distant, including characteristics of the midwives that shaped these relationships. They cited dimensions of the midwives that they most valued, attaching worth to the interpersonal interactions. Women in this study readily identified the attributes of the midwives that had an impact on their childbirth experience, categorizing midwives as either 'good' or 'bad'. The women contested that 'good' midwives treated them with respect: they were approachable, understanding and supportive, findings that concur with other studies (Churchill and Benbow, 2000; Fleming, 1998; Holroyd *et al.*, 1997; Oakley *et al.*, 1996; Walker *et al.*, 1995). These midwives were able to form a rapport and engaged in 'ordinary' conversation; women felt the relationship was of a social nature – 'they [midwife] were more of a friend' (Maheera, 19-year-old woman) as opposed to a 'professional' (Farzana, 20-year-old woman). Non-verbal and verbal aspects of social interaction were seen as helpful, as one 21-year-old woman asserted:

The way they [midwives] spoke to me, the way they explained... and very warm and welcoming and you know they would say we are here anytime you want us. Making you feel that you are safe, and don't be afraid of asking of anything you want. Just giving this feeling to the patient is just very helpful for a patient and I guess they did a good job of that and I guess that made me feel more at home. (Eiliyah)

Attributes of good midwives that were important to Pakistani women have been echoed by many other worldwide studies, for example Berg *et al.* (1996); Halldorsdottir and Karsldottir (1996); Kennedy (1995); Kirkham (1989); McCrea *et al.* (1998). In a recent integrative review, Nicholls and Webb (2006) affirmed that attributes of a good midwife important to all childbearing women were those within the affective domain; that is, midwives who are friendly, kind, smiling, caring, approachable, non-judgemental, have time for the women, are respectful, good communicators, provide support and companionship.

Some of the negative attributes of the midwives, cited in Nicholls and Webb's (2006) review, are those of being unhelpful, insensitive, abrupt, officious, not listening and lack of concern. Similarly, Pakistani women in Bharj's study labelled some midwives as 'bad' because they were 'ignorant' (Ghazala, 21-year-old woman), 'not responsive' and 'rude' (Khatiza, 22-year-old woman). Some women professed that some midwives were 'ignorant' (Bilqis, 25-year-old woman), lacking knowledge of the women's needs. 'Bad' midwives, they asserted, failed to respond to women's support needs and they behaved disrespectfully. For example, Khatiza stated:

> Not speaking nicely and being ignorant. You know, when you call for them [midwives], they take time coming. Fair enough, there are plenty of patients there, but there are plenty of staff there, at the same time. And when they do come, they look at you and speak to you in the way, as if to say why are you calling me again, sort of thing. You know they just don't want to know and they just don't want to help. (Khatiza)

Those midwives who did not engage in conversation were perceived as uninterested. Women who had negative encounters with the midwives did not feel part of the birthing process. They felt 'undermined, marginalised, and angry' (Ghazala) and 'less confident' (Bilqis). Whilst these midwives provided physical care, the women did not get to know them. These findings concurred with those of other studies (Anderson, 2000). The Pakistani women were able to compare the differences between their relationships with different midwives, particularly when they had been cared for by more than one midwife:

> She [midwife on night-duty] was okay, I was a bit scared to talk to her because she was answering and then full stop and not explaining things... They [midwife and the student midwife on day duty] were bubbly and nicer than the other lady [midwife on night duty]. They

just come in [delivery room] and talk to you. You asked her [midwife on night duty] a question, she would just answer and walk back out again. It was just... She was not friendly and nice... They [midwife and the student midwife on day duty] make you feel at home and stuff. The first lady was not like that, she was not horrible or anything, but she wasn't nice either. But the other ladies you could tell as soon as they came, they smiled at me, they were asking me how I am, joking about with me, being lovely and that was the difference, totally different, I could tell straight away. (Farzana)

Pakistani women in this study developed a typology of the midwives as being either 'good' or 'bad', and identified the characteristics that underpinned the way in which they reached such decisions. Similarly, in other studies women have described midwives as 'caring and empowering' as opposed to 'uncaring and discouraging' (Halldorsdottir and Karsldottir, 1996) or 'warm professional' versus 'cold professional' (McCrea *et al.*, 1998). Those midwives who displayed the attributes of kindness, connection, companionship and a good relationship were typed as caring midwives and those who were unsupportive, operated within rules and routines and were cold and harsh were seen as uncaring (Halldorsdottir and Karsldottir, 1996). Similarly, women in McCrea *et al.*'s study (1998) indentified attributes of a warm professional as being friendly, treating women respectfully and valuing women, whereas the cold professionals were emotionally distant and lacked empathy, understanding and compassion.

Literature of women's accounts and personal experience confirms that midwives develop relationships with the women which extend from being good to that of a therapeutic benefit (Anderson, 2000; Berg *et al.*, 1996; Davies, 2000; Halldorsdottir and Karsldottir, 1996; Kirkham, 2000; McCrea and Crute, 1991). Although this is the case in the majority of instances, there are some situations where the relationships between the midwives and the women are not therapeutic and are not good. Good relationships between women and midwives are defined as those which 'do not involve open conflict or bad feelings and indeed often involve co-operation' (McCrea and Crute, 1991: 184). However, in many cases relationships between women and midwives go beyond this level, becoming emotionally involved to develop a therapeutic relationship encompassing 'authenticity of being', 'conscience', 'commitment', 'presence', 'compassion', 'empathy' and 'empowerment' (Siddiqui, 1999: 111–13). That said, every woman's relationship with her midwife differs from that of a professional or a friend. Midwives assert that when they are unable to form an emotional relationship with a woman then they develop a professional relationship, where 'they would simply do what was necessary physically, but would not become emotionally involved' (McCrea and Crute, 1991: 188).

Quality of relationship: Midwives' ways of working

The findings of Bharj's study suggest that the quality of Pakistani women's relationships with their midwives is intertwined with the quality of midwives' interaction and communication and the impact of these on women's experiences of maternity services. In addition, evidence highlights that Pakistani women, among other minority ethnic communities, have poor clinical outcomes in circumstances where they are unable to engage with maternity services and where communication is of poor quality (Lewis, 2004, 2007). Therefore good relationships are fundamental to enhancing women's experiences as well as to clinical safety.

The Pakistani women (Bharj, 2007) had varied experiences of childbirth, some 'good' and some 'less good', but all their reflections were insightful. Similar findings have been echoed by other studies where it is reported that women have either profoundly good or profoundly poor experiences (Hirst and Hewison, 2002; Hirst et al., 2002). Evidence suggested that Pakistani Muslim women's birth experiences were influenced by the quality of the relationship they had with their midwives. Those women who did describe their relationship with their midwives as not being 'good' did, however, value and appreciate the care they received from them:

> In hospital... It was brilliant. It was really good. It was all new to me and I couldn't believe all the things they [midwives] did – running around, cleaning you up – that was new to me as well. They were brilliant and they [midwives] are doing an excellent job... It was really good yeah. They were brilliant. Yeah. (Inayat, 20-year-old woman)

The variation in the way midwives are perceived to operate is of interest and a number of possible explanations are provided. Some commentators have argued that midwives provide maternity care to meet the needs of the obstetricians and not the women (Oakley, 1984) and others claim that midwives maintain the 'status quo' by toeing the line and not upsetting the routines of clinical settings (Niven, 1994). There is another suggestion, that 'professionalization' which is accompanied by increased authority leads to a greater distance between the care-giver and the service user (Isherwood, 1992). It is possible, therefore, that with the constraints of professionalization, hierarchy and the current NHS culture, the midwives' encounters with the women are brief and midwives may appear to be aloof (Davies, 1995,1996), such that the midwives are unable to develop relationships with women in a meaningful manner and fail to be 'with women' (Isherwood, 1992: 14) or may be 'absently present' (Berg *et al.*, 1996). Or it may be that because they have to 'juggle priorities' (Kirkham and Stapleton, 2001), midwives develop coping strategies to manage their occupational stress by minimizing the development of relationships and saving time by 'mass-processing' (Lipsky, 1980).

Pakistani Muslim women are possibly another source of stress for the midwives. Having to meet informational needs and communicate with women who are not proficient in English requires more time, placing extra demands on the midwives. Midwives are possibly pressurized into 'doing it to the women' and 'getting the job done' rather than 'being with the women' and meeting their needs. Midwives therefore employ coping strategies of looking 'busy', employing 'routines and rituals' and becoming 'task-oriented', which all lead to controlling women and reducing direct contact with them (Menzies, 1970). It is possible that when midwives have to prioritize all the demands placed on them, the needs of those in a more powerful position take precedence over those in a lower hierarchical position. Thus the individual needs of women do not remain central to care provision (Kirkham and Stapleton, 2001). It is therefore likely that, having to work within the culture of managing competing demands, compounded by current recruitment and retention issues, the midwives may have little time to spend attending to the women's needs.

'Bad care days'

The operating environment where midwives have little time to address or meet the needs of Pakistani women who are not fluent in English and the development of strategies to get the job done bring me, Margaret Chesney, to reflect on a time in my midwifery career in the late 1980s, when I worked as a community midwife in a wholly Pakistani practice in Rochdale (Chesney, 2004).

In what I glibly described as 'bad care days', I vividly remember that during my working week Tuesday was the 'clinic day' and it was just impossible to give the women the time they deserved. The antenatal care began at 1 p.m. and finished around 6 p.m. As I had to assist at another clinic at 9 a.m., there was precious little time to fit in eight or so home visits. At this time the concept of selective visiting had not been born, so twice daily for the first three days and daily until the baby was ten days old was the requirement.

My strategy for Tuesdays was first to pray on the doorstep of a woman's house that there would be no problems. If it was a visit for a colleague's non-Pakistani practice, I would hope that the woman would not be in; although I did not stoop to knocking lightly, I was relieved when there was no answer. On the other hand, the Pakistani women would always be in. I would breeze in chirpy and cheerful, with the pidgin 'OK thiak hai', 'no problems' an effective blocker for any problem. The obligatory top-to-toe examination of mother and baby was conducted using *my* agenda, at a speed that I hoped the woman would not judge as rushed. If I had a student this was wonderful, as both 'top to toes' could be conducted simultaneously. If there was a problem that I had 'looked through' on arrival or that arose during my swift record keeping, I would move into super-efficient mode and deal with it quickly, with little thought.

On reflection, I was using what Foucault (1980) describes as the 'professional gaze'. According to the time available, I would use the 'gaze' to enable or disable the women. As the women were always pleased to see me, I used to kid myself that I did not need an interpreter; when my conscience told me otherwise, I would rationalize that it was the way the women wanted it. The women, however, knew no different. They did not have an expectation of me being able to understand. Speed certainly does not allow for true listening or for the assessment and provision of vital psychosocial care. On further reflection, I had nothing to listen to, because I could not understand. On non-clinic days, I tried to make up for the shortfall in care. This must have been very confusing for the women, as I probed and actively 'listened' to their body language one day and was professionally distant the next.

Interpreters: A three-way relationship

In the four years I spent working in this practice I had developed a 'patter' of pidgin Punjabi, and talked with my hands, face and body. This was developed entirely on a trial-and-error basis: if it served *my* purpose it was reinforced, and if not I tried a different approach or often just gave up. The effectiveness of this one-sided communication was based entirely on my getting the answers I wanted. It is only in retrospect and with embarrassment that I recognize this and other strategies I employed on busy days and always on Tuesdays, with women who did not know the words to tell me how they felt.

Although we had the good fortune to have an interpreter on staff in the hospital and in the clinic, there was no regular availability during home visits. On rare occasions I would arrange for a 'volunteer' on-call interpreter to meet me at the woman's home. This was not always successful: if the interpreter was a stranger she may not have beeen trusted or, worse, she may have been known to the women, who would be afraid of her gossiping.

The role of the interpreter, in most codes of ethics, upholds neutrality as a key component (Kaufert and Putsch, 1997). Whether neutrality is a realistic expectation for interpreters is debated by Soloman (1997). However, the interpreters I have worked with have not shown any degree of neutrality. One particular story, told to me by a Pakistani student midwife, involved an interpreter telling a woman to 'have the baby taken away as it would only be a burden on her family' and that she 'could always have another baby'. One of my first experiences of working with an interpreter (for details see Chesney, 2000) highlighted that without appropriate insights some interpreters treated the women as objects (to gain respect) and adopted an authoritarian approach to communicating with women. On challenging such behaviour the interpreters became withdrawn and unhelpful. Their power in the triad relationship showed itself clearly as they failed to facilitate communication between me and the women.

I also have direct experience of teaching a group of interpreters 'woman centredness', in a bid to get them to sit with the women in the waiting room and come through the clinic with them. Sad to say this did not happen: the interpreters wanted to be 'with' the doctors and midwives servicing the rooms at the clinic. The role of sitting with the women was, they said, a 'relative's place'. It is perhaps understandable that some of the interpreters identified with the higher status of the health-care professionals. This further emphasizes the disparate elements of class. The major issue that sets interpreters, midwives and doctors apart is education, which ultimately accords all of them occupational access to the health system; a freedom denied to most Asian women generally (Hayes, 1995). There is also the ever-present possibility that there may not be a linguistic equivalent for the interpreter to use, which presents a dilemma. This is especially important if it is superimposed on a total lack of understanding of the true meaning in one language. Tests for screening fall into this category.

Freidson, as far back as 1985, focused on issues of power and dominance in clinical communication. Although he was referring to health-care providers and clients rather then interpreters and professionals, the principles apply. There is much value to be gained from morally sensitive people in a particular situation, bridging the cultural gap. It should be remembered, however, that the right to the moral high ground must always remain in question, especially cross-culturally.

Policies that restrict the role of the interpreter and emphasize cultural neutrality and invisibility may ignore the other important dimension that should be brought to the role of interpreter, that of broker or mediator. There are many important issues that surface when the interpreter takes on this role, not least the ethical dimension.

In my naïveté and ignorance, I believed and trusted that interpreters would interpret my words verbatim. However, this did not appear to be the case; interpretation is a complex process which involves more than word-for-word translation. It requires decoding of linguistic codes where each language has its own rules and the time this involves is further complicated by the three-way relationship. The interpreters interviewed in Kuldip Bharj's study (2007) asserted that interpretation 'is not about translating word for word, in some cases it is not possible to just translate words because there are no words in Urdu for an English word' (Shabana, interpreter). To ensure that the women fully understand the message and the progress of their pregnancy or labour, the interpreters sometimes had to explain the context so that the women understood all the necessary information when making decisions about consent, care and treatment. This point is echoed by Kaufert and Putsch (1997), who state that interpreters often need to extend or adapt the message so that it is understandable in a different language or culture. This is frequently conducted in a mediating way to prevent conflict or to protect both parties. Managing the information to the benefit of both parties involves what Schott and Henley (1996) identify as cultural brokerage. However, there is suspicion (from either the giver or receiver) around cultural adaptation (Bharj, 2007). The interpreter as the carrier of the message may suspect that direct translation is inappropriate, or the owner of the message may suspect the interpreter of altering the meaning of the message. Nevertheless, many interpreters in Kuldip's study found that many midwives and doctors were uncomfortable with the process of interpretation. In particular, it was in those circumstances where the health-care professional had asked a question and the interpreters had to enter into a dialogue with the women, explaining the issue in detail, that the health-care professionals were casting doubts on the interaction and appeared to be mistrusting of them.

Acknowledging that straight verbatim interpretation might not get the message across, however, Kaufert and Putsch (1997) found that some interpreters possibly introduced a bias into the message. It was only after I had worked with different interpreters and had myself studied Punjabi and the Islamic culture that I saw the truth in this: straight verbatim interpretation is not possible when there are no parallel words in both languages. However, neither the interpreters nor I had received any training for this part of our role, and I often asked why it took many more words to effect translation.

Notwithstanding the above, trust is needed on both sides. The interpreter, who has usually worked and lived in both cultures, with a working knowledge of the topic and hopefully possessing skills as a communicator, may be the best person the make a judgement on how the information is best managed. There are also other factors to be considered: the interpreter's standing in the community, personality, gender, religion, dress and attitude all have the potential to make or break the vital link to effective communication.

The literature emphasizes language and cultures as 'barriers'. Kaufert and Koolage (1984) found that interpreters or bilingual health workers were usually represented by ancillary members of the health-care team. Thus despite the importance of the interpreter's role, the power structure, the culture of the health service and the low status and pay of the interpreter can easily lead to marginalization.

While acknowledging the contribution that interpreters make to enhance communication with women whose competence in speaking English is low, some midwives expressed concern about the quality and standard of interpretation by the interpreters (Bharj, 2007). Midwives in that study were concerned about the accuracy of the content and not knowing what was communicated. Although they were unable to confirm this, they based these assumptions on the non-verbal cues, body language and lengthy communication between the woman and the interpreter that preceded only short feedback. Other studies have reported similar concerns among health-care professionals (Gerrish, 2001; Pharoah, 1995). Another explanation may be that when using interpreting services, the midwives do not remain in 'control' of the communication and feel 'alienated' and 'marginalized', leading midwives to mistrust the communication process (Chesney, 2000). Clearly, in three-way communication the midwives are not holding the same power base as in two-way communication with the women. It is likely that most midwives prefer 'word-for-word' translations and do not focus on the content of the consultation. However, word-for-word translation is difficult and sometimes unachievable because of linguistic differences.

Conclusion

Midwives are central to women's experiences of childbirth. Evidence from Kuldip Bharj and Margaret Chesney's studies suggest that women's birth experiences are grounded in the relationships that they developed with their midwives. These relationships were built on respect, and women's voices corroborated that it was the midwives, together with their qualities and behaviours, their continuing concern, the manner in which they cared and their respect for the women, that were the underpinning ingredients to how the women viewed their birth experiences. There is a growing body of knowledge highlighting attributes of midwives which facilitate positive relationships between them and the women, in particular Pakistani Muslim women. A positive relationship facilitates a safe environment where women are able to engage with midwives in determining their care as well as have a positive experience of maternity services.

However, caring for women who are not fluent in speaking English creates a challenge in delivering responsive care. Communication and linguistic issues are major factors which either facilitate or hinder the provision of effective services. Midwives acknowledge that it is difficult to communicate information and develop relationships with the Pakistani women, especially those who are not proficient in English. Whilst interpreting services are available to overcome communication and linguistic challenges, these services are not always accessible and in many circumstances neither the midwives nor the interpreters are trained in managing the process of interpretation. Furthermore, the business of three-way communication is a highly skilled process and both the midwives and the interpreters need education and training in developing that competence. Such skills need to be taught; until excellent role models are widely available, they cannot simply be left to be caught.

So that midwives can be 'with' the women, serious consideration needs to be given to the development of midwives' attributes within the affective domain. It is these that women, in particular Pakistani Muslim women, appreciate and value.

References

Anderson, T. (2000) Feeling safe enough to let go: The relationship between a woman and her midwife during the second stage of labour, in Kirkham, M. (ed.), *The Midwife–Mother Relationship*, London: Macmillian.

Berg, M., Lundgren, I., Hermansson, E. and Wahlberg, V. (1996) Women's experience of the encounter with the midwife during childbirth, *Midwifery*, 12(1): 11–15.

Bharj, K.K. (2007) Pakistani Muslim women birthing in northern England: Exploration of experiences and context, unpublished thesis, Sheffield Hallam University.

Chesney, M. (2000) A three-way relationship, in Kirkham, M. (ed.), *The Midwife–Mother Relationship*, Basingstoke: Macmillan.

Chesney, M. (2004) Birth for some women in Pakistan: Defining and defiling, unpublished PhD thesis, University of Sheffield

Churchill, H. and Benbow, A. (2000) Informed choice in maternity services, *British Journal of Midwifery*, 8(1): 41–7.

Davies, C. (1995) *Gender and the Professional Predicament in Nursing*, Buckingham: Open University Press.

Davies, C. (1996) Cloaked in a tattered illusion, *Nursing Times*, November 6, 92(45): 44–6.

Davies, J. (2000) Being with women who are economically without, in Kirkham, M. (ed.), *The Midwife–Mother Relationship*, London: Macmillan.

Edwards, N. (2005) *Birthing Autonomy: Women's Experiences of Planning Home Births*, London: Routledge.

Fleming, V.E.M. (1998) Women-with-midwives-with-women: A model of interdependence, *Midwifery* 14(3): 137–43.

Foucault, M. (1980) *Power/Knowledge: Selected Interviews and Other Writings 1972–1977*, New York: Pantheon.

Freidson, S.E.T. (1985) Approaches to the measurement of explanation and information giving in medical consultations: A review of empirical studies, *Social Sciences and Medicine* 18: 571–80.

Gerrish, K. (2001) The nature and effect of communication difficulties arising from interactions between district nurses and South Asian patients and their carers, *Journal of Advanced Nursing* 33(5): 566–74.

Halldorsdottir, S. and Karsldottir, S.I. (1996) Journeying through labour and delivery: Perceptions of women who have given birth, *Midwifery* 12(2): 48–61.

Hayes, L. (1995) Unequal access to midwifery care: A continuing problem, *Journal of Advanced Nursing* 21: 702–9.

Hirst, J., Green, J., Khan, M., Ashrafi, K. and Mortimer, J. (2002) *The Evaluation of a Postnatal Listening Service for Pakistani, Bangladeshi and Chinese women*, Leeds: Mother and Infant Research Unit, University of Leeds.

Hirst, J. and Hewison, J. (2002) Hospital postnatal care: Obtaining the views of Pakistani and indigenous 'white' women, *Clinical Effectiveness in Nursing* 6(1): 10–18.

Holroyd, E., Yin-king, L., Pui-yuk, L.W., Kwok-hong, F.Y. and Shuk-lin, B.L. (1997) Hong Kong Chinese women's perception of support from midwives during labour, *Midwifery* 13(2): 66–72.

Isherwood, K.M. (1992) Are British midwives 'with women'? The evidence, *A.R.M. Midwifery Matters* 54(Autumn): 14–17.

Kaufert, J.M. and Koolage, W.W. (1984) Role conflict among culture brokers: The experience of native Canadian medical interpreters, *Social Sciences and Medicine* 18: 3283–6.

Kaufert, J.M. and Putsch, R.W. (1997) Communication through interpreters in health-care: Ethical dilemmas arising from differences in class, culture, language and power, *Journal of Clinical Ethics* 8(1): 71–87.

Kennedy, H.P. (1995) The essence of nurse-midwifery care: The woman's story, *Journal of Nurse-Midwifery* 40: 410–17.

Kirkham, M. (1989) Midwives and information-giving during labour, in Robinson, S. and Thompson, A.M. (eds) (1989) *Midwives, Research and Childbirth,* Vol. 1, London: Chapman and Hall.

Kirkham, M. (ed.) (2000) *The Midwife–Mother Relationship,* Basingstoke: Macmillan.

Kirkham, M. and Stapleton, H. (eds) (2001) *Informed Choice in Maternity Care: An Evaluation of Evidence-based Leaflets,* NHS Centre for Reviews and Dissemination, Report 20, York: University of York.

Lewis, G. (2004) *Confidential Enquiry into Maternal and Child Health: Improving the Health of Mothers, Babies and Children, 'Why Mothers Die' (2000–2002),* The Sixth Report of the Confidential Enquiry into Maternal Deaths in the United Kingdom, London: RCOG Press.

Lewis, G. (ed.) (2007) *The Confidential Enquiry into Maternal and Child Health (CEMACH). Saving Mothers' Lives: Reviewing Maternal Deaths to Make Motherhood Safer – 2003–2005.* The Seventh Report on the Confidential Enquiry into Maternal Deaths in the United Kingdom, London: CEMACH.

Lipsky, M. (1980) *Street-level Bureaucracy: Dilemmas of the Individual in Public Services,* New York: Russell Sage Foundation.

Lundgren, I. and Berg, M. (2007) Central concepts in the midwife–woman relationship, *Scandinavian Journal of Caring Services,* 18: 368–75.

McCrea, B.H., Wright, M.E. and Murphy-Black, T. (1998) Differences in midwives' approaches to pain relief in labour, *Midwifery* 14(3): 174–80.

McCrea, H. and Crute, V. (1991) Midwife/client relationship: Midwives' perspectives, *Midwifery* 7(4): 183–92.

Menzies, I.E.P. (1970) *The Functioning of Social Systems as a Defence against Anxiety: A Report on a Study of the Nursing Service of a General Hospital,* London: Tavistock Institute of Human Relations.

Nicholls, L. and Webb, C. (2006) What makes a good midwife? An integrative review of methodologically-diverse research, *Journal of Advanced Nursing* 56(4): 414–29.

Niven, C. (1994) Coping with labour pain: The midwife's role, in Robinson, S. and Thomson, A.M. (eds), *Midwives, Research and Childbirth,* Vol. 3, London: Chapman and Hall.

Oakley, A. (1984) *The Captured Womb: A History of the Medical Care of Pregnant Women,* Oxford: Basil Blackwell.

Oakley, D., Murray, M.E., Murtland, T., Hayashi, R., Andersen, F., Mayes, F. and Rooks, J. (1996) Comparisons of outcomes of maternity care by obstetricians and certified nurse-midwives, *Obstetrics and Gynaecology* 88(5): 823–9.

Pharoah, C. (1995) *Primary Health Care for Elderly People from Black and Minority Ethnic Communities,* London: HMSO.

Schott, J. and Henley, A. (1996) *Culture, Religion and Childbearing in a Multiracial Society: A Handbook for Health Care Professionals,* Oxford: Butterworth-Heinemann.

Siddiqui, J. (1999) The therapeutic relationship in midwifery, *British Journal of Midwifery* 7(2): 111–13.

Soloman, M.Z. (1997) From what's neutral to what's meaningful: Reflections on a study of medical interpreters, *Journal of Clinical Ethics* 8(1): 88–93.

Walker, J.M., Hall, S. and Thomas, M. (1995) The experience of labour: A perspective from those receiving care in a midwife-led unit, *Midwifery* 11(3): 120–29.

Walsh, D. (1999) An ethnographic study of women's experience of partnership caseload midwifery practice: The professional as friend, *Midwifery* 15(3): 165–76.

CHAPTER 10

Midwifery Relationships with Childbearing Women at Increased Risk

MARIE BERG

A pregnant woman who gets to know that there is an increased risk of herself or her child being afflicted with complications is more exposed and vulnerable compared to other women (Berg and Dahlberg, 2001). Simultaneously, the transition into motherhood is one of the main transitions in life. Every pregnant woman is worried for the well-being of her child and a main question for the midwife is how the situation of increased risk influences women and their growth into motherhood. Another important question is: What comprises ideal midwifery caring for women at risk?

These questions have been essential for me ever since I became engaged in the care of women at increased risk. I worked on a ward which had alternative birth care (ABC) at one side, and antenatal and postpartum care for women at increased risk on the other side. The ABC side emphasized trust in the physiological, bodily process and in women's strength and resources in giving birth in a natural way without any chemical pain relief. At the other side we cared for a wide range of conditions but all signified as increasing risk, some during pregnancy, others after a complicated childbirth for the women themselves or their baby. I asked myself: What is the challenge for me as a midwife in addition to giving medically safe care? This was the start of my journey of identifying the characteristics of midwifery in the care of women at increased risk in relation to childbearing, here defined as the period of pregnancy, childbirth and infancy.

Normality and risk in relation to childbearing

Historically there was a lack of knowledge about both the aetiology and treatment of different conditions of risk in relation to childbearing; a fear of nature dominated. As knowledge increased and treatment options developed, the fear was replaced by trust in developments in technology, which led to more and more control over nature. Today, conditions that previously did not allow women to go through pregnancy and childbirth with a healthy outcome are manageable due to medical developments, including diagnostic and therapeutic procedures directed at both the woman and her foetus. Further obstetric risk factors are continuously being identified. Additionally, the number of interventions – especially of a technical nature – is continuously increasing. Complications during pregnancy and delivery are being and will in the future continue to be explained, and treatments are improving. Thanks to better knowledge, many women who earlier could not give birth to a healthy child can do so today. Women with diabetes mellitus exemplify this. Less than 100 years ago, such mothers and babies mostly died in pregnancy or childbirth. Improved care, effective insulin treatment and knowledge about what constitutes a good lifestyle leading to normal blood glucose levels has improved the statistics to near 'normal outcomes' in terms of an uncomplicated childbirth and neonatal period for both mother and child. Many other chronic high-risk conditions are now compatible with giving birth to a healthy child as a result of developments in medical techniques. The same improvement has occurred in the treatment of pregnancy-related complications, although the aetiology of many conditions is still unknown. Pre-eclampsia and its manifest form eclampsia provide such an example.

The concept of 'increased risk' mostly means an increased probability for the woman herself or her child-to-be to get complications related to pregnancy or childbirth. The proportion of childbearing women defined as being at high risk is constantly increasing. However, it is a question of doubt whether the higher frequency of high-risk women corresponds to a real increase. The reason is probably that modern maternity care is organized from a biomedical perspective, which is committed to detecting and treating diseases and complications, and deals with risks even when relatively low. This perspective increases the frequency of medical controls and interventions. It may also contribute to the fact that the definition of the concepts 'normal pregnancy and childbirth' has been narrowed over the years and is often changed to 'low-risk pregnancy and childbirth'. This is a consequence of the culture of modern society, which focuses on risk rather than the person (c.f. Giddens, 1991). Health care in relation to childbearing has become more specialized and divided according to risk level: care of women with normal pregnancy and childbirth, 'low-risk care', and care of women with increased risks, 'high-risk care'. Everything is considered as 'risk', only at different levels. In what way, then, has this risk focus influenced midwifery care? In Sweden, ever since the first midwifery regulation in 1711, midwives are expected to be responsible for 'normal' childbearing women, while physicians are responsible when pathologic and complicated conditions occur. A crucial question, also articulated by the midwife and researcher Soo Downe (1996), is whether this risk dimension in health science has caused midwifery practice to be even more narrowly circumscribed. On the other hand, even in the care of women at risk, midwives have a responsible role; specialized in various risk-related fields, they are given delegated responsibility. One such example in Sweden is midwives specialized in diabetes. However, it is important to gain more knowledge about the overall motive, feature and meaning of midwives' care of women with increased risk conditions. Here 'caring' is defined as 'good and ideal caring' and, thus, is separated from 'uncaring', which is defined as a lack of caring or care that causes suffering (Eriksson, 2001). Of course, high-risk childbearing women are not a homogeneous group in dealing with the challenges they face, but some general conditions exist. In order to get the most relevant knowledge we have to go to the women themselves and explore their needs.

Women's experiences of pregnancy and type 1 diabetes

Let us start with pregnant women with type 1 diabetes mellitus who get intensive medical care, but for whom only a paucity of qualitative studies describe their experiences and how they deal with the resulting challenges. One such study, performed in Sweden, describes how, in order to optimize the possibilities for the birth of a healthy child, they are controlled by blood-glucose levels and efforts to normalize those levels. Blood glucose was experienced as a personified object, constantly reminding the mother of the coming child who made demands from the very beginning of pregnancy. The women expressed a loss of control and an awareness of having an unwell, high-risk body. This was defined as objectification; an abstract word for not being integrated in one's own body. Another central mood identified was 'exaggerated responsibility', including constant worry, pressure and self-blame. In summary, pregnant women with type 1 diabetes mellitus are, in their transition from woman to mother, largely influenced by the living conditions demanded by their disease (Berg and Honkasalo, 2000). Their dealings with life circumstances are summarized as a construct of duality: 'to master or to be enslaved'. The overall experience of challenges and managing is understood to depend on the individual woman's identity, attitude and resources, which also include health-care professionals and special environment (Berg, 2005b).

Women's experiences of a complicated childbirth

In another study women were interviewed concerning their experience of childbirth, which for all of them was defined as complicated. A broad spectrum of risks was present, such as diabetes mellitus, previous renal transplantation, severe pre-eclampsia, delivery ending in emergency caesarean section or vacuum extraction, postpartum haemorrhage, severe perineal rifts, manual removal of placenta and birth of a premature baby. The essence of their descriptions was not focused on the complications as such but on their need to be affirmed. If this happened, they felt good enough as birthing women and as mothers. The affirmation included being seen as a unique person with unique needs, being listened to and getting support. It included being trusted and accepted, for example in how they tolerated pain.

Central to affirmation was a continuous dialogue with health-care professionals, including continuous information. The need for information was very great and was a prerequisite for feeling participative. Through affirmation the woman could feel in control over labour and her body. She could feel trust in health-care professionals and thus more easily surrender herself into their hands, being a tool for the birthing process. The closeness to her newborn child promoted her feelings of motherhood and tempered a traumatic experience. Lack of affirmation by the care-giver, especially by the midwife, gave way to feelings of stress, insecurity, disappointment, worse pain management and difficulty in accepting motherhood. It also led to feelings of guilt for giving the baby a brutal birth when obstetric interventions were necessary. Women who did not feel accepted were discouraged and did not trust themselves or their capacity for giving birth. They felt a loss of control, had feelings of unreality and became a depersonified object (Berg and Dahlberg, 1998).

A midwifery model of care for childbearing women at high risk: Genuine caring in caring for the genuine

In order to promote ideal midwifery care, a synthesis was performed of the above two studies together with an interview study with midwives caring for childbearing women at high obstetric risk or who had obstetric care (Berg and Dahlberg, 1998, 2001; Berg and Honkasalo 2000). The aim was to create a theoretical model of midwifery care based on the lived experiences of both childbearing women and midwives, and ultimately to raise the quality of evidence-based care in the field of childbearing.

The resulting midwifery model of ideal care is structured with three constituents: a dignity-protective relationship; embodied knowledge; and a balancing of the natural and medical perspectives. The model is labelled 'Genuine caring in caring for the genuine'. Here the word *genuine* expresses the nature of midwifery care including the midwife's genuineness to herself, as well as to the nature of each pregnant woman being cared for as a unique individual. I will now describe the three constituents further with quotations by the interviewed women (W) and midwives (M). The model was originally presented in the *Journal of Perinatal Education* (Berg, 2005a).

A dignity-protective relationship

An essential component of midwifery care is to protect the woman's dignity. The basis for this component is a caring relationship where each pregnant woman is treated as a unique person. Five overlapping elements are included in the constituent labelled 'a dignity-protective relationship': mutuality, trust, ongoing dialogue, enduring presence and shared responsibility.

Mutuality

The ideal caring relationship is expressed as a mutual process between the midwife and the pregnant woman, which develops when both the midwife and the woman encounter each other in openness. The opposite of mutuality is one-sidedness, each one encountering the other only from the perspective of oneself.

> A meeting cannot just be one-sided. It must be mutual... The most important thing is to build a relationship, to build a bridge. Mutuality includes confirmation of the other. Make it plain that I see her. (M)

Mutuality is not established as a technique but as a way of being. However, it may be expressed in a concrete manner by affirming a woman in pain during labour: 'It was nice to get the confirmation, that you don't just imagine your pain' (W in labour). On the other hand, lack of confirmation or disconfirmation violates the woman's dignity. It paves the way to feelings of stress, insecurity, disappointment and ineffective pain management, and may also support feelings of failure and guilt: 'I felt as if they found me troublesome' (W in labour).

Trust

The midwife should trust the woman: her feelings, capacity to give birth and ability as a mother-to-be. Trust needs to be reciprocal. In order to perform caring, the midwife needs to feel that the woman trusts her, in both her professionalism and her attributes as a person. A pregnant and birthing woman who feels that the midwife receives her, dares in return, to receive and to trust the midwife's care and, thus, to relax:

> Create reliability and security out of chaos... I must establish a line of communication so that she can learn to trust and understand me, feel safe with what I've got to offer and trust in it so that we can work together, that it is a mutual trust. (M)

> I wasn't worried that anything would happen. They have to know their job. I have left myself in their hands. (W)

Ongoing dialogue

Dignity is also protected through an ongoing dialogue. This is a way of showing respect for the childbearing woman. It includes continuously informing the woman about what has happened and what is going to happen, even when the woman herself has difficulty in communicating:

> So that one knew what to expect. (W in labour)

> Lack of respect violates dignity: I know that I looked through a mist. I didn't understand. They talked beyond my control. (W during labour)

Enduring presence

Enduring presence is a necessary element in the dignity-protective caring of women at risk. The midwife should be present with the woman, near and available in both an emotional and a physical sense:

> I give her my time, show her that I have time for her. I stop and sit down... This is quality time that you are working with, as so many others are making demands upon you. (M)

Enduring presence, for example in the care of a hospitalized pregnant woman with complications, also means that all midwives together form a collective. By coordinating with and complementing each other, a midwife is always at hand for the woman. The best situation is that a woman is treated by as few midwives as possible: 'by minimizing the number of persons around every woman' (M). When the woman feels that the midwife is either emotionally or physically absent, she expresses violated dignity: 'It was a real disappointment to feel alone. I found that this midwife just wasn't there' (W in preparation for an emergency caesarean section).

Shared responsibility

Although childbearing women at high risk are in great need of expert care, they need to be involved in the process. The ideal condition occurs when responsibility is shared with the health-care providers, including the midwife. A midwife who takes over the situation by being too dominant may provoke feelings of objectification and of violated dignity: 'It had to be done her way, just lie still. I was not allowed to say anything' (W). This behaviour may pave the way for feelings of unreality, as for this woman who had an emergency caesarean section: 'It was almost like being at the cinema. It wasn't me lying there' (W). A feeling of shared control, on the other hand, promotes a feeling of being in control, even when health professionals guide the process, as experienced by another woman who went through an emergency section:

> You are able to control the decision of leaving the control to other people. I am the thing that must be used to obtain what they want. You must leave your body. You don't look at yourself, but at the course of events. I saw somebody with a green dress. You look at an operating theatre... You make an image for yourself. (W)

Embodied knowledge

The second identified constituent of genuine care is embodied knowledge, the kind of knowledge the midwife uses as the most important tool in caring for at-risk women. The word 'embodied' focuses on the fact that the knowledge is deep-rooted and integrated within the midwife. The midwife *is* her knowledge: 'One learns new things all the time that sink in, leaving room for more learning. This is deep-rooted knowledge' (M). Midwives' knowledge is lived out through all their senses: sight, hearing, smell, taste, touch and the so-called sixth sense, intuition. Embodied knowledge consists of five integrated elements: genuineness towards oneself, theoretical, practical, intuitive and reflective knowledge.

Genuineness towards oneself

For embodied knowledge to be a reality, it is essential for the midwife to be open and genuine towards herself. This includes acceptance of one's own personality and feelings, and the courage to live those out. Caring for a woman with pre-eclampsia may exemplify this. When the woman's symptoms become aggravated, midwives observe her more often, measuring blood pressure and conducting blood tests. Here the midwife's challenge is to promote security and trust while at the same time being honest by showing her own feelings: 'She is worried anyway... It is better to be forthright and explain what we are feeling, why, and what we are doing about it' (M).

Theoretical, practical, intuitive and reflective knowledge

Sound *theoretical knowledge* about various complicated conditions and diseases that may interfere is essential in the care of pregnant and labouring women at high risk, both to give feelings of security and safety, and to presuppose guidance through a natural course of events and the avoidance of pathologization:

> We need more knowledge of all these complications, how they affect childbearing, in order to emphasise the normal. (M)

Knowledge is also obtained through *practical experience*. There are no short cuts; the midwife must experience repeated, diverse situations with women to obtain knowledge rooted in practical experience. As one midwife expressed it:

> Working as a midwife and meeting so many people and having these short, intensive meetings, and sometimes slightly longer relationships with patients – it's obvious that it provides me with experience of how to get to know a person.

Intuition is a more integrated level of embodied knowledge which can develop as professional experience increases. It is an excellent tool for understanding and determining a woman's condition and needs. Intuitive knowledge is often used in a midwife's first encounter with a woman, and may be experienced as a sense of worry or uneasiness, or a feeling that things are not quite right:

It has something to do with experience and sensitivity; which I also think has something to do with intuition, midwife-intuition, midwife-sense.... I do not think we should be afraid of trusting these feelings. We often feel things long before anyone else notices anything. (M)

Embodied knowledge presumes *reflective knowledge*; that is, to reflect continually both about care already given and about the actual caring situation. The work of a midwife is independent and often lonely, undertaken together with the pregnant or birthing woman and her partner/family. Essential reflections, made both within oneself and together with colleagues, function as guidance and as the basis for a growing knowledge and an increased sense of professional security. As one midwife said: 'One needs to reflect on things with one's colleagues.'

A balancing of the natural and medical perspectives

The third and final constituent in the model focuses on how midwives should strive to reach a balance between the natural and the medical perspectives in their care, especially by promoting the natural perspective, including each woman's inborn capacity to be a mother and to give birth in a natural manner even when increased risk exists. Its elements are *supporting normalcy* and *exhibiting sensitivity for the genuine*.

Supporting normalcy

Childbearing women who are at increased risk need to be treated as normal. This is exemplified by women with diabetes mellitus, who often have aversion to actions and items of equipment that identify them as special and at risk: 'Simply that everything was so special-special' (W). Midwives should view childbirth as a normal life process and strive to 'help the mother get through pregnancy and birth with as little sickness and complications as possible' (M). However, a risk of 'pathologization' or 'the worst-scenario image' is embedded in the organization. The care of childbearing women at risk is based on close collaboration between midwives and obstetricians. Sometimes their different caring perspectives clash. A midwife's balancing act implies finding a level where both the natural and the medical perspectives may exist side by side. It does not mean counteracting special treatment; rather, it includes a struggle 'to let nature take its course, to see childbirth and maternity care from the point of view of the normal' (M). Midwives are convinced that 'every woman has an inborn strength that we support so that natural process is promoted' (M). Their challenge, in the care of women at high risk, is to treat childbearing as a genuine, normal process. Midwives may even raise the limit for normalcy:

> I have reconsidered my views as to what sickness is and what health is. One would have thought that one would become fixated with the complicated, but it has been rather the opposite. I have raised the limit for what I consider as normal. (M)

Exhibiting sensitivity for the genuine

Midwifery caring includes openness and sensitivity to the genuineness of every woman. This is also a dignity-protective action, stressing the importance of keeping the woman in focus, keeping her in view:

> She is not the complication in itself, but rather the person who has complications. (M)

> Focus and see the woman more – not just the machines, tests and everything surrounding her. (M)

Pregnant women at increased risk in relation to the well-being of the child are frequently filled with self-accusations. This is exemplified both by women going through a more complicated childbirth, and by women with diabetes mellitus who struggle to reach normal blood-glucose levels to give the foetus the best conditions for a healthy start in life:

> If anything is wrong with the child or if something had shown up at the ultrasound, you would easily have blamed yourself a lot. (W)

The midwife's sensitivity for the genuine comprises affirmation of these feelings. This also empowers the woman's capacity as a mother. The genuine includes the process of moving into motherhood, and the challenge is to empower each woman to feel a good enough mother for her child, even in the case of severe complications. There are numerous possibilities for midwives to provide space for parenthood in different situations of risks and complications. One such challenge is in the care and preparation for a caesarean section of a mother with advanced cervical cancer:

> They were both so happy because suddenly they were to be parents, it was not just all about cancer. (M)

Another situation is in the postpartum care of a mother who has a premature child, when physical closeness between mother and child should be promoted:

They came on to me with the incubator and took her [the baby] out of it. Then they put her on my tummy. And I thought it was lovely, yes very nice and cozy... I think it was the mother in me at once. (M)

A further example is breastfeeding, which the midwife will support even if the child has little chance of survival. Midwifery care when a baby is stillborn is a challenge, but yet there is parenthood to be confirmed:

So that they have a child they can mourn – to help parents meet their child. (M)

Final reflections and practical applications of the resulting midwifery model

The results of the present analysis share similarities with central concepts in other midwifery theories (Kennedy, 2000; Lehrman, 1988; Swanson, 1991; Thompson *et al.*, 1989). However, these results are original in that the focus is on midwifery care for pregnant women at high risk.

Several years ago, Oakley (1989: 217) posed an important question: 'If technology is the obstetrician's weapon, what is a midwife's anyway?' The present synthesis of research offers one answer: The midwife's weapon is genuine caring in caring for the genuine; that is, a dignity-protective, caring relationship based on embodied knowledge and a balance between the medical and natural perspectives.

The results show that midwifery care indeed has a central value in the care of women at high risk. In today's health culture with obstetric care focused on risk, this ongoing struggle for balanced care is necessary and is probably not limited to the Swedish context but valid in all modern societies. A Norwegian midwifery researcher has described modern midwifery as practised at the point of intersection between medical science, which emphasizes that all births have the potential of pathology, and traditionally based knowledge, which includes a natural view of child-bearing (Blåka-Sandvik, 1997). This synthesis indicates that the midwives' struggle is not for the legitimacy of their profession but, rather, for women's rights to remain in the natural process connected with pregnancy and childbirth. Childbearing women at high risk live in an extremely vulnerable situation. For the women's sake, it is crucial that midwifery and medical care exist on equal terms. Balanced care of women at high risk is of the utmost importance, satisfying both their medical needs and promoting the inherent right to be mothers and to give birth in a natural manner.[1] The focus on the natural process of pregnancy and birth does not mean that reasonable and imperative medical treatment should be avoided. However, it may reduce the misuse and overuse of a variety of interventions, just as models of midwifery care for women at low obstetric risk have demonstrated significantly lower rates of interventions without compromising safety (Harvey *et al.*, 1996; Linder-Pelz *et al.*, 1990; Waldenström *et al.*, 1996).

The basis for genuine midwifery caring is mutual respect and confidence between different health-care professionals, with all striving for the same goal to promote mothers' well-being during pregnancy and childbirth with as little sickness, complication and intervention as possible (Berg and Dahlberg, 2001). Midwives, physicians and other health professionals in antenatal care have a special responsibility to give care that not only optimizes the biological possibility for a healthy child to be born, but also supports the woman with type 1 diabetes mellitus to master her situation rather than experience enslavement and, thus, promote her health, well-being and motherhood (Berg, 2005b).

Genuine caring focuses on the very nature of a midwife's way of being. Caring for every woman in her genuineness focuses on her value. Respect for the absolute dignity of the human being has been found to be the deepest ethical motive in caring (Edlund, 2002), and this includes midwifery care (Kennedy, 2000; Thompson *et al.*, 1989). The starting tool for this action is the caring relationship, which has been frequently emphasized in the literature on caring (Eriksson, 2001; Paterson and Zderad, 1988). The relationship should be characterized by mutuality,[2] trust,[3] ongoing dialogue,[4] enduring presence[5] and shared responsibility,[4] respecting the high-risk pregnant woman in her uniqueness, performed through the midwife's use of deep-rooted knowledge.[6]

Notes

1. The childbearing woman is foremost meant to be a mother. The developed model emphasizes that a childbearing woman at risk often feels insufficient as a mother. Therefore, the midwife's duty is to help strengthen the woman by confirming her needs and empowering her identity as a mother. An enormous, intrinsic power exists

in motherhood. The support for normalcy includes trust in mother-hood as well as in the woman's body, shown in both my own (Berg and Honkasalo, 2000) and other research (Bergum, 1997; Kennedy, 2000).

2. The element of 'mutuality' in the dignity-protective relationship is a human responsibility identified by several philosophers (Buber, 1979; Lévinas, 1988; Løgstrup, 1956). It is something originally abstract that becomes tangible when one sees the other's face (Lévinas, 1988). Mutuality eliminates the space between two encountering persons, as in a caring relationship between a midwife and a woman, and places them in a no-man's land where nobody predominates and both persons give and take. Such an authentic encounter includes vulnerability but paves the way for a close connection, which is a prerequisite for a caring, empowering rela-tionship (Halldórsdottir, 1996). Although the initiative and responsi-bility for such a caring relationship are placed on the midwife, a caring relationship is not possible without the woman's willingness to face the midwife. Bergum (1997) has stated that the midwife and pregnant woman affirm each other when they collaborate as two living 'I' beings.

3. Reciprocal trust is another essential element in the dignity-protective relationship. Reciprocal trust is a necessary component of a satisfy-ing, effective health-care relationship (Thorne and Robinsson, 1988). Women need to trust the midwife, both as a person and as having professional competence (Halldorsdottir, 1996; McCrea and Crute, 1991). In turn, the midwife should trust the woman. Enduring presence constitutes another dimension of the fundamen-tal nature of caring for high-risk women. As a collective midwives provide an enduring presence for women, of special importance in high-risk care which is often long-lasting and engages many special-ist care-givers.

4. The need to create a genuine dialogue includes continuous informa-tion in order for the pregnant woman to feel part of the process. Numerous researches have recognized that women's sense of partic-ipation when giving birth has a great impact on their childbirth expe-rience, and the midwifery model reveals that women at risk want to maintain a sense of control, even when it is necessary to allow profes-sionals to take charge. The element of shared responsibility focuses on this aspect. In other literature, shared responsibility is described as 'shared control' and 'entrusted control' (Corbin, 1987).

5. Presence has been shown to be central in caring (Gilje, 1992;

Paterson and Zderad, 1988; Swanson, 1991), including midwifery caring (Berg *et al.*, 1996; Fleming, 1998; Hunter, 2002). Presence means closeness in a physical, psychological, emotional and spiritual sense and includes nearness in time, space and amount (Paterson and Zderad, 1988). In the sense of serving and being accessible, presence means to value the patient's dignity. Demonstrating presence is eminently subjective and cannot be taught theoretically. From this awareness of oneself, demonstrating presence to others can be learned (Donna *et al.*, 1997). The midwife learns presence when she is present to herself. In this synthesis the element of enduring presence constitutes another dimension of the fundamental nature of caring for high-risk women.

6. Midwives' genuineness, i.e. openness and knowledge of self, is of great importance both for ideal caring and for developing embodied knowledge. According to philosophy, all real human knowledge (e.g. understanding, memory, perception, and emotional and cognitive relations to the world) is embodied knowledge. In accordance with a philosophy of phenomenology, individuals live as subjects in and through their bodies (Heidegger, 1998; Husserl, 1970; Merleau-Ponty, 1995). The present findings are largely similar to Benner's (1984) description of the development of nursing knowledge. Embodied knowledge is probably essential in caring, no matter what profession. Because childbearing has risks, focusing on the embodied knowledge of complicated conditions and diseases seems extraordinarily important. Embodied knowledge may function as a tool for midwives to raise the limit for normalcy and protect the natural process during pregnancy and childbirth, which is so easily downplayed in favour of a focus on the risk itself. Thus, embodied knowledge may reduce the risk of pathologization.

References

Benner, P. (1984) *From Novice to Expert*, Menlo Park, CA: Addison-Wesley.

Berg, M. (2005a) A midwifery model of care for childbearing women at high risk: Genuine caring in caring for the genuine, *Journal of Perinatal Education* 14(1): 9–21.

Berg, M. (2005b) Pregnancy and diabetes: How women handle the challenges, *Journal of Perinatal Education* 14(3): 23–32.

Berg, M. and Dahlberg, K. (1998) A phenomenological study of women's experiences of complicated childbirth, *Midwifery* 14: 23–9.

Berg, M. and Dahlberg, K. (2001) Swedish midwives' care of women who are at high obstetric risk or who have obstetric complications, *Midwifery* 17: 259–66.

Berg, M. and Honkasalo, M.-L. (2000) Pregnancy and diabetes – a hermeneutic phenomenological study of women's experiences, *Journal of Psychosomatic Obstetrics and Gynaecology* 21: 39–48.

Berg, M., Lundgren, I., Hermansson, E. and Wahlberg, V. (1996) Women's encounter with the midwife during childbirth, *Midwifery* 12: 11–15.

Bergum, V. (1997) *A Child on Her Mind: The Experience of Becoming a Mother*, London: Bergin & Garvey.

Blaka-Sandvik, G. (1997) *Moderskap och födselarbeid* (Motherhood and labour), Bergen-Sanviken: Fagbokforlaget.

Buber, M. (1979) *I and Thou*, trans. W. Kaufman, New York: Scribner, originally published as *Ich und Du*, 1923.

Corbin, J.M. (1987) Women's perceptions and management of a pregnancy complicated by chronic illness, *Health Care for Women International* 8: 317–37.

Donna, M.E., Haggerty, L.A. and Chase, S.K. (1997) Nursing presence: An existential exploration of the concept, *Scholarly Inquiry for Nursing Practice* 11: 3–16.

Downe, S. (1996) Concepts of normality in maternity services: Applications and conse-quences, in Frith, L. (ed.), *Ethics and Midwifery*, Oxford: Butterworth-Heinemann.

Edlund, M. (2002) Human dignity. A basic caring science concept (originally in Swedish: Människans värdighet. Ett grundbegrepp inom vårdvetenskapen), doctoral thesis, Åbo Akademi, Finland.

Eriksson, K. (2001) Caring science in a new key, *Nursing Science Quarterly* 15: 61–5.

Fleming, V. (1998) Women-with-midwives-with-women: A model of interdependence, *Midwifery* 14: 137–43.

Giddens, A. (1991) *Modernity and Self-Identity: Self and Society in the Late Modern Age*, Stanford, CA: Stanford University Press.

Gilje, A. (1992) Being there: An analysis of the concept of presence, in Gant, D.A. (ed.), *The Presence of Caring in Nursing*, New York: National League for Nursing.

Halldórsdóttir, S. (1996) *Caring and Uncaring Encounters in Nursing and Health Care – Developing a Theory*, Medical dissertations no 493, Linköping, Sweden: Linköping University.

Harvey, S., Jarell, J., Brant, R., Stainton, C. and Rach, D. (1996) A randomised controlled trial of nurse-midwifery care, *Birth* 23: 128–35.

Heidegger, M. (1998) *Being and Time*, trans. J. Macquarried and E. Robinsson, Oxford: Blackwell, originally published 1927.

Hunter, L.P. (2002) Being with woman: A guiding concept for the care of labouring women, *Journal of Obstetric, Gynecologic and Neonatal Nursing* 31: 650–57.

Husserl, E. (1970) *The Crisis of European Sciences and Transcendental Phenomenology: An Introduction to Phenomenological Philosophy*, trans. D. Carr, Evanston, IL: Northwestern University Press, originally published 1936.

Kennedy, H.P. (2000) A model of exemplary midwifery practice: Results of a Delphi study, *Journal of Midwifery and Women's Health* 45: 4–19.

Lehrman, E.J. (1988) A theorethical framework for nurse-midwifery practice, unpub-lished doctoral dissertation, University of Arizona.

Lévinas, E. (1988) *Etik och oändlighet (Ethics and Infirmity)*, Stockholm: Almqvist & Wiksell, originally published 1927.

Linder-Pelz, S., Webster, M.A., Martins, J. and Greenwell, J. (1990) Obstetric risks and outcomes: Birth centre compared with conventional labour ward, *Community Health Study* 14(1): 39–46.

Løgstrup, K.E. (1956) *Den etiske fording (The Ethical Demand)*, Copenhagen: Gyldendalske Boghandels Nordisk Forlag.

McCrea, H. and Crute, V. (1991) Midwife/client relationship: Midwives' perspectives. *Midwifery* 7: 183–92.

Merleau-Ponty, M. (1995) *Phenomenology of Perception*, trans. C, Smith, London: Routledge, originally published 1945.

Oakley, A. (1989) Who cares for women? Science versus love in midwifery today, *Midwives Chronicle*, 102: 214–21.

Paterson, J. and Zderad, L. (1988) *Humanistic Nursing*, New York: National League for Nursing.

Swanson, K.M. (1991) Empirical development of a middle range theory of caring, *Nursing Research* 40: 161–6.

Thompson, J., Oakley, A., Burke, M., Jay, S. and Conklin, M. (1989) Theory building in nurse-midwifery: The care process, *Journal of Nurse-Midwifery* 34: 120–30.

Thorne, S.E. and Robinsson, C.A. (1988) Reciprocal trust in health care relationships, *Journal of Advanced Nursing* 13: 782–9.

Waldenström, U., Borg, I.M., Olsson, B., Sköld, M. and Wall, S. (1996) The childbirth experience: A study of 295 new mothers, *Birth* 23: 144–53.

Midwives' Personal Experiences and their Relationships with Women: Midwives without Children and Midwives who have Experienced Pregnancy Loss

CHRIS BEWLEY

In this chapter, I revisit some of the work I have carried out in relation to how midwives' own pregnancy-related losses affect their relationships with women. The different pieces of work span more than 20 years, with some initial thoughts arising during my own midwifery training in 1983. The first piece of research was completed in 1995 and the latest in 2005 (Bewley, 2000a, 2000b, 2008).

At some point in a midwife's professional relationship with a pregnant woman, the question 'Have you got children?' is almost inevitably asked. As a midwife who does not have children, I found myself thinking about how best I could answer the question without losing credibility and without feeling that I had to justify my childless state. When I was younger, people's responses were generally that I had plenty of time, or they speculated as to whether seeing many women in labour had put me off. As I got older, and it became obvious that I was of an age when pregnancy was unlikely, I noticed that women responded in a different way when I answered 'no' to their question. I could almost see them wondering why, and sometimes it was difficult for me not to feel I had to tell them why. I also noticed that the nature of the question changed as I got older, and was more likely to be 'How many children have you got?' – the assumption obviously being that I was a mother.

Once the question had raised itself to me and I noticed the effects it had on my relationships with women, even if only on a temporary basis, I began to observe how other midwives reacted in response to the question. I was particularly interested since many of my midwife colleagues had quite sad obstetric and reproductive histories. One had a long history of infertility and desperately wanted a family. Another, after many years of infertility, conceived only to find that she had an ectopic pregnancy. Yet another had a termination of pregnancy for gross foetal abnormality; another had a baby with a chromosomal abnormality who only lived a few hours. On one occasion I was with a community midwife whose preterm baby had died at only a few hours old and we were visiting a woman who had given birth to twins, one of whom had died. The midwife was extremely supportive, and at one point in the conversation the woman asked her: 'Have you got children?' The midwife replied 'no', but I wondered how she felt and I realized what a loaded question 'Have you got children?' is. How do midwives respond when they have had a baby and something has happened to it? Do they spend their days being constantly reminded of their loss? Do they feel they have to tell women that they have shared the birth experience but that their baby died? How do they relate to women and what happens to that relationship when such intense emotions are involved?

I also contemplated the often heard statements, 'you can't be a good midwife until you've had your own baby' and 'I am a much better midwife now I have had my own baby'. I wondered how anyone could know without asking whether a person had children, or whether a midwife was 'better' or otherwise. I wanted to know what signs there would be of the effects of that experience.

These initial thoughts led to three research projects, all of which have now been published (Bewley, 2000a, 2000b, 2008). The first was a small, phenomenological study of six midwives who did not have children (Bewley, 1995, 2000a), the second was a larger questionnaire and follow-up interview study of 184 midwives who did not have children (Bewley, 2000b) and, finally, there was a replication of the second study using a slightly different sampling technique, an analysis of 40 narrative accounts and 10 follow-up interviews in a grounded theory approach (Bewley, 2005, 2008). All the studies received ethical approval.

I also carried out extensive reviews of the relevant literature, to gain insight into how midwives' own experiences of pregnancy and pregnancy-related loss influence their work with women. I explored concepts of loss, depression, why aspects of loss might be different for midwives as opposed to non-midwives, returning to work following pregnancy loss, self-disclosure, and shared experience in the development of the midwife–mother relationship. This chapter concentrates on these as they apply to the findings from the studies rather than the study designs, but in each case brief details of study design and method are given. Some of the supporting literature may seem dated when judged by its year of publication, but is retained because of its importance and sustained relevance to midwives' relationships with women. Finally, the chapter closes with some recommendations.

Background literature and findings from the studies

Whilst the life-changing experiences of pregnancy, pregnancy loss and childbirth are reasonably well documented (Bartlett, 1994; Kent, 2000; Rogan *et al.*, 1997), there is little available research-based literature about midwives' personal experiences of pregnancy and pregnancy loss, and how these affect their work and relationships with women. Gaskin (1994) suggests that midwifery training does not place sufficient emphasis on the midwife's personal life experiences and their potential effects on the midwife–mother relationship. Thomas (1994: 2) asks 'What do midwives bring to the birth arena?', observing that life experiences which affect a proportion of women, such as eating disorders, sexual abuse, depression, domestic abuse, stillbirth and homosexuality, must, by their widespread existence, have an impact on the personal lives of some midwives. She comments that very little work has been done on the psychodynamic nature of the midwife–mother relationship, speculating that failure to explore oneself conceals good or bad influences that midwives may bring to their practice.

Further, Flint (1989) suggests that some midwives treat women insensitively and that much of this thoughtless treatment arises from the unresolved grief of childless midwives. She also offers this as a reason for the unkind treatment of young midwives by their older, childless colleagues. Walton (1994: 113) comments that 'women on the whole, prefer the midwife to be a mother'. These sweeping statements are made confidently by Flint and Walton, women who have children, operating from an apparent power base of knowledge and privilege. They may be sincere and compassionate in their call for midwives to be supportive of one another, but they imply that midwives who do not have children are somehow lacking, with little or no research to support, refute or balance their views.

With these thoughts in mind, my first study (Bewley, 1995) used phenomenology to explore the experiences of a self-selected group of six midwives who did not have children. Recruitment was by letter of invitation sent to all 17 midwives in team practice, whose individual reproductive circumstances and history were unknown to me. I asked for respondents who did not have children, and all but one of the participants were young women, who had not yet 'tested' their fertility (Bartlett, 1994) and who fully expected to have children at some point in the future. One respondent had been diagnosed with infertility. My sampling strategy had not produced the group I had really wanted to study, but nevertheless, the findings provided insight into the previously unresearched topic of midwives who do not have children. It also revealed, among other things, that the issue of being a midwife without children is important, not only to those who have had adverse reproductive experiences but also to those midwives who have not yet tested their fertility. All the midwives were asked regularly whether they had children, and all felt that sometimes the question challenged their legitimacy as a midwife. They used various responses to convey to women and their families that they were qualified and experienced midwives, who were caring and empathetic, even though they had no personal experience of pregnancy and childbirth (Bewley, 2000a). However, the form of their answers troubled them and some were clearly unhappy at issuing a direct and unqualified no to the question 'have you got children?' and felt they had to justify their childlessness. One said: 'I usually say, no, not yet, I feel too young.' Another was also unhappy at just saying no, but was unsure what else to say: 'I feel sometimes I should make a bit of a joke, but I think, no, that's not the right answer.'

However, for some of the midwives, making a joke or giving a light-hearted answer was exactly how they dealt with the need to say more than just no. One of them said: 'I say no, I've got enough babies here, I don't need any more, and they take that as a funny gesture and laugh.' The one midwife who knew she could not have children cited instances of aggressive attacks on her credibility as a midwife because she did not have children. One concerned the mother of a labouring woman:

> She was very forceful and direct... she says 'How can you look after women in labour without any children?'... she went on and on for twenty minutes, half an hour... really personal, really digging.

Their struggle to respond to that question, and my desire to gain information from a wider range of experiences, informed my next, much larger study in 1998 (Bewley, 2000b), for which 184 participants responded to an advertisement in the *Royal College of Midwives Journal*. The sample was again aimed at midwives who did not have children, but included those who had experienced pregnancy loss, or a pregnancy-related loss, such as a diagnosis of infertility. Data was initially collected using questionnaires, which were based on the findings from the first study. The study design allowed for ten follow-up, in-depth interviews from randomly selected participants. Clearly the participants wanted to tell their stories, as 150 of the 184 respondents wanted to participate in further interviews.

In common with the midwives in the first study, they were often asked if they had children, and they showed a strong inclination to answer in ways which suggested that they would have children in the future, or that they were experienced and empathic midwives who would support their client regardless of their own situations. Again, some used humour to deal with the question, giving responses such as 'I want to sleep all night, thanks!' or 'no children but I've got four cats…' Five participants found the question so problematic that they 'invented' a child; one said she realized that women lost confidence in her when she said she didn't have children, so she told a 'white lie' and said that she had. Another interviewee quoted a childless colleague who said she had two grown-up children at university, saying she thought this was done to 'protect her battered heart'. Many told of their frustration when it was suggested that it was impossible to be a good midwife without having had children, and one said: 'I know midwives [who have had children] who I wouldn't let deliver my post, let alone my child.'

Like the midwives in the first study, they differentiated between the experience of pregnancy and birth, and the expertise gained by a midwife who had attended many women in labour. They too tried to emphasize their credibility as midwives, and would call on others' experience when imparting advice which may otherwise have invited scepticism, saying things like: 'I don't have children myself, but other women have told me that…' They stressed that whether practice became 'better' after the personal experience of childbirth was dependent on the midwife being capable of empathy and compassion in the first place (Bewley, 2000b).

Those who had experienced pregnancy loss, or fertility problems, also found it difficult to phrase their response. They dealt with probing, personal questions, sublimating their own emotions, particularly at times when they were dealing with their own feelings about their losses. Some found it difficult to be with women who they felt jeopardized their pregnancies by taking drugs or smoking, or who showed signs of rejecting their babies (Bewley, 2000b). Some simply found it difficult to be around pregnant or newly delivered women, and one said: 'I was distraught... I hated to see them [mothers] postnatally caring for their babies, and the love between them.'

However, many of them felt that their relationships with women remained positive, and they did not allow their own feelings to impinge on the woman's experience. Many also described their journey towards resolution when they felt they had come to terms with their loss. Many said how therapeutic they had found it to write about their experiences for the study. Some respondents, however, said they felt depressed, and some had been diagnosed with depression. Some had also left midwifery specifically because their own personal experiences made it difficult to be around other women's pregnancies (Bewley, 2000b).

Again, this study provided valuable new information, although once again the concentration was on midwives who did not have children, and I realized that midwives who may have experienced pregnancy-related losses then gone on to have children, or who may have had children then experienced pregnancy loss, would not have responded to my invitation advertisement. I then formulated another study, using the findings from the second to construct a questionnaire, with open questions, which generated narrative accounts under specific headings. I also modified the inclusion and exclusion criteria in order to attract the wider sample I sought (Bewley, 2005). I wanted to explore midwives' experiences during everyday contact with women and babies, whilst dealing with their own reproductive circumstances.

In the meantime, other writers were looking at the same and similar topics, for example Rowan's (2003) phenomenological study of midwives without children reported findings from interviews with 15 midwives who did not have children. These were similar to my previous studies (Bewley 1995, 2000a, 2000b) and are written up under similar theme headings, suggesting that despite the small size the experiences of the participants were similar. Rowan concluded that personal experience of childbirth does not necessarily improve quality of care for women, although this is difficult to confirm without input from the clients concerned.

Mander (1996) wrote specifically about what she termed voluntarily childless (or child-free) midwives, focusing mainly on the consequences for midwives and midwifery of the increasing number of women in the UK who will choose not to have children. Her observations about the probing and personal nature of questions asked of child-free midwives echo the findings of previous writers (Bartlett, 1994). She also recognized the well-documented negative stereotypes surrounding child-free women suggesting they are selfish and somehow 'abnormal' (Bartlett, 1994;

Morrel, 1994). However, Mander's (1996) article was largely speculative, without in-depth exploration of the events which may lead a woman to describe herself as child free. Bartlett (1994) interviewed 50 women who called themselves child free, suggesting that they had made a conscious decision not to have children. However, some were infertile and some had miscarried, suggesting that the term 'child free', with its positive connotations about choice, is perhaps a misnomer. Mander's (1996) work, and its tentative links to midwives without children, is cited here as it is one of the few articles which look at the issue of being childless or child free and how this may affect midwives. This general lack of literature on the subject confirmed my decision to conduct a further study.

The aim of the most recent study, therefore, was to explore the experiences of midwives who were having problems with any aspect of reproduction, and relate this to their approach and attitude to their work with pregnant and childbearing women and to their colleagues (Bewley, 2005, 2008).

A grounded theory approach used written data from 40 narrative accounts and 10 in-depth, follow-up interviews with randomly selected participants. The sample was self-selected and included female midwives, ex-midwives and students, who responded to a letter in *Midwives* (Bewley, 2003) which gave details of the research and asked interested parties to respond. The sample included those who had experienced miscarriage, termination of pregnancy, infertility (with or without treatment), those who had experienced stillbirth or neonatal death and those who were not in a relationship where they could have children. The analysis acknowledged the variety of experiences and that there was no one universal response. However, the unifying factor is that of loss, which crosses all the experiences at some level.

Concepts of pregnancy loss

The midwives wrote and talked of their experiences of loss and how this affected their dealings with pregnant and newly delivered women. I explored what was similar and what was different to other women who had also experienced loss.

Kohner and Henley (1997) used letters, other written accounts and interviews to document the experiences of parents who had experienced the loss of a pregnancy. Each loss is unique, however the bereaved parents have much in common. They describe feelings of emptiness, isolation, guilt that they might have contributed to their baby's death, failure and pain. Importantly, they describe their responses of jealousy and envy of others who have had babies. Seeing pregnant women and babies in pushchairs often triggered these feelings, and they were angry at the thought of pregnant women who risked harm to their unborn babies by smoking, drinking or taking drugs. Moulder (2001) found similar responses from women who had had miscarriages.

Much of the literature on grief and loss relating to pregnancy suggests that negative feelings are so frequently reported by bereaved parents as to be considered normal. In fact, Kohner and Henley (1997) suggest that parents worry that their feelings are abnormal and unnatural, and their book provides supportive evidence that others feel just the same. In the current study, participants avidly read literature on loss and bereavement, to assure themselves that what they were feeling was not 'abnormal'.

Work on grief and loss traditionally supposes that grief is resolved at some point, with an unspoken assumption that resolution involves acceptance that the lost loved one will never return and the assimilation of that loss into their own lives, enabling the bereaved person to 'let go' and 'move on' (Bowlby, 1991; Parkes, 1998). Walter (1999) challenges this last task of mourning and, whilst not dismissing the concept of resolution, offers another view of resolution, which is that some people simultaneously 'keep hold' and 'move on'. For me, this is exemplified by a survivor of the Hillsborough football disaster, in which she lost friends and relatives, and who was asked at one point if her life was back to normal. Her response was that things would never be back to normal, as her own personal normal was now different to her pre-Hillsborough normal (Taylor *et al.*, 1995).

For some participants in my study, the journey to resolution involved a period of depression, which further complicated their ability to function as midwives.

Loss and depression

A number of participants experienced clinical depression after their losses, and one said, 'I became severely depressed... developed an eating disorder and could not perform my job adequately.' At times this was noticeable to colleagues, as another participant pointed out: 'I said to someone, I think I was a bit depressed... and she said "a bit depressed" as if – God, I was awful.'

The links between loss, grief and depression have been described and researched by a number of authors (Cooper and Murray, 1998; Wheatley *et al.*, 2003), with postnatal depression receiving considerable attention. However, Evans *et al.* (2001) suggest that 10–20 per cent of pregnant women are depressed antenatally, and that high scores on antenatal assessment instruments are predictive of postnatal depression (Hughes *et al.*, 1999, 2002). Other researchers who specifically explored links between depression and pregnancy loss (Chambers and Chan, 2004) suggest that that one in five mothers will experience what they call (but without definition) 'prolonged psychological morbidity' after perinatal death. This shows itself as morbid fixation on the baby or foetus, anger directed at clinical staff or family, self-directed guilt or a sense of failure, desperate searches for explanations and negative feelings towards other babies. Once again, whilst these feelings are common in bereaved parents, the difficulties of functioning as a midwife when experiencing similar thoughts were clearly evident from the participants in my study.

Although there is no acknowledged specific or consistent link with clinical depression, one or more participants in the current study (Bewley, 2005) and both previous studies (Bewley, 1995, 2000a, 2000b) revealed momentary thoughts about abducting a baby in their care. However, they immediately realized the grief they would cause to the parents and the consequences for their professional lives. One who had a hysterectomy after miscarriage and other reproductive problems said:

> I cared for a baby once in the nursery who was awaiting social services collecting him. I fantasized about walking out with him... could I get away with it. I even thought about approaching the Mum and asking if I could have him (I didn't, of course).

Another felt she was discriminated against during her interview for midwifery training because her baby had been stillborn. She was accepted on the course, but her Neonatal Intensive Care Unit placement coincided with a storyline in a popular television series about a baby who was abducted by a woman whose own baby had died. The participant felt she was closely watched and under suspicion. Such thoughts were also documented by women who told their stories to Kohner and Henley (1997). Rabun's (1995) analysis of baby abductions in the UK and in North America suggests that in stranger abduction, whilst the perpetrator may have experienced pregnancy loss and may impersonate a nurse to achieve abduction, there was no evidence of depression in the abductors and nor were there cases of abduction by a nurse or midwife (Rabun, 1995).

Participants in the second and third studies were reticent about disclosing depression, because of the links between depression and the harmful behaviour towards patients/clients by nurses such as Beverly Allit and Amanda Jenkins, both of whom murdered or otherwise harmed patients. These cases led to closer monitoring of the mental health status of nurses and midwives (Bullock, 1997; Clothier, 1994). It became difficult for students and practitioners to disclose a potential need for counselling or treatment for depression (Dimond, 1997) in case their training programmes, or indeed their careers, were at risk. However, Brooks (2000) describes the positive experience of disclosing depression during her student nurse training. She received appropriate support and counselling, which helped her recover and successfully complete her training.

Being a midwife and being a woman

Although the participants experienced similar emotions to non-midwives in situations of pregnancy loss, there were certain issues which were unique to being a midwife as well as being a woman who had undergone loss. For example, in common with many midwives and health professionals, some participants talked of having preferential treatment, such as having earlier appointments and being able to chose who looked after them. Although this seemed beneficial, there were drawbacks. One midwife who had a termination of pregnancy for foetal abnormality said:

> I shouldn't have been rushed, I should have been given some time. The consultant meant well, and was looking after me, and he was going away for the weekend, and in the end he didn't, he stayed around because of me. It would have been better to have left me till the Monday to let me have the weekend to let me have the idea of saying goodbye really.

Some also felt there was an expectation that they would be well informed about their own pregnancies because of their midwifery knowledge and experience. However, they found it difficult to be objective when the knowledge and experience assumed such a personal context. Another participant who had rupture of membranes following amniocentesis, and subsequently had termination of the pregnancy, said, 'I felt I was not given good information, it was assumed that as a midwife I should know.'

Thus the midwife as client brings a whole new dimension to the concept of the midwife–mother relationship. There is the potential for role confusion as midwives caring for midwives and midwives being cared for by midwives struggle to function within their ascribed roles, and sometimes to move between them. For those returning to work following reproductive loss, perhaps the blurring of those roles created particular issues.

Returning to work after pregnancy loss

As described earlier, participants sometimes found it difficult to return to work in a job where they were continually exposed to other women's fertility and motherhood, and where they were expected to resume the role of midwife rather than (potential) mother:

> I am acting all day pretending to be pleased and happy about patients' 'good news'... being a midwife at the moment is making me very stressed because it is highlighting every minute of every day that I am not pregnant... there could not be a worse job when trying to conceive – I feel a failure. It is in my face all day long, but I know I have developed good ways of hiding it.

Many participants talked of hiding their feelings, because their love of midwifery and their desire to provide good care to women made them sublimate their own emotional needs.

This accords with Hochschild's (1983) work on professional groups, such as airline stewardesses, who adopt techniques associated with acting to maintain a calm and emotionally manageable atmosphere. She proposed that while some of the techniques distanced them from the emotional reality of their work, others were deeply internalized and became part of their reality. However, as Smith (1992) observes, some situations challenge the emotions so strongly that they bring about almost complete emotional shutdown, as demonstrated by the midwife who said, 'I am surprised none of them [the women she cared for] complained about me being distant and aloof.' For many midwives, the division of their lives into professional and personal enabled them to function. They would assume the role of the midwife, and save their true emotions for the privacy of areas away from the public eye such as the sluice and their own cars. As Hochschild (2008) observes, feelings may be natural, but the recognition and management of them by the midwife is anything but natural, it is rather an additional skill, which she terms emotional art.

The findings from my three studies and the associated literature suggest that, in common with many professionals and others who deal face to face with the public, midwives adopt a professional façade, as they conceal aspects of their own experiences which may alarm the client, or which may expose their own, sometimes very new and raw feelings. Many of the midwives experiencing pregnancy-related loss were returning to the place of work where they had received care or treatment for infertility, been booked for their antenatal care, or indeed where they had lost their baby. Some specific issues for midwives frequently related to how they were treated by their own colleagues, which directly or indirectly affected their relationships with women and their performance as midwives. Many participants expressed dismay that despite the emphasis now placed on supporting bereaved parents, midwifery colleagues were often less than supportive to their peers. Whilst participants could forgive lay people who made insensitive comments, they felt that midwives should know better. Sensitive approaches included being asked where they wanted to work and being able to change their minds at short notice if a situation became difficult, although there seemed to be a fine line between sensitivity and lack of sensitivity. This extract shows how important it is to check with the person what the appropriate action should be, rather than making assumptions, however well meant:

> instead of the shift leader asking me how I felt about caring for mothers with problems or pregnancy losses, they would assume that either it was good for me to come to terms with my loss, and that I could not avoid it forever, or limit it to the extent that these mothers would not be discussed in my presence.

Others were also surprised at what they perceived as thoughtless comments from their midwifery colleagues. I had asked if there was anything participants could specifically remember that was helpful:

> I really can't remember anyone saying anything that was helpful. Most people were sympathetic to start with, but trotted out the supposedly helpful statements – you are young, it was for the best etc.

Despite some difficulties, there were many positive comments, often relating to the personal qualities of individual colleagues and managers who exhibited care and concern, and who were emotionally and practically supportive. Participants valued having their wishes about where they wanted to work taken note of, and appreciated flexibility of placement according to their feelings. Anticipation of difficult dates and locations on their behalf by caring colleagues and managers was also greatly valued. Participants wanted to be seen as people with individual needs, not just names on off-duty rotas whose work needed to be covered in their absence.

Self-disclosure and sharing experiences

As women, all the participants in the studies had experiences which impinged on their knowledge and attitudes to midwifery and which may have affected their practice and their interactions with clients. Many participants confirmed how they wanted to use what were potentially negative experiences to improve the outcome for others. They described how they formed support groups, and entered fundraising and other positive activities. They updated literature in their own workplace to support parents, and acquired specific knowledge around particular areas, such as pregnancy following IVF and miscarriage, which informed their work with their clients. Some shared their stories with clients, but there were mixed feelings; some were unhappy with the outcome, and in some cases so were their clients. Pope *et al.*'s (1998) UK study of what contributed to being a 'good midwife' suggested that women valued sharing of personal experience by the midwife. However, the researchers do not make clear exactly what aspects of personal experience, other than that relating to ante- and postnatal experiences. Despite the potential for shared experience, the midwife must disclose this, as there is nothing which immediately marks out the mother from the non-mother, or the grieving mother. Self-disclosure is an important part of developing relationships and those who self-disclose are generally well liked, as long as what they disclose is socially acceptable (Argyle, 1990).

One participant in the third study had a termination of pregnancy for foetal abnormality. She disclosed her experience to couples in her care, but only after carefully judging what she thought their views of termination of pregnancy might be. A student midwife participant kept her own termination of pregnancy to herself, as in class discussions her peers were remarkably unrestrained in their criticism of abortion (Bewley, 2005). The Nursing and Midwifery Council does not specifically advise on self-disclosure; rather, it promotes the safeguarding of all aspects of the patient's (sic) interests, including emotional well-being. This is in contrast to the Nurses' Registration Board of New South Wales, Australia (2004), which acknowledges that self-disclosure can be helpful for patients, but that disclosure used to deal with a practitioner's own unresolved issues is inappropriate and can be harmful to the client. It particularly emphasizes that self-disclosure should only occur within an established therapeutic relationship.

Current work suggests that discussion and memory work around personal experiences and how they affect relationships is now being acknowledged as a valid source of evidence about events and experiences, and a number of birth-oriented publications now use the medium of story telling (Browne, 2003) and creative writing to capture experience (Bolton, 2000). Leaman (2004) examines how structured reflective activities can be used to help practitioners come to terms with puzzling or traumatic events, although the emphasis is on appropriate disclosure with an experienced facilitator, with an encouragement to reflect privately on personal events.

In the midwife–mother relationship there are a number of factors to consider. The current organization of maternity care in the UK means that there are two ways in which clients and midwives may meet and form relationships. First, and particularly in a hospital situation, the midwife may encounter a number of different women and not see any of them more than once. In these short encounters, as Kirkham (2000: 245) suggests, there is little motivation for the midwife to move beyond the most superficial greetings before proceeding to the business at hand. In these circumstances, the midwife may feel it is not worth the emotional distress involved in self-disclosure if she is unlikely to see the woman again. However, when women's questions about whether or not the midwife has children are brushed aside with humour or one-line responses, the woman may seek other signs that she can trust the midwife. In the absence of any personal knowledge about the midwife, and in the somewhat impersonal hospital setting, the woman may respond in a way which the midwife, who may already be in an emotionally compromised state, finds hurtful. This is damaging to both parties. Women are afraid of alienating their care-givers, and afraid of the consequences of non-compliance (Edwards, 2004). Furthermore, if the woman is in labour, the physiological consequences may even prevent her labour progressing. If the woman were in her own environment or workplace she would probably act in a different way, and exhibit the same emotional temperance and control the midwives did, when they steeled themselves to deal with pregnancy and birth in the face of their own losses.

Edwards (2004) suggests that trust is an essential component of a relationship; however, trust must be built, and midwives are not always able to convey that they are to be trusted. I return to the example quoted earlier of midwives engaging in deceptive behaviour and saying that they had children when they did not. One midwife commented on the timing of her deception, which was at the woman's transition from the first to the second stage of labour. Mander (2002) observes that this is a crucial moment when a woman presents 'a frank and honest articulation of her likes and dislikes at this time... which can be interpreted as rudeness' (Mander 2002: 10). In the case I highlighted, the midwife was untruthful because she felt the woman wanted assurance that she had shared and could identify with her pain. Similarly, a midwife experiencing infertility was asked by the labouring woman's partner if she had children and she received the following angry response from the woman: 'then how the **** can she look after me?' (Bewley, 2000a: 175).

In both cases the midwives were dealing with women whom they had never met before. The dishonest answer left both parties superficially satisfied, but the honest one left the midwife feeling devalued; though we have no way of knowing how the woman felt, we may suppose she felt cheated at what she perceived was a lack of personal experience and therefore a lack of understanding of her pain. Both midwives looked forward to situations where they could develop relationships which would enable them to disclose their personal circumstances in a less emotionally charged atmosphere, and when their skills and experiences as midwives who had supported many mothers would transcend their lack of experiential knowledge. The types of relationships between midwives and mothers which are promoted in one-to-one schemes and home birth teams facilitate disclosure and encourage the personal investment of the midwife.

For the midwives in my studies, the ability to form good relationships may have been compromised (perhaps temporarily) by their own reproductive experiences. Like any grieving person, they needed to work through the processes to reach a stage where they could use their experience to enrich the midwife–mother relationship. Within the relationship, the mother must remain the central focus. She is the client, and her pregnancy and labour are the sole reason for her engagement with the midwife. However, in order for midwives to be supportive, they need to be supported and nurtured themselves. There are a number of potentially supportive strategies which could be helpful for midwives dealing with their own pregnancy-related losses, and which may influence their ability to form caring and fulfilling relationships with women. Some which emerge as important are:

- Midwives who do not have children need to think about how they are going to deal with the often asked question in a way that makes them feel comfortable and that does not alienate the women.
- Midwives who have experienced pregnancy-related loss value a pre-return to work meeting with managers to discuss flexible ways of working.

- Midwives returning after pregnancy loss or after diagnosis and/or treatment of infertility may not be able to function in the full role of the midwife. However, their sensitive treatment at this time may enable them to remain in the profession, and at some time in the future resume the full role.
- Talking through or writing about personal experiences can be helpful for midwives, as can counselling, preferably outside the workplace.

Conclusion

The midwife–mother relationship is complex and is affected by the individual experiences of each one, as well as the environment and time frame over which the relationship develops. For midwives who do not have children, and those who have experienced pregnancy-related losses, there are many positive approaches to maximizing the skills and experiences they bring to the relationship. However, like any bereaved person, they may need practical and emotional support as they work through their losses to reach their own resolution.

References

Bartlett, J. (1994) *Will You Be Mother: Women Who Choose to Say No*, London: Virago.

Bewley, C.(1995) Midwives without children: A phenomenological study of relationships, unpublished Master's dissertation, Royal College of Nursing/University of Manchester.

Bewley, C. (2000a) Midwives' personal experiences and their relationships with women: Midwives who do not have children, in Kirkham, M. (ed.), *The Midwife–Mother Relationship*, Basingstoke: Macmillan.

Bewley, C. (2000b) Feelings and experiences of midwives who do not have children about caring for childbearing women, *Midwifery* 16: 135–44.

Bewley, C. (2003) Letter to editor, *Royal College of Midwives Journal* 6(2): 86.

Bewley, C. (2005) unpublished PhD thesis, Middlesex University.

Bewley, C. (2008) Midwives' experiences of personal pregnancy related loss, in Hunter, B. and Deary, R. (eds), *Emotions in Midwifery and Reproduction,* Basingstoke: Palgrave Macmillan.

Bolton, G. (2000) *The Therapeutic Potential of Creative Writing*, London: Jessica Kingsley.

Bowlby, J. (1991) *Attachment and Loss, Volume III Loss: Sadness and Depression*, Harmondsworth: Penguin.

Brooks, A. (2000) I don't want to cause distress, *Nursing Times* 96(23): 24.

Browne, J. (2003) Bloody footprints: learning to be 'with woman', *Royal College of Midwives Evidence Based Midwifery* 1(2): 42–7.

Bullock, R. (1997) *Report of the Independent Enquiry into Major Employment and Ethical*

Issues Arising from the Events Leading to the Trial of Amanda Jenkinson (the Bullock Report), Nottingham: North Nottinghamshire Health Authority.

Chambers, H.M. and Chan, F.Y. (2004) Support for women/families after perinatal death (Cochrane Review), in *The Cochrane Library Issue 2*, Chichester: John Wiley and Sons.

Clothier, C. (1994) *The Allitt Inquiry: Independent Inquiry Relating to Deaths and Injuries on the Children's Ward at Grantham and Kestevan General Hospital during February to April 1991*, London: HMSO.

Cooper, P.J. and Murray, L. Postnatal depression, *British Medical Journal* 316(7148): 1884–6.

Dimond, B. (1997) Safe practice or prejudice, *Modern Midwife* 7(9): 20–22.

Doan, H.M. and Zimmerman, A. (2003) Conceptualising prenatal attachment: Toward a multidimensional view, *Journal of Prenatal and Perinatal Psychology and Health* 18(2): 109–29.

Edwards, N. (2004) Protection – regulations and standards: Enabling or disabling, *Midwives* 7(4): 160–63.

European Council (1993) *European Working Time Directive, Council Directive No 93/104/EC*, 23 November, Brussels: European Council.

Evans, J., Heron, J. and Francomb, H. (2001) Cohort study of depressed mood during pregnancy and after childbirth, *British Medical Journal* 323(7307): 257–60.

Flint, C. (1989) *Sensitive Midwifery*, London: Heinemann.

Gaskin, I. (1994) Beyond spiritual midwifery, *AIMS Journal* 6(3): 6–9.

Hochschild, A.R. (1983) *The Managed Heart: Commercialisation of Human Feeling*, Berkeley, CA: University of California Press.

Hochschild, A.R. (2008) Foreword, in Hunter, B. and Deary, R. (eds), *Emotions in Midwifery and Reproduction*, Basingstoke: Palgrave Macmillan.

Hughes, P.M., Turton, P. and Evans, H. (1999) Stillbirth as a risk factor for depression and anxiety in the subsequent pregnancy: Cohort study, *British Medical Journal* 318(7200): 1721–4.

Hughes, P., Turton, P., Hopper, H. and Evans, C.D.H. (2002) Assessment of guidelines for good practice in psychosocial care of mothers after stillbirth: A cohort study, *Lancet* 360: 114–18.

Hunter, B. (2001) Emotion work in midwifery: A review of current knowledge, *Journal of Advanced Nursing* 34(4): 436–44.

Kent, J. (2000) *Social Perspectives on Pregnancy and Childbirth for Midwives, Nurses and the Caring Professions*, Buckingham: Open University Press.

Kirkham, M. (ed.) (2000) *The Midwife–Mother Relationship*, Basingstoke: Macmillan.

Kohner, N. and Henley, A. (1997) *When a Baby Dies: The Experience of Late Miscarriage, Stillbirth and Neonatal Death*, London: Pandora Press.

Leaman, J. (2004) Sharing stories: What can we learn from such practice? *MIDIRS Midwifery Digest* 14(1): 13–16.

Mander, R. (1996) The childfree midwife: The significance of personal experience of childbearing, *Midwives* 109(1302): 186–8.

Mander, R. (2001) *Supportive Care and Midwifery*, Oxford: Blackwell Science.

Mander, R. (2002) Care in labour in the event of perinatal death, *Practising Midwife* 5(8): 10–13.

Morell, C.M. (1994) *Unwomanly Conduct: The Challenges of Intentional Childlessness*, London: Routledge.

Moulder, C. (2001) *Miscarriage: Women's Experiences and Needs*, London: Routledge.

Nurses' Registration Board of New South Wales (2004) *Guidelines for Registered and Enrolled Nurses Regarding the Boundaries of Professional Practice,* Sydney: Nurses' Registration Board of New South Wales, www.nursesreg.nsw.gov.au/bounds/guidlin.htm, accessed 12 April 2004.

Parkes, C.M. (1998) *Bereavement: Studies of Grief in Adult Life,* Harmondsworth: Penguin.

Pope, R., Cooney, M., Graham, L., Holliday, M. and Patel, S. (1998) Aspects of care 4: Views of professionals and mothers, *British Journal of Midwifery* 6(3): 144– 7.

Rabun, J. (1995) Are there ways to recognize potential infant abductors, and what strategies can prevent abduction? *AWHONN Voice* 3(6): 9.

Ritsher, J.B. and Neugebauer, R. (2002) Perinatal Grief Scale: Distinguishing grief from depression following miscarriage, *Assessment* 9(1): 31–40.

Rogan, F., Schmied, V., Barclay, L., Everitt, L. and Wyllie, A. (1997) 'Becoming a mother' – developing a new theory of motherhood, *Journal of Advanced Nursing* 25: 877–85.

Rowan, C. (1998) Midwives without children, *British Journal of Midwifery* 11(1): 28–33.

Sarantakos, S. (1998) *Social Research,* 2nd edn, Basingstoke: Macmillan.

Smith, P. (1992) *The Emotional Labour of Nursing,* London: Macmillan.

Strauss, A. and Corbin, J. (1998) *Basics of Qualitative Research: Techniques and Procedures for Developing Grounded Theory,* 2nd edn, London: Sage.

Taylor, R., Ward, A. and Newburn, T. (eds) (1995) *The Day of the Hillsborough Disaster: A Narrative Account,* Liverpool: Liverpool University Press.

Thomas, P. (1994) Accountable for what? New thoughts on the midwife–mother relationship, *AIMS Journal* 6(3): 1–5.

Toedter, L.J., Lasker, J.N. and Janssen, H.J.E.M. (2001) International comparison on studies using the perinatal grief scale: A decade of research on pregnancy loss, *Death Studies* 25: 205–28.

Walter, T. (1999) *On Bereavement: The Culture of Grief,* Buckingham: Open University Press.

Walton, I. (1994) *Sexuality and Motherhood,* Cheshire: Books for Midwives Press.

Wheatley, S.L., Brugha, T.S., Shapiro, D.A., and Berryman, J.C. (2003) PATA PATA: Midwives' experiences of facilitating a psychological intervention to identify and treat mild to moderate antenatal and postnatal depression, *MIDIRS Midwifery Digest* 13(4): 523–30.

CHAPTER 12

Midwifery Partnership: A Professionalizing Strategy for Midwives

SALLY PAIRMAN

It is now some 20 years since legislative changes in 1990 reinstated professional autonomy for midwives and thereby provided the impetus for a complete redesign of New Zealand's maternity system. Over this time the system has moved from a doctor-led and hospital-centred model to a midwife-led and women-centred model of care. In the old model doctors provided most of the antenatal care and took overall responsibility for maternity care. Women mostly gave birth in hospitals, where midwives provided all the continuous care and assessments over eight-hour shifts, and women remained in the postnatal wards for about five days before returning home. Most women received no postnatal follow-up in the home, returning to their general practitioner for a six-week postnatal check. Child health nurses visited the home in the first month; their focus was on the baby. Women knew their general practitioner, but generally did not know the midwives who provided care through labour and the postnatal period. The organizational needs of hospitals and their employees generally took priority over the needs of individual women and families, and women experienced fragmented pregnancy and birth care dominated by routine. They expressed frustration in a 'one size fits all' maternity system (Dobbie, 1990; Strid, 1987). This model of maternity service is common and will be recognized by readers in many parts of the world.

New Zealand's current midwife-led and women-centred maternity service sets out to provide a very different experience for women and their families. This vision was articulated by the Department of Health (1998: 11) when it stated:

Each woman and her whanau [family] will have every opportunity to a have fulfilling outcome to her pregnancy and childbirth, through the provision of services that are safe and based on partnership, information and choice. Pregnancy and childbirth are normal life stages for most women, with appropriate additional care available to those who require it. A Lead Maternity Carer chosen by the woman with responsibility for assessment of her needs, planning care with her and the care of her baby and being responsible for ensuring provision of Maternity services, is the cornerstone of maternity care in New Zealand.

The maternity service today takes an integrated approach to the provision of care for each woman and her family. It starts from the premise that pregnancy and birth are normal life events and therefore sit in the primary health arena. Each woman is entitled to choose a Lead Maternity Carer (LMC), generally a midwife but they can be an obstetrician or general practitioner, who is responsible for providing and coordinating all care throughout pregnancy, labour, birth and up to four to six weeks after the birth. The LMC is required to develop a plan of care with each woman, recognizing each woman's right to make informed decisions and to have a maternity experience that meets her specific needs.

This primary health service is centrally funded by the state and is free to all women. If the woman requires additional medical, obstetric or in-hospital care, her LMC can provide the care, arrange consultation and provision of collaborative care with an appropriate specialist, or transfer care to an obstetric team. If the woman chooses a doctor as her LMC the doctor will need to ensure that midwifery care is provided. The percentage of women choosing midwives as their LMCs has increased since this model commenced in 1996 and now some 76 per cent of LMCs are midwives (NZHIS, 2007). Women are also able to choose the place of birth and all options from home birth to tertiary centres are funded by the government and free to women.

New Zealand's current maternity system is unique for its individualized women-centred focus, for its integration of primary, secondary and tertiary maternity services and for its personal, one-to-one continuity of care model. It is a system that relies on and respects interpersonal relationships – those between midwives and women, between midwives and their midwifery colleagues, between midwives and medical colleagues and between women and medical practitioners. At a system level it relies on co-operation, communication and respect between individual practitioners, professional groups, consumer support groups, organizations such as hospitals and government agencies such as the Ministry of Health.

Because it is designed to provide an integrated, continuous and seamless maternity service to women, the maternity system relies on midwives working autonomously and within the Midwifery Scope of Practice. The boundaries for practice for New Zealand midwives encompass the provision of midwifery care, on their own responsibility, throughout pregnancy, labour, birth and the postnatal period up to six weeks after the birth (Midwifery Council of New Zealand, 2004).

The shift to a woman-centred and midwife-led maternity service did not happen overnight, but has evolved since the 1990 Nurses Amendment Act and in the previous decade of political activity by women and midwives in partnership that brought about the legislative change. Midwives established the New Zealand College of Midwives (NZCOM) in 1989 to lead the development of midwifery as a profession, and recognized the reciprocal relationship between midwives and women by claiming partnership as a central tenet within their foundational Midwifery Philosophy, Standards of Midwifery Practice and Code of Ethics (New Zealand College of Midwives, 2008).

The reinstatement of midwifery autonomy and the subsequent redesign of the maternity system gave midwives the opportunity to work with women in a close relationship underpinned by continuity of care. In 1994 Karen Guilliland and I wrote *The Midwifery Partnership: A Model for Practice* as an exploration and description of the midwife–woman relationships that we were experiencing in practice and observing around us. We identified common characteristics and components of these relationships and developed a set of principles and a model to guide midwives in their practice of partnership (Guilliland and Pairman, 1995). The model was descriptive and was designed to provide a framework within which other midwives could examine their relationships with women if they chose. Key to the model is the premise that each midwife–woman relationship is unique and will be different, because each partner makes a unique contribution and because their interaction is negotiated to meet the needs of both partners (Guilliland and Pairman, 1995). In 1998 I undertook further exploration of midwife–woman relationships through qualitative research that resulted in further development of the model (Pairman, 1998, 2006; Pairman and McAra-Couper, 2006). A key finding was the notion of partnership as 'professional friendship' (Pairman, 1998, 2000). Coined by participants in the study, 'professional friendship' was used to describe a professional relationship that was experienced as a friendship between women rather than traditional models of client–health professional relationships with inherent power differentials.

The concept of partnership has influenced midwifery's development as a profession (Pairman, 2005a). This chapter explores how partnership is expressed in individual woman–midwife relationships, how the practice of partnership has led to an alternative model of midwifery professionalism and how the practice of partnership has affected New Zealand's maternity services and outcomes for women and babies.

Background to legislative changes and partnership

By legislating in 1990 that only medical practitioners *or* registered midwives could take responsibility for the care of women in pregnancy or childbirth, the New Zealand Government provided women with a choice of maternity care provider for the first time since 1971. Through this legislation the government, on behalf of the public, established doctors and midwives as practitioners of equal status in relation to the provision of maternity services. The amendments to the principal Act also resulted in amendments to other legislation, enabling midwives to order laboratory tests, prescribe drugs, admit women to hospital under their care and be paid for their work in the same way (and at the same rate) as doctors (Department of Health, 1990). The New Zealand College of Midwives (NZCOM) was recognized as the professional organization representing midwives, with the same right to negotiate fees for maternity care as the New Zealand Medical Association (NZMA). For the first time since 1971, midwives could work autonomously in the full scope of midwifery practice.

Lack of midwifery autonomy, medical control of childbirth, centralization and institutional control of maternity services and the consequent lack of control and autonomy for women were key triggers for the political activism by women and midwives that led to the legislative changes of 1990 (Pairman, 2005b). From the early 1920s onwards, women became more and more discontented with New Zealand's maternity services (Coney, 1993; Kedgley, 1996). Women and their families had little control over their care. Maternity services were centralized to main centres, midwifery education was downgraded and midwifery was seen as a specialism of nursing rather than a discipline in its own right. In this obstetric-dominated system, midwives lost their traditional 'with women' role and many lost sight of themselves as specialists in normal childbirth. Politicized through the international women's health movement and the second wave of feminism, maternity consumer groups such as Parents Centre New Zealand, the Home Birth Association and Save the Midwife set out to reinstate the autonomous midwife so that women could choose an alternative to the medical model of childbirth (Strid, 1987).

The leaders of these maternity consumer groups understood the risk of a system in which the midwife's role was restricted and had faith in the role that midwives could play. These women had a vision of what the maternity service could be, particularly if women, midwives and doctors could work together. Mary Dobbie (1990: 130) expressed this vision when she said:

> The ideal of mother, midwife and medical practitioner conferring as equals in a health partnership, pooling their knowledge and resources, is not an impossible goal. As a better informed public persists with its questioning, and as women share decision-making, that ideal will come closer to reality.

While women struggled with lack of choice and lack of control over their birth experiences, midwives struggled with their loss of identity and loss of professional autonomy. Legislative changes removing midwifery autonomy, downgrading midwifery education, removing the word 'midwife' from legislation and reducing midwifery to a specialist area of nursing practice were key triggers to the politicization of midwives. Through the 1980s midwives joined with women in political action, led collaboratively by maternity consumer organizations and the Midwives Section of the Nurses Association. In 1989 midwives established the New Zealand College of Midwives to give them a professional voice separate from nursing and the College provided strong leadership in political action.

It was recognition by both midwives and women that their objectives were complementary that led to the groups working together on a political strategy that would ultimately bring about the legislative changes that reinstated midwifery autonomy. And it was the reinstatement of midwifery autonomy that provided women with the opportunity to choose midwifery care, a key trigger to reshaping New Zealand's maternity services.

Evolution of a maternity system

With midwifery able to provide maternity services, significant changes to the organization and provision of maternity services took place. These were also within a context of four major health restructurings between 1983 and 2000 (Gauld, 2001). The maternity service, perhaps more than any other, has reflected these wider contextual changes, which provided both opportunities and threats for midwifery and for the consolidation of a women-centred service. I will focus here mainly on how funding of maternity services influenced their development.

By giving doctors and midwives the same social mandate in relation to the autonomous provision of maternity services, and by paying both groups the same for primary services, the government effectively set midwives and general practitioners in competition with each other. This had a number of consequences. First, doctors objected to being paid the same as midwives; their objections were heard by a Maternity Benefits Tribunal established by the Minister of Health in 1992. The Tribunal upheld the principle of equal pay for work of equal value and until 1996 midwives and doctors continued to be paid from the Maternity Benefit payment schedule. The Maternity Benefit schedule provided for a 'one-off' payment equivalent to one and half hour's work in labour and birth and for a higher half-hourly rate for time thereafter. Midwives, of course, provided considerably more than one and half hour's work during a labour and birth, but in the absence of any other payment schedule they received the high half-hourly payments.

This fee-for-service model was replaced by a capped funding budget for a specified set of services. In 1993 health funders (Regional Health Authorities) initiated a joint maternity service project which aimed to improve maternity services through a focus on quality, access, information and resource allocation (Coopers & Lybrand, 1993). The project involved extensive consultation with consumer groups, maternity service providers and professional bodies. The result was an integrated maternity services framework in which funding would be for specified services and consumers would be entitled to make choices about the service they would receive (Coopers & Lybrand, 1993). This framework was adopted by the Regional Health Authorities and from 1993 to 1996 negotiations were held with NZCOM and NZMA that resulted in service specifications that established the minimum level of care that all women should receive. These service specifications and accompanying payments were incorporated in legislation (Section 51 of the Health and Disability Services Act, 1993 and, later, Section 88 of the New Zealand Public Health and Disability Act, 2000).

The cornerstone of the 1996 change was the introduction of the concept of Lead Maternity Carer (LMC), which I referred to earlier. Instead of being able to choose care from a midwife or a doctor or both, women now had to choose a single LMC as the person with overall clinical responsibility for their primary maternity care (National Health Committee, 1999). In the earlier model, women could choose care provided by a midwife who attended her at home or in the hospital and consulted with an obstetrician if complications arose. They could also choose care from a general practitioner or obstetrician, but in these cases they either received midwifery care from a known 'self employed' midwife or from hospital-employed midwives working in birthing suites and post-natal wards. Women could also choose 'shared care' where their general practitioner (GP) and a midwife both shared the antenatal care, the midwife attended the woman in labour but called the doctor for the birth and then the midwife provided the postnatal care with some visits by the GP. If midwives and GPs wanted to provide shared care, they were expected to share the fee.

In 1999 midwives made up 66 per cent of LMCs while 20 per cent were general practitioners (Ministry of Health, 2001). By 2004 (the most recent published data) the percentage of midwife LMCs had risen to 76 per cent while general practitioners had dropped to 4.5 per cent (NZHIS, 2006).

While there have been a number of reviews of the maternity system and its services since the LMC model was introduced in 1996, there have been no major changes. The National Health Committee carried out an extensive review in 1999. The findings generally supported the LMC model, but made a number of recommendations designed to improve the implementation and monitoring of the model, such as the establishment of a co-ordinated perinatal database and improved access to services for Māori, Pacific and rural women. Variations to Section 51 and Section 88 notices for primary maternity services were made in 1998, 2001, 2005 and 2007. Each was preceded by public consultation and each resulted in relatively minor variations to the service specifications or to the payment schedule. A review of regulations governing how LMCs access publicly funded maternity units was carried out in 2006 and resulted in minor changes. In 2008 a review of maternity services in one main centre was undertaken, sparked by an unexpected baby death in a primary maternity unit. This review has also recommended only minor changes, most of which were already under way before the review was completed (Crawford et al., 2008).

The public support for New Zealand's maternity service model is also reflected in a series of consumer surveys conducted in 1999, 2002 and 2007 (Health Services Consumer Research, 2008; Ministry of Health, 2003; National Health Committee, 1999). The percentage of women overall satisfied with their maternity service rose from approximately 88 per cent in 1999 to 96 per cent in 2007. While levels of satisfaction are high, the 2007 survey showed an increase from 11 per cent in 2002 to 19 per cent in 2007 of women who had difficulty finding an LMC of their choice. This is likely to reflect current shortages in the midwifery work-force in parts of New Zealand and the recent unanticipated rise in the birth rate.

Midwives are now the main maternity providers in New Zealand. They do not work only with 'low-risk' women but provide care to the full range of women with medical, obstetric and social risk factors. When women require additional medical and specialist care, midwives work collabora-tively with obstetricians to provide a full and integrated maternity serv-ice. General practitioners have indicated that they do not wish to provide maternity care and the priority for the maternity system is to ensure a stable and sufficient midwifery and obstetric workforce. For midwives this means practising in a way that aligns with their philosophy and with their notions of professionalism. And that brings us back to partnership.

Midwifery professionalism

It was essential for midwifery to regain its professional status if midwives were to do anything to challenge medicine's domination of maternity services and society's understanding of childbirth as a medicalized and hospitalized event. Midwifery needed to achieve professional status so that it could control the setting of birth and develop an alternative body of knowledge about childbirth that could challenge the dominance of the medical paradigm in childbirth services. American sociologist Barbara Katz Rothman noted as long ago as 1984:

> I have come to see that it is not that birth is 'managed' the way that it is because of what we know about birth. Rather, what we know about birth has been determined by the way it is managed. And the way childbirth has been managed has been based on the underlying assumptions, beliefs, and ideology of medicine as a profession. (Katz Rothman, 1984: 304)

This view holds true today. But, as we shall see later, New Zealand midwives understood the need to regain professional autonomy if they were to develop a women-centred body of knowledge about childbirth and be able to support women to take back control of birth.

However, midwives and women were concerned about what profes-sionalism might mean, particularly as lay understandings of models of profession emphasized the authority of the professional, the power of the professional over the client, barriers to entry to the profession and educational and regulatory mechanisms that separated professions from their client base (Donley, 1989). These traits of professions were antithetical to midwives who, by the mid-1980s, were beginning to see themselves as a group aligned to women. Women consumers also did not want midwives merely to replicate the authority and dominance of medicine. A new model of a profession had to be developed.

From as early as 1986, midwives discussed and articulated their core values as they attempted to shape their concepts of a profession. Important early work was an extensive consultation process that led to the articulation of a philosophy, a set of practice standards and a code of ethics (New Zealand College of Midwives, 1992). The central philosophical stance relates to midwifery's relationship with women. This states: 'Midwifery care takes place in partnership with women. Continuity of care enhances and protects the normal process of childbirth' (NZCOM, 1992: 2). This philosophy of partnership was also articulated in the Code of Ethics and Standards for Practice (NZCOM, 1992: 5, 12). Midwifery's understanding of itself as a profession *in partnership with women* became the central definition of its professional project.

Through shared political activity with women, midwives increasingly understood that 'the only real power base we have rests with the women we attend' (Guilliland, 1989: 14). Midwifery did not want to establish a structure that created barriers between midwives and women. Midwifery also recognized that the sociopolitical context was changing and that traditional models of a profession were no longer appropriate in a climate that valued the rights of people to information and input into their own health care.

Coincidentally but symbolically, the last midwifery conference held under the auspices of the nursing professional organization opened in Auckland in 1988, on the same day that the Cartwright Report on the Cervical Cancer Inquiry was published. This landmark inquiry of 1987–88 into the denial of women's rights to informed consent at the National Women's Hospital in Auckland resulted in wide-reaching changes in relation to consumer rights and professional–client relationships (Committee of Inquiry into Cervical Cancer, 1988).

By the time the college was established in 1989, its inaugural President, Karen Guilliland, stated: 'midwives in New Zealand have come to acknowledge the pivotal role the consumer plays in the protection of their profession' (1989: 14). The founding constitution of the NZCOM provided for consumer participation at both regional and national level (Donley, 1989; Guilliland, 1989). It also recognized that feminist processes such as consensus decision making were appropriate for a nonhierarchical organization that valued the participation of all members and a collaborative and inclusive approach to all its activities, emancipatory and otherwise (Eldridge Wheeler and Chinn, 1991). From its beginnings the New Zealand College of Midwives has claimed that it is a feminist profession (Guilliland and Pairman, 1995; Pelvin, 1990). As a gendered profession, midwifery works to support both childbearing women and midwives to claim their own power and liberation (Guilliland and Pairman, 1995).

Liz Tully's doctoral work on the professionalism of New Zealand midwifery identified that midwifery partnership is a form of feminist professional practice that was used as a cultural resource in midwifery's struggle to obtain and consolidate professional autonomy (Tully, 1999). She said:

> By redefining the professional–client relationship as one of 'partnership', in which each partner contributed knowledge and experience, it also embraced feminist criticism of the hierarchical power relations involved in the doctor–patient relationship and the consequent devaluing of women's knowledge. (Tully, 1999: 165)

The way in which New Zealand midwifery uses its power in support of women is through its organizational structure and processes and through its relationships with women. Through negotiated partnerships, midwives recognize the realities of the life of each woman they work with and aim to encourage and support each woman's agency and autonomy. Midwifery partnership has been recognized as a distinctly feminist form of professional practice, because it uses 'particular constructions of gender and expertise... as discursive resources in the struggle to obtain and consolidate autonomous status' (Tully, 1999: 220).

As the college has evolved it has developed other mechanisms to give life to its commitment to women and to its practice of partnership. For example, the Midwifery Standards Review (MSR) is the central quality assurance process in which all midwives, no matter how they work, must participate every two years (Midwifery Council, 2008). It is a confidential, educative and supportive process whereby each midwife reflects on her previous year's practice with a panel of one consumer and one midwifery peer. Among other features, it considers feedback from women clients. By including women as panel members and by gathering feedback from women about their midwifery care, the MSR process gives effect to midwifery's women-centred and partnership philosophy and practice.

While MSR is a process for midwives, the college also offers resolution committees specifically for women. Any woman who has concerns about the care she received from her midwife can use the resolutions process. One midwife and one consumer make up each committee and also participate in a national training programme to prepare them for the role. The committee helps a woman to resolve her issues, sometimes through facilitating a meeting with the midwife or by providing a forum in which a woman can have her concerns heard and discussed. If resolution is not possible, the committee assists the woman to access other available avenues.

By claiming partnership as a central tenet and through its professional organization and activities, New Zealand midwifery is an example of 'new professionalism', whereby both the midwife (professional) and the woman (client) have recognized expertise and work together in reciprocal and equitable relationships (Davies, 1995; Health Workforce Advisory Committee, 2005; Pairman, 2005a; Tully, 1999). By redefining traditional notions of professionalism, New Zealand midwifery has established itself as a profession that recognizes that its primary commitment is to the women it attends and consciously works to put control over childbirth into the hands of women (Donley, 1989; Guilliland, 1989; Pairman, 2005a).

> When articulating midwifery as a partnership of equal status midwives have redefined the accepted view of professionalism. Instead of seeking to control childbirth, midwifery seeks to control midwifery, in order that women can control childbirth. Midwifery must maintain its women-centred philosophy to ensure that its control of midwifery never leads to control of childbirth (Guilliland and Pairman, 1995: 49)]

Public support from women, along with a number of other contextual influences such as sociopolitical support for women's issues and expectations of professional accountability, enabled midwifery's claim for professional autonomy to succeed. Women, therefore, had the right to expect that midwives would deliver on their promises. These meant that midwives had to action their autonomy and begin to practise independently of doctors:

> Women gave midwives a social mandate for practice thereby redefining midwifery as an independent profession. This professional identity carries with it a moral obligation to provide the service women called for and which only midwives can provide. Without independent prac-

tice provided throughout the whole maternity experience, midwifery reverts to an occupation, midwives lose their 'with women' status and women lose the opportunity for an alternative childbirth service. (Guilliland and Pairman, 1995: 39)

The ability to work on a one-to-one basis with women over eight to ten months has provided New Zealand midwives with a unique opportunity to explore the relationships they have with childbearing women and to create sustainable models for practice that reflect the values of the profession. In defining their relationships with women as partnerships, New Zealand midwives have actively worked to equalize their relationships with women and to shift power to those women so that they can control their own childbirth experiences (Pairman, 2005a; Tully, 1999).

Midwifery partnership

The notion of 'partnership' for midwifery evolved not only from the relationships between midwives and women, but also from experiences as citizens in a bicultural nation (Guilliland and Pairman, 1995). New Zealand's constitutional foundation is the Treaty of Waitangi, a formal agreement made between New Zealand's indigenous peoples, Māori, and the British Crown representing new settlers who came to establish a new British colony. The treaty was signed in 1840 to ensure a rightful place for both in New Zealand and to govern the relationship between Māori and the Crown. Partnership is an important principle of the treaty, and is understood to be mutually defined and negotiated on an equal basis, with full participation of both partners, ensuring the protection of each (Ramsden, 1990).

Although signed in 1840, the treaty is still relevant today. 'Partnership' is part of everyday language in New Zealand and is used to describe a variety of social, political, cultural and economic relationships. Increasingly, it is used to describe relationships in which imbalances in power and status are recognized and attempts are made to redress these imbalances through negotiation between both partners. It was these kinds of relationships that midwives and women wanted to exemplify by integrating partnership into midwifery's professional identity.

Through writing *The Midwifery Partnership: A Model for Practice*, Karen and I were attempting to articulate our understanding of the meaning of partnership in day-to-day midwifery practice with women (Guilliland and Pairman, 1995). We stated that midwifery partnership was:

A relationship of 'sharing' between the woman and the midwife, involving trust, shared control and responsibility and shared meaning through mutual understanding. It is this sharing relationship which constitutes midwifery and it is one which spans the life-experience of pregnancy and childbirth. Because of the individual nature of the relationship, midwifery's practice of partnership is a personal one between the woman and the midwife... Because midwifery recognises the social context of all women, the partnership is also a political one at both a personal and organisational level. (Guilliland and Pairman, 1995: 7-8)

The Midwifery Partnership Model identified a framework for practice with elements of recognition and understanding of pregnancy and childbirth as normal life events; that midwifery is professionally independent of other disciplines; that midwifery works in a continuity of care model providing care to women throughout the entire childbirth experience; that midwifery is about ensuring that women are in control of their own birth experiences; and that midwifery services meet women's needs (Guilliland and Pairman, 1995). What identified these midwife–woman relationships as partnerships was the equality of partners who make different but equally important contributions to the relationship. We considered that working together in a partnership relationship could be empowering for both women and midwives.

The theoretical concepts we identified in the partnership model and its refinements (Guilliland and Pairman, 1995; Pairman, 1998, 2000, 2006; Pairman and McAra-Couper, 2006) were intended as guidelines or a framework through which midwives might examine their relationships with women. Midwifery is practised in relationships between childbearing women and midwives. Women and midwives come together for a purpose and share the life events of pregnancy, labour, birth and new parenting. To work with each other in an equal relationship, or partnership, requires willingness, self-knowledge, well-developed communication skills, honesty, trust, generosity and time. Continuity of care throughout the childbearing continuum provides time for both partners to get to know each other, to share information, to discuss issues, to make informed decisions and to clarify expectations and responsibilities. When midwives and women engage in partnership relationships, they equalize the balance of power between them in a way that is empowering for them both.

Critique of partnership

While Midwifery Partnership is central to New Zealand midwifery's identity and professionalism, it was the subject of some critique in the early years of midwifery's professional project (Pairman, 2005a). The concept of equality between partners (the midwife and the woman) was challenged on the grounds that different social and educational backgrounds created an inevitable power imbalance in the relationship, such that the midwife and woman enter a contract rather than participate in a partnership relationship (Skinner, 1999). The underpinning philosophy that pregnancy and childbirth are normal life events and that midwifery is defined by how midwives practise autonomously across the childbirth continuum was seen as prescriptive, self-limiting and exclusionist, because the model 'assumes that normal birth is something for which all women should strive and that midwives only function as midwives in such [partnership] environments' (Fleming, 2000: 201). Another study concluded that equality was not necessary for a partnership relationship (Freeman *et al.*, 2004).

These criticisms appear to be based on misunderstandings of the Midwifery Partnership Model (Guilliland and Pairman, 1995). The model does not require the partners to be equal in the sense of 'being the same'. Rather, it contends that both partners have equal status and work together on equal terms (equality). Indeed, the model emphasizes the different expertise that both partners bring to the relationship. It does not deny the midwife's expertise, as after all that is the basis of her involvement with women – it is her professional expertise that she offers to women. However, the model gives equal weight to the contribution that the woman makes in terms of her knowledge of her self, her own health, her needs and wishes as appropriate to her own circumstances and context. Successful midwifery care relies on participation from the woman and co-operation in her own health care.

If midwifery is to achieve its aim of empowerment and self-determination for each birthing woman, then it needs birthing women to take part and exercise their personal power. This participation is unlikely to be achieved in relationships where the midwife uses authoritarianism. The Midwifery Partnership Model identifies a process of negotiation as the partners address issues of their respective roles and responsibilities, decision making and power sharing to come to mutual understanding and agreement. The balance of power between the midwife and the woman will be influenced by differences in education, class, culture, socialization and gender that have the potential to destabilize or inhibit partnership if they are not acknowledged and addressed. It is therefore essential that midwives recognize and understand their professional power in relation to the birthing woman and their responsibility for working to facilitate the woman's empowerment. When midwives work with women who are not used to exercising their personal power, it is the midwife's responsibility to find ways to work with the woman that will encourage her to begin to make decisions and take responsibility for these. The midwife and the woman may not reach the point where they feel they are working on equal terms, but even making small shifts in the balance of power can be empowering for both.

The Midwifery Partnership Model is a framework, not a prescription. Like all frameworks, it rises and falls on the way in which it is understood and the way it is implemented. Because it sets out principles and recognizes that each midwife–woman partnership will be different, there is wide scope for midwives and women to practise their partnerships howsoever they wish and in whichever setting they wish. As long as both partners participate and their decisions are mutually agreed without coercion, it can still be defined as a partnership.

International perspectives on partnership

As independent models of midwifery have been established in countries such as the United States, Canada and the United Kingdom, a small but growing body of international research has provided support for the Midwifery Partnership Model. Canadian midwife Deborah Harding (2000) reported a small exploratory study undertaken in British Columbia soon after midwives gained legislative autonomy in 1993. She interviewed a small group of midwives to explore how they experienced and implemented shared decision making in their practice.

These midwives identified the midwife–client relationship as the foundation of a shared decision-making process. They described the relationship as one of trust, respect and commitment that facilitated communication and enhanced care. Continuity of care was important, as mutual trust developed over time. Harding called the relationship one of 'reciprocal caring': the caring promoted the relationship and the relationship promoted the caring. The midwife and client were described as partners and shared decision making reflected 'the equal, collaborative nature of the midwife–client relationship wherein the professional context and the specific expertise of the midwife can be situated as a resource rather than a directing factor' (Harding, 2000: 83).

American midwife Holly Powell Kennedy has completed several studies into women's experiences and midwifery practice in continuity of care models (Kennedy, 1995, 2000, 2002, 2004). Her findings reflect concepts similar to those seen in New Zealand and Canada, such as trust, continuity of care, time and informed decision making. Midwives were 'present' with the labouring woman in relationships of mutuality, equality and respect. Midwives created an environment in which the woman's wishes were met, where she was kept safe along the way and where normalcy was supported and protected. Interventions were used selectively on the basis of clinical judgement and women's wishes, and the midwives talked about 'the art of doing nothing'. Midwives described transformative experiences for women as well as their own growth and learning, and at times humility. Kennedy concluded that such models of care had the potential to improve health outcomes and thereby reduce health-care costs (Kennedy, 2004). Kennedy's studies all identified the midwife–woman relationship as foundational to midwifery practice which is participatory, seeks to support and enhance normalcy and works to encourage women's self-determination. She does not term these midwife–woman relationships 'partnerships', but they easily could be as they are characterized by equality, mutuality, reciprocity and power sharing.

Women's perceptions and experiences of labour and birth within a caseload model of midwifery care were explored by UK midwife Denis Walsh (1999). The relationship between the midwife and the woman emerged as the primary theme. These relationships were informal, personal and reciprocal; the midwives were seen by the women as 'enabling' and, as found in my 1998 research, were described as 'friends' (Pairman, 1998, 2000).

An innovative model of midwifery care, known as One-to-One Midwifery, was established in London in 1993. Midwives worked with midwife partners, carrying a caseload for whom they provided continuity of midwifery care on their own responsibility, similar to the self-employed LMC midwifery practice of New Zealand midwives. Evaluations of this model of care demonstrated, among other things, reduced intervention rates and increased satisfaction from women (McCourt and Page, 1996). Extensive research to explore women's responses to their care showed that women felt confident and in control of their experiences. The personal nature of their relationship with the midwife and the development of this relationship through continuity of care enabled effective communication, information sharing and supportive care (McCourt and Page, 1996; McCourt *et al.*, 2006).

These relationships share some key elements with partnership. Page stated that 'bringing childbearing woman and midwives together in relationships in which the midwife "works with" rather than "doing to or for"' can have a profound effect on care that is 'greater than the sum of the parts... where women learn about their own capacity to love and care for the baby, and about their own strength and knowledge in the process of pregnancy and birth and the early weeks of the baby's life, and where joy rather than anxiety is the dominant emotion' (Page, 2003: 124). In order to 'work with', it is necessary to establish a relationship of equality, reciprocity and power sharing, such as a midwifery partnership.

The first edition of this book brought together perspectives from a number of midwives in the UK and elsewhere who were attempting to work with women in more collaborative ways (Kirkham, 2000). Key themes that emerged in this collection of research included support, continuity of care, trust, relationship skills, the place of self and taking power. The context of midwifery practice can assist or block the development of women-centred relationships (*Ibid.*).

The importance of context is highlighted by McCourt *et al.* (2006) in their review of research evidence on continuity of care. These authors recognized that continuity of care or carer may enhance or facilitate aspects of the midwife–woman relationship such as autonomy, confidence and decision making, and provide important clinical and psychosocial benefits to women, but that the environment or context of care may also limit these effects (McCourt *et al.*, 2006).

Whilst most of the international research discussed above does not identify the midwife–woman relationship as a 'partnership', there are a number of concepts common to all models. It is possible to conclude that when midwives and women can get to know each other in a one-to-one relationship over time, midwifery practice takes on certain characteristics in response to the personal nature of the relationship. Midwives' commitment moves from the profession or the employer to focus instead on the woman and her individual needs. Midwives who work in this way express a similar set of values and beliefs: a woman's right to self-determination in her childbirth experience; that childbirth is physiological and needs technological intervention only occasionally; that midwives and women share a reciprocal relationship in which trust and power are shared; and that the midwife's role is one of guardian and facilitator of a life-changing process that has far-reaching effects.

On the basis of her findings, Kennedy (1995) concluded that the midwifery profession should operate from a philosophy that emphasizes women's rights to determine their care and share power and responsibility in the midwife–woman relationship. By defining itself as a profession *in partnership with women,* New Zealand midwifery has developed an alternative model of midwifery professionalism over two decades that puts this philosophy into practice. And the practice of partnership has reshaped

New Zealand's maternity services and improved outcomes for women and babies.

Outcomes of midwifery care

While there are no New Zealand studies that formally link the partnership model of care with clinical outcomes for women and babies, evidence is beginning to emerge showing that care provided by LMC midwives is having a positive impact. In 1997 the New Zealand College of Midwives established the Midwifery and Maternity Provider Organisation (MMPO) as a practice management and quality assurance infrastructure to support self-employed midwives based in the community and paid by government via the Section 51 (later Section 88) schedules. A key component of the MMPO is the provision of a standardized set of maternity notes that simultaneously operate as documentation of care, claims for service provision and a database of clinical care. Through this process the MMPO has built a large dataset of midwifery care and its first report has been released (MMPO, 2008).

This first report provides data about 9953 mothers who gave birth to 10,064 babies between 1 January and 31 December 2004 and who were under the care of 390 midwife members of the MMPO. Some 47.2 per cent of the midwives were located in the South Island, where the MMPO has been established for longest. Nationally approximately 19 per cent of all midwives (including 24 per cent of LMC midwives) are located in the South Island and provide care for 20.7 per cent of all births (Midwifery Council, 2004; NZHIS, 2007). Further reports on MMPO data for 2005, 2006 and 2007 are expected and these reports will cover a wider spread of midwives across New Zealand.

Across a variety of outcome measures, the MMPO midwives provided care that was as good as or better than that reported from the national dataset for the same period. Unlike many other countries, midwives in New Zealand are not restricted to caring for women deemed to be 'low risk'. In 2004 almost 45 per cent of the women cared for by MMPO midwives had one or more 'risk factors' such as being over 39 years of age or giving birth for the first time over the age of 37 years. A small number (0.5 per cent) had multiple pregnancies. Many (41.6 per cent) had a co-existing medical condition such as diabetes or asthma and almost 9 per cent had experienced a previous caesarean section. Smoking in pregnancy was reported for 23.6 per cent.

Differences in practice between MMPO midwives and the wider

maternity workforce nationally can be seen in a comparison of outcome measures. MMPO midwives induced women in labour less frequently at 16.5 per cent, compared with 20.4 per cent of women nationally (NZHIS, 2007). A total of 20 per cent of all women (including those who gave birth by caesarean section) had an epidural compared with 28 per cent of all women in the national data (excluding those who had caesarean sections). Some 70 per cent of women under the care of MMPO midwives had no anaesthetic procedures (general, epidural, spinal or local) during labour. Episiotomy was used for 6.9 per cent of women compared with the national episiotomy rate of 13 per cent (NZHIS, 2007).

Just over 13 per cent of women gave birth in a primary maternity facility and 7 per cent at home, while 43.5 per cent gave birth in a secondary unit and 35.5 per cent in a tertiary unit. Approximately 45 per cent of births took place in a rural location. These birth locations to some extent reflect the spread of midwives in this cohort, as there are more rural maternity facilities in the South Island. Only 4.8 per cent of women were required to transfer during labour from their planned place of birth.

Most women (71.9 per cent) had a normal vaginal birth, 7.9 per cent had operative vaginal births and almost 20 per cent had caesarean sections. Only 0.5 per cent of births were breech and of those only the primiparous women (0.1 per cent) required operative assistance. The national data for the same year reported that 66.5 per cent of women had a normal vaginal birth, 23.7 per cent had a caesarean section, 9.6 per cent had operative births and 0.3 per cent had spontaneous breech births (NZHIS, 2007).

Most babies were live born (99.2 per cent) and without congenital abnormalities (97 per cent). The majority of babies were born between 37 and 41 weeks of pregnancy, with 8.6 per cent over 42 weeks and 13.3 per cent at less than 36 completed weeks. Just over 65 per cent of babies weighed between 3000 and 3999 grams at birth, while 1.2 per cent weighed less than 1000 grams, and 4.9 per cent weighed between 1000 and 2500 grams. Almost 78 per cent of 2004 MMPO babies were exclusively or fully breastfed at two weeks. Babies born at home had the highest rate, at 91.5 per cent.

Perhaps the most unexpected aspect of the report is the information provided about the management of the third stage of labour and postpartum blood loss. Active management of the third stage was conducted for 61.6 per cent of women, with a further 3.4 per cent requiring additional ecbolic treatment for haemorrhage. Physiological management was conducted for 30.3 per cent of women and a further 4.6 per cent required follow-up treatment with ecbolic. Those women who had 'active management with an ecbolic' during the third stage experienced higher blood loss, with 21 per cent having lost more than 500 ml, compared to 8 per cent for those women who experienced a physiologically managed third stage. Those who had active management of the third stage also had the highest rate of ragged membranes. These findings suggest that the way in which the third stage is managed physiologically by these MMPO midwives results in less blood loss than where active management is used. Current research recommends active management to reduce blood loss (Prenderville *et al.*, 2000). It will be interesting to see whether these findings from MMPO data are repeated in later analysis of larger groups of midwives and more births, and whether New Zealand midwifery can offer fresh evidence in relation to the management of the third stage.

A contribution that New Zealand midwifery is now making is evidence that midwife-led continuity of care is safe for women and babies and that outcomes are good. Whether Midwifery Partnership improves outcomes further is yet to be researched.

Conclusion

It was the loss of identity and threat of extinction that drove New Zealand midwifery to seek professional status through legislative change. In seeking professional status, midwifery sought autonomy of practice in the area of normal childbirth (in line with the International Confederation of Midwives' Definition of a Midwife) and self-determination as a profession in order to control its education, set standards of practice and code of ethics, and establish its regulatory mechanisms. However, it was the political partnership with women that helped midwives achieve these goals and through which midwives came to understand their interdependency with women.

By claiming partnership as foundational to its professional identity, New Zealand midwifery has developed an alternative model of a profession. In this model midwifery's first allegiance is to women and the midwife–woman relationship is more equitable, reciprocal and personal than those represented by traditional authoritarian models of a profession (Ehrenreich and English, 1973; Katz Rothman, 1991; Kirkham, 2000; Page, 2000; Pairman, 2005a).

The opportunity to practise within the full scope of practice and in partnership with women has influenced how New Zealand midwives have shaped their practice and this practice has in turn shaped the wider maternity system (Pairman, 2005a). There is cohesion between the Midwifery Scope of Practice and the maternity system, in that pregnancy and childbirth are seen as life events that require primary health services, continuity of care, seamless access to secondary and tertiary services when required and a focus on the needs and choices of each pregnant woman. New Zealand really has been able to develop a maternity system that is women centred and midwife led. We are in a unique position to develop midwifery knowledge about midwife–women relationships and about autonomous midwifery practice within a caseload model. We can provide an example of 'new professionalism' and of midwifery partnerships in action. Emerging data shows that autonomous midwifery care provides positive outcomes for mothers and babies on a national scale.

Midwifery Partnership provides a framework for a new way for midwives and women to work together. It not only benefits both women and midwives, it also provides a framework for re-establishing women's control over childbirth and bringing about long-lasting change in maternity services.

References

Committee of Inquiry into Allegations Concerning the Treatment of Cervical Cancer at National Women's Hospital and into Other Related Matters (1988) *The Report of the Cervical Cancer Inquiry 1988*, Auckland: Government Printing Office.

Coney, S. (1993) *Standing in the Sunshine: A History of New Zealand Women Since They Won the Vote*, Auckland: Penguin Books.

Coopers & Lybrand (1993) *First Steps Towards an Integrated Maternity Services Framework: A Report by Coopers & Lybrand for the New Zealand Regional Health Authorities*, Wellington: Coopers & Lybrand.

Crawford, B., Lilo, S., Stone, P. and Yates, A. (2008) *Review of the Quality, Safety and Management of Maternity Services in the Wellington Area*, Wellington: Ministry of Health.

Davies, C. (1995) *Gender and the Professional Predicament in Nursing*, Buckingham: Open University Press.

Department of Health (1990) *Nurses Amendment Act: Information for Health Providers*, Wellington: Department of Health.

Department of Health (1998) *Maternity Services Notice pursuant to Section 51 of the Health and Disability Services Act 1993*, Wellington: Department of Health.

Dobbie, M. (1990) *The Trouble with Women: The Story of Parents Centre New Zealand*, Whatamongo Bay: Cape Cately.

Donley, J. (1989) Professionalism: The importance of consumer control over childbirth, *New Zealand College of Midwives Journal*, Sept.: 6–7.

Ehrenreich, B. and English, D. (1973) *Witches, Midwives and Nurses,* London: Writers and Readers Publishing Cooperative.

Eldridge Wheeler, C. and Chinn, P. (1991) *Peace and Power: A Handbook of Feminist Process,* New York: National League for Nursing.

Fleming, V. (2000) The midwifery partnership in New Zealand: Past history or a new way forward? in Kirkham, M. (ed.), *The Midwife–Mother Relationship,* London: Macmillan.

Freeman, L., Timperley, H. and Adair, V. (2004) Partnership in midwifery care in New Zealand, *Midwifery* 20: 2–14.

Gauld, R. (2001) *Revolving Doors: New Zealand's Health Reforms,* Wellington: Victoria University of Wellington.

Guilliland, K. (1989) Maintaining the links: A history of the formation of the NZCOM, *New Zealand College of Midwives Journal,* Sept.: 14.

Guilliland, K. and Pairman, S. (1995) *The Midwifery Partnership: A Model for Practice,* Monograph Series 95/1, Wellington: Department of Nursing and Midwifery, Victoria University of Wellington.

Harding, D. (2000) Making choices in childbirth, in Page, L. (ed.), *The New Midwifery: Science and Sensitivity in Practice,* London: Harcourt Publishers.

Health Services Consumer Research (2008) *Maternity Services Consumer Satisfaction Report,* Auckland: Health Services Consumer Research.

Health Workforce Advisory Committee (2005) *Fit for Purpose and for Practice: A Review of the Medical Workforce in New Zealand,* Wellington: Health Workforce Advisory Committee.

Katz Rothman, B. (1984) Childbirth management and medical monopoly: Midwifery as (almost) a profession, *Journal of Nurse-Midwifery* 29(5): 300–6.

Katz Rothman, B. (1991) *In Labour: Women and Power in the Birthplace,* New York: W.W. Norton.

Kedgley, S. (1996) *Mum's the Word: The Untold Story of Motherhood in New Zealand,* Auckland: Random House.

Kennedy, H.P. (1995) The essence of nurse-midwifery care: The woman's story, *Journal of Nurse-Midwifery* 40(5): 410–17.

Kennedy, H.P. (2000) A model of exemplary practice: Results of a Delphi study, *Journal of Midwifery and Women's Health* 45(1): 4–19.

Kennedy, H.P. (2002) The midwife as an 'instrument' of care, *American Journal of Public Health* 92(11): 1759–60.

Kennedy, H.P. (2004) The landscape of caring for women: A narrative study of midwifery practice, *Journal of Midwifery and Women's Health* 49(1): 4–19.

Kirkham, M. (2000) How can we relate? in Kirkham, M. (ed.), *The Midwife–Mother Relationship,* London: Macmillan.

McCourt, C. and Page, L. (1996) *Report on Evaluation of One-to-One Midwifery,* London: Thames Valley University, Centre for Midwifery Practice.

McCourt, C., Stevens, T., Sandall, J. and Brodie, P. (2006) Working with women: Developing continuity of care in practice, in Page, L.A. and McCandlish, R. (eds), *The New Midwifery: Science and Sensitivity in Practice,* 2nd edn, London: Churchill Livingstone.

Midwifery and Maternity Providers Organisation (2008) *Report on New Zealand's MMPO Midwives: Care Activities and Outcomes 2004,* Christchurch: New Zealand College of Midwives.

Midwifery Council of New Zealand (2004) *Midwifery Scope of Practice*, rwww. midwiferycouncil.org.nz/main/Scope/, accessed September 2008.

Midwifery Council of New Zealand (2008) Letter to midwives with updated Recertification Programme, unpublished.

Ministry of Health (2001) *Report on Maternity, 1999,* Wellington: Ministry of Health.

Ministry of Health (2003) *Maternity Services Consumer Satisfaction Survey,* Wellington: Ministry of Health.

National Health Committee (1999) *Review of Maternity Services in New Zealand,* Wellington: National Health Committee.

New Zealand College of Midwives (1992) *Midwives Handbook for Practice,* Christchurch: New Zealand College of Midwives.

New Zealand College of Midwives (2008) *Midwives Handbook for Practice,* Christchurch: New Zealand College of Midwives.

New Zealand Health Information Service (NZHIS) (2006) *Report on Maternity: Maternal and Newborn Information 2003,* Wellington: Ministry of Health.

New Zealand Health Information Service (NZHIS) (2007) *Report on Maternity: Maternal and Newborn Information 2004,* Wellington: Ministry of Health.

New Zealand Government (1990) *Nurses Amendment Act,* Wellington: Government Printer.

Page, L.A. (ed.) (2000) *The New Midwifery: Science and Sensitivity in Practice,* London: Harcourt Publishers

Page, L.A. (2003) One-to-one midwifery: Restoring the 'with woman' relationship in midwifery, *Journal of Midwifery and Women's Health* 48(2): 119–25.

Pairman, S. (1998) The Midwifery Partnership: An exploration of the midwife/woman relationship, unpublished master's thesis, Victoria University of Wellington.

Pairman, S. (2000) Women-centred midwifery: Partnerships or professional friendships? in Kirkham, M. (ed.), *The Midwife–Mother Relationship,* London: Macmillan.

Pairman, S. (2005a) Workforce to profession: An exploration of New Zealand midwifery's professionalising strategies from 1986 to 2005, unpublished doctoral thesis, University of Technology, Sydney.

Pairman, S. (2005b) From autonomy and back again: Educating midwives across a century, Part 1, *New Zealand College of Midwives Journal* 33(Oct.): 4–9.

Pairman, S. (2006) Midwifery partnership: Working 'with' women, in Page, L.A. and McCandlish, R. (eds), *The New Midwifery: Science and Sensitivity in Practice,* 2nd edn, Edinburgh: Churchill Livingstone.

Pairman, S. and McAra-Couper, J. (2006) Theroretical frameworks for midwifery practice, in Pairman, S., Pincombe, J., Thorogood, C. and Tracy, S. (eds), *Midwifery: Preparation for Practice,* Sydney: Elsevier.

Pelvin, B. (1990) Midwifery: The feminist profession, *Proceedings of the New Zealand College of Midwives National Conference,* Dunedin: New Zealand College of Midwives.

Prenderville, W.J., Elbourne, D. and McDonald, S. (2000) Active versus expectant management in the third stage of labour. Cochrane database of Systematic reviews 93) Art No: CD000007 DOI: 101002/14651858.

Ramsden, I. (1990) *Kawa Whakaruruhau: Cultural Safety in Nursing Education in Aotearoa,* Wellington: Ministry of Education.

Skinner, J. (1999) Midwifery partnership: Individualism, contracturalism or feminist praxis? *New Zealand College of Midwives Journal* 21: 18–20.

Strid, J. (1987) Maternity in revolt, *Broadsheet* 153: 14–17.

Tully, E. (1999) Doing professionalism differently: Negotiating midwifery autonomy in Aotearoa/New Zealand, unpublished doctoral thesis, University of Canterbury, New Zealand.

Walsh, D. (1999) An ethnographic study of women's experience of partnership caseload midwifery practice: The professional as a friend, *Midwifery* 15: 165–76.

CHAPTER 13

The Midwife as Container

MEG TAYLOR

This is not an academic work: it is what occurred to me when I considered the concept of the midwife–mother relationship. I am writing as a retired midwife and psychotherapist, the mother of two sons and with experience as a member and chair of my local Maternity Services Liaison Committee. I have been retired now for many years and am essentially housebound with multiple sclerosis, but I have maintained an interest through membership of the ukmidwifery egroup; I have a close friend who is a practising independent midwife; and I have a carer who had her first baby in November 2007. This gives me a particular viewpoint. I have some theoretical knowledge and I think that my distance from current practice might give me an advantageous perspective.

Between 1982 and 1987 I worked as a community midwife in a district in inner London. My work involved all aspects of midwifery, but in distinctly unequal proportions. I had two antenatal clinics a week in a local health centre and I made occasional antenatal home visits; I did very little intrapartum work because the part of London where I was working lacked that specific stratum of middle-class women who wanted home births, and domino births were only just beginning to be established there. There had not been any history locally of GPs providing cover for home births, unlike other pockets in north London (it was around this time that midwives who wanted to provide home births began to do so under the aegis of the local hospital maternity department rather than general practitioners). The greatest bulk of my work was providing postnatal care. There was very little continuity of care because, for geographical reasons, most women gave birth in a hospital outside my specific district. Although I might see the same women antenatally and postnatally, I missed a very important part of the process. I was frustrated about the lack of intrapartum work, but the area, like many in inner London, consisted of an ethnically diverse population comprising very affluent families, a well-established white working-class community with smaller subgroups of people from Caribbean and South Asian backgrounds, and some very poor people, including the homeless. While this cultural mix implies a lack of interest in home births (the affluent women had private obstetric care and the poorer women were quite happy to accept what was on offer), it certainly provided a lot of sociopolitical interest. While I would have liked more continuity and intrapartum work, especially home births, I appreciated the fact that the balance of my work was similar to that of childbearing women. We are pregnant for around 40 weeks, in labour for maybe 24 hours, but mothers for the rest of our lives.

I believed, and still believe, that postnatal work is very important. At the time the practice was that if any woman was at home within the first three days after giving birth she was visited twice a day, and then every day until the baby was ten days old. Most mothers and babies were discharged then into the care of the health visitor and GP, but we could continue to visit for up to 28 days if we considered either the mother or the baby needed it. Before I started working on the community I had worked in a central London hospital where, although I considered the labour ward procedures abysmal, the postnatal care was, I think, about as good as hospital postnatal care could be.

I was, and remain, a passionate supporter of breastfeeding and I devoted whatever time I felt necessary to supporting women in this. Breastfeeding produces nutrition which is ideally suited to a human child. Because of the inevitable physical closeness of mother and child and the way in which the child initiates the feed and responds to the mother's let-down reflex, the whole process is much more physically intimate and conversational than that of being bottle fed. It is the quality of this communication which, it is thought, contributes on a level other than merely the physiological to the child's subsequent neurological development (Schore, 1994; Sunderland 2006). This is one factor among numerous others affecting the better quality of health of breastfed babies; an improvement which lasts far longer than childhood.

The World Health Organization recommends that babies be given nothing but their own mother's milk for the first six months of life, with a gradual introduction of other foods during the second six months, and that breast milk remain a significant part of the diet until the child is at least two years old. In the context of a country where most babies are being fed formula by six weeks this advice may seem extreme, but in the world's population as a whole most babies are breastfed for between two and five years.

Given these advantages, if as part of postnatal care a midwife's work is to help the foundation and maintenance of breastfeeding, this, in itself, is profoundly important work. Because we live in a society where most babies are bottle fed, the advantages of breastfeeding are never adequately described in order to avoid alienating most mothers. Nevertheless, I maintain that breastfeeding is important not only physiologically, but because it enhances the quality of attachment, the quality of security which a child feels as its foundation psychologically and socially. What follows will suggest the profound importance of the quality of this primary attachment as the basis of subsequent mental health.

I soon noticed that a substantial part of my postnatal work was not the detection and treatment of pathology. It is true that there was quite a bit of this, particularly dealing with perineal breakdown. But in addition to supporting breastfeeding, I found I was listening to women talking about the pattern of their days and nights with a new baby, and I came to believe that this simple act of listening was in itself very important. While for first-time mothers the newness of this task is evident, even for mothers of subsequent babies it seemed necessary. The intensity of their involvement with their existing children seemed to mean that they had forgotten the reality of a newborn.

What was this listening providing for these mothers? Why did I come to feel that it was so important?

I was practising midwifery in a context where many first-time mothers had never held or seen a newborn baby. Much of my postnatal work was to reassure them that their experiences were normal. New mothers did not need to be poorly educated to be naive about this. I visited one couple where the father was a paediatric consultant and the mother an experienced paediatric nurse. Both were totally inexperienced in the ways of the normal newborn. Both needed the same kind and level of support and reassurance.

Before I became a midwife I had studied psychology for five years and had a first degree in social psychology and a Master's in psychopathology. As a student of psychology I was told that postnatally, new mothers were in a state unlike any other. Some authors referred to it as a critical period, others as a sensitive period. But whether critical or sensitive, the theorizing was that there was a specific window of opportunity for mother and baby to relate to each other with a strength and quality unique to this particular time. Midwifery tutors referred to this as' 'bonding". It was even occasionally referred to in clinical notes, although I was critical that this concept had not been sufficiently well understood and that a particular behavioural style was expected; this misunderstanding allowed opportunities for judgement and condemnation. For example, a mother may be described as "not bonding properly", but there was seldom any recommendation about how this situation, if indeed it was the case, may be improved. And it seemed that much maternity care fostered judgement and condemnation while precluding the conditions for autonomous relationships, either between professional and client or between mother and baby. Ironically, although the psychological theorizing was postulating an instinctive response, it seemed to me that the instinct must be based on autonomy.

In psychotherapy the word 'holding' is often used, as is the word 'container'. Both refer to something psychotherapists do for their clients: they apprehend and accept what is often feared and denigrated, and the simple fact of acceptance enables the client to live with what was previously felt to be intolerable. In this particular context the word 'holding' is especially pertinent. It might be said that the midwife metaphorically holds the mother so that she can both literally and metaphorically hold her baby. It is obvious that when women are in labour they need a high level of care and attention, but I think that a particular quality of attention continues to be required in the postnatal period. I think that when I was listening to the stories mothers were telling about their new experiences with their babies, I was providing this kind of holding.

I feel it is necessary to state something about the academic status of psychotherapeutic, and particularly psychodynamic and psychoanalytic, concepts. Within academic psychology such theories are frequently derided because they are considered unscientific. I agree that they are unscientific, although I do not think that this means that they are useless. Not all phenomena are amenable to scientific analysis and quantification. Some, such as the phenomenon of labour, are simply too complex and multifarious to be subdivided into the easily quantifiable. Others are just too subjective. An entomologist is clearly very different from his subject matter; this is not true of psychologists, sociologists or anthropologists. I think that psychodynamic concepts are useful because they offer an imaginative explanation of subjectivity and particularly irrationality. In the context of childbirth I think they are particularly relevant because they emphasize the strength and importance of early childhood experience and therefore imply a depth of importance to the mother–child relationship. They also therefore imply a commensurate importance to the work of the midwife. They also include the concept of the parallel process, and I shall be suggesting that the midwife–mother relationship is in some ways parallel to that of the mother and child. The particular psychodynamic concepts I shall be focusing on here are those of attachment theory and primary maternal preoccupation.

When I was an undergraduate we learnt the famous experiment of

Harlow's monkeys (Harlow, 1958). The rationale for this experiment was to test the behaviourist tenet, which now seems unbelievably naive to me, that the only positive reinforcements or rewards experienced by any animals, including humans, are those which meet very basic drives. In other words, we are only motivated by the most basic of instincts. Harlow disagreed with this and theorized that if he could demonstrate that animals other than humans can be motivated by needs other than the most basic, this must apply to human beings also. He took baby rhesus monkeys, separated them from their mothers and gave them two options. One was a wire contraption which provided milk and the other consisted of soft terry towelling. Both contraptions had pretend and very unconvincing faces with eyes. Behaviourist theory would predict that the baby monkeys would prefer the option which provided food. We were taught that the baby monkeys, while they would go to the milk-producing contraption when they were hungry, much preferred the terry towelling one; in other words they preferred the sense of tactile quality to that of being fed. I learnt this theoretically from a textbook, but later actually saw a film of the experiment and wept when I saw the terrified little monkeys desperately clinging to this lifeless and unresponsive pseudo-mother. When these baby monkeys grew up they were unable to rear their own young because they themselves had not been adequately mothered. They had been removed from their kinship group and therefore had not seen other adults mothering and, possibly more significantly, had not experienced being mothered subjectively themselves.

Attachment theory is based on the work of John Bowlby who, starting in the 1950s, wrote three books entitled *Attachment, Separation* and *Loss* (Bowlby, 1971, 1975, 1981). As his theorizing became more focused on the concept of attachment, he published a book called *A Secure Base* (Bowlby, 1988). His work was descriptive, essentially ethological. He maintained that babies need a single, primary carer with whom they develop a particularly strong relationship and that it is only after the development of such a relationship that they are able to tolerate separation without finding it traumatic. Of course, degrees of separation must be age appropriate: a separation of a few minutes is all that a newborn can tolerate; when children can walk they can mitigate separation by following their primary carer: it is noticeable how children can appear to be playing quite separately while their mother is in the room but as soon as she leaves, they will notice and follow her. As children grow older the length of separation which can be tolerated grows commensurately. Loss or bereavement, is unusual in childhood in affluent societies; but while it is statistically unusual, it is not abnormal in the sense of pathological.

For most children their primary carer is their mother. There will be important significant others in the immediate and extended family. In the West where small nuclear families are the norm, it is probable that the numerical extent of significant others is underestimated.

Feminists have strongly disapproved of Bowlby's theories. However, I always thought that this was unfair criticism. First, it seemed to me that all Bowlby was doing was describing an inevitable reality. It is only women who can gestate and give birth. Secondly, while other mothers can nurse an infant, and this is quite common in some societies, all mothers of newborns will produce milk and as an advocate of breastfeeding it therefore seemed appropriate that a child's primary carer should be his or her mother.

However, while attachment theory describes the setting up of secure foundations, it does not describe the parallel process that a midwife provides to a mother. For that I should like to evoke the work of Winnicott and the concept of primary maternal preoccupation (Winnicott, 1975).

Winnicott was a consultant paediatrician at Paddington Green Children's Hospital in central London. He used this work as the basis of his theory and practice as a psychoanalyst. Like Bowlby, his work was descriptive and ethological. The fact that Winnicott was a paediatrician, unlike most psychoanalysts who were either psychiatrists or neurologists, I consider very important. He was not dealing with children who were psychiatrically ill or whose families were particularly dysfunctional, and he therefore experienced a range of normal family environments unusual for a psychoanalyst. He is famous for his concept of 'good enough mothering', for his realistic description of a family environment where children experience their parents' human failings and, indeed, where such experiences are necessary for a child to develop a realistic sense of self and others.

When Winnicott described his concept of primary maternal preoccupation, he was referring not only to the critical or sensitive period immediately after childbirth, but to a longer period which starts during pregnancy when a mother begins to relate to her unborn baby. This relationship will involve fantasy to some extent and each woman's personal history and will alter irrevocably when the child is born. Yet Sigmund Freud saw that 'there is much more continuity between intra-uterine life and earliest infancy than the impressive caesura of the act of birth allows us to believe' (Freud, 1936: 109).

Psychoanalysts such as Winnicott, who focus on early experience and relationship, are referred to by the ugly term 'object-relations theorists' and their focus was on the psychic reality of young babies, but this reality does not include a concept of self separate from that of the other. The birth of the psyche could be considered to occur when the child is able, in Bowlby's terms, to tolerate separation. The length of this time will vary according to each individual relationship.

When Winnicott was writing about primary maternal preoccupation, he said that in any other context this degree of focus would be described as an illness (Winnicott, 1975). He did not elaborate because his concern was to demonstrate that primary maternal preoccupation was a normal part of new motherhood, but the psychiatric terms which occur to me are obsession, monomania and psychosis, in the sense of having loose boundaries to the self (Symington, 1986). Primary maternal preoccupation is not only normal in the sense of being statistically usual, it is positively healthy for the baby's subsequent development. It provides the maternal template on which the secure base is founded.

I should like to make some comments on Winnicott's use of the word 'illness'. He was clearly referring to psychiatric illness. I am critical of the medical model of both mental illness and childbirth. I do not believe that postnatal 'illness' can be reduced to the hormonal. While the fact of new motherhood is no doubt crucial, new motherhood involves more than just the hormonal; it involves the social, political and spiritual, to say nothing of each woman's personal history. I believe, on the basis of my own experience as a mother and a psychotherapist, that when mothers are dealing with children too young to speak they need to empathise on a non-verbal level, and that by doing so they relive on an unconscious level their own childhoods; when these have been problematic or traumatic they are more vulnerable to postnatal 'illness'.

There was an edition of the *AIMS Journal* (2007) in which mothers were saying that they felt they could not speak freely about their mental state to health professionals in case their children were taken into care. I think it is statistically normal for new mothers to have 'mad' thoughts. These thoughts are specific to new motherhood, but are rendered pathological by the fact that our society is not accepting of the state of primary maternal preoccupation. The mothers of new babies are socially isolated at a time when they are having to come to terms with this unique condition.

I should like to describe some of the mad thoughts I had when I first became a mother to illustrate which ones I think are intrinsic to the condition of motherhood and which ones I think are distinctly personal to me. It is a cliché of feminism that the personal is political and by being autobiographical here I would like to express the normality of these supposedly mad thoughts. By including the personal I think it should be possible to make similar distinctions for others.

When I gave birth to my older son I was a midwife; I was used to the phenomenon of birth; I understood newborn babies. None of this theoretical and practical knowledge prevented me from being shocked by the sight of my son. I was so used to experiencing him as a mobile being inside me and through palpitating myself that the distinction between the visual and tactile had never occurred to me. I had not been able to imagine him as separate from myself. He was evidently normal and healthy, but was so distinctly an individual: skinny, redheaded and half bald – and male. I had been convinced I was going to give birth to a dark-haired girl. Nowadays most women have scans which indicate the sex of their babies and it is my impression that most mothers are keen to know this in advance. I had not wanted this. I had not wanted a professional to tell me about my baby; I had wanted the uncertainty which would only be resolved at the time of birth. Even so, I was not able to apprehend the reality at all. Dealing with him initially was easy; I knew how to handle newborn babies. When he had problems latching on I took the advice I would have given any other new mother and it worked. Because I had mild relaxing remitting MS and knew that mothers with MS were most at risk of acute episodes postnatally, my partner had taken four weeks off work to support me and everything was happening within an intense bubble as I got to know the reality of living with a newborn. As soon as my partner went back to work, the bubble broke and I became terrified. I was terrified that I had now become totally vulnerable: the most precious thing in the world was outside me and it was my duty to protect him and the world seemed a terrifying place. He was born the day after *The Herald of Free Enterprise* had sunk off Zeebrugge harbour with massive loss of life – in fact, my waters had broken as I was watching the news bulletin. I found watching the television news intolerable. I found the world outside my house very frightening. When I went out I used to carry my son in a sling and I had fantasies of somebody running towards me and smashing his skull with some sharp object. My partner used to attend meetings of a particular political group and I was convinced he was going to be arrested under the Prevention of Terrorism Act, that he would go out and I would never see him again, that he would go out and I would not know when or whether he would return.

I think the shock of seeing your baby for the first time is very common, in spite of the way in which ultrasound tries to make visible what is internal and tactile. I think most new mothers are in a state of shock, both in the colloquial sense and in the psychological sense. Psychotherapists use the word 'shock' to describe a state different from but analogous to physical shock: with physical shock the body shuts down peripheral systems to maintain the viability of the vital core. With psychological shock the mind shuts off thoughts and perceptions which are threatening or irrelevant to the matter in hand and in this case the matter in hand is learning about one's new baby.

I think the degree of shock may relate to some extent to factors intrinsic to labour. My son was born two and half weeks early; maybe if my pregnancy had lasted 40 or 42 weeks I might have been better prepared psychologically for the sight of him. And I know that women who experience rapid labour also experience shock which, in that case, probably has a considerable physiological component. (I am not concerned here with psychological aspects of what is unusual or abnormal. Everything I write is intended to relate to what is within the bounds of the physiologically normal, in other words the province of midwifery expertise.)

I also think it is very common for new mothers to find the outside world threatening and to find themselves particularly sensitive to others. When I attended conferences of the Marce Society, it was a truism that postnatal depression was different from other sorts of depression because it included aspects of agoraphobia. And I think the way in which the boundaries of the self become fluid in pregnancy and new motherhood can often lead to unbearable empathy with others. In pregnancy one's body is accommodating a completely different human being in development, yet in the early stages this completely different person is utterly physically dependent on one. I remember as a student reading that psychoanalytic descriptions of pregnancy stress that the psychological task for the mother is first to accept the dependence and indivisibility of the relationship with the baby, and then to conceive of the baby as a separate being. This indivisibility is the basis of primary maternal preoccupation, attachment. If attachment is a state of specific hormonal as well as psychological characteristics, then I think the state of heightened empathy has a physical basis. (Maybe midwifery knowledge is that which integrates the hormonal and the emotional. Tricia Anderson was researching the relationship between oxytocin and trust.). I remember my partner delightedly telling me how much he was enjoying watching me fall in love with my baby: this is what the 'babymoon' is all about, and it is not specific to humans. It is well known that any mammal with a new offspring can be dangerous. I think that my fantasy of a lethal attack on my baby was possibly a reflection of my own capacity to defend him lethally if necessary.

'Mad' thoughts are not limited to the postnatal period. An article on antenatal depression in the *Guardian* (2008) quoted a number of women who considered their feelings and responses in pregnancy abnormal. One was so concerned about causing damage to her unborn child that she went from ensuring that she used no artificial chemicals in toiletries and make-up to feeling a need to go home and wash after a stranger had accidentally brushed against her while out shopping. This woman's previous pregnancy had ended in miscarriage. She went on insightfully to say, 'I knew I was being irrational, but the behaviour also seems logical to me. The fears were layered onto one another – the fear of harming the baby, the fear of the baby dying, the fear that I was going mad.' Another said, 'I have read that being pregnant is the closest you will ever get to the other side... with the soul inside of you straddling the worlds of darkness and light.'

Winnicott says that primary maternal preoccupation begins in pregnancy. I find both of the women quoted above perfectly comprehensible. The first's response was exaggerated terror, a concern which had been coloured by previous loss; and much compulsive behaviour is to do with cleanliness. It would be interesting to know whether this behaviour was cured by the birth of a healthy baby. The second is speaking from the position of 'psychosis' as psychoanalysts use the term, from the state where the boundaries of the self are loosened.

I think all the above is generic to primary maternal preoccupation. Adam Phillips in his book on Winnicott wrote: 'it was no longer sexuality or the death instinct that constituted the unacceptable in Winnicott's version of psychoanalysis, it was the early dependence and the terrors involved both its full acknowledgement and in its possible insufficiency' (Phillips, 1988). Early psychoanalytic theory articulated and made conscious what, at the time, was considered unacceptable. The reference to sexuality as something taboo is obvious; the reference to the death instinct is somewhat arcane and I would consider the word 'aggression' to be more appropriate. What early psychoanalytic theory did was to make clear that all of us embody sexuality and aggression, whether we choose to express this or not. Phillips here is emphasizing the total acknowledgement of dependency and its insufficiency. Much of the above can be seen in this light. Many new mothers' experience of shock is concerned with the realization that this baby needs looking after 24 hours a day, 7 days a week, 52 weeks a year. When I was a midwife I used to have discussions with health visitors about whether it was possible to tell pregnant women the reality of new motherhood. I was never sure and used to wonder whether the health visitors' certainty that it was impossible was because they didn't want to make the attempt. However, at the time I wasn't a mother. Recently one of my carers has had a baby. During her pregnancy I said that with a very small baby I had sometimes found it difficult to make time to brush my hair. She couldn't imagine that until after her baby was born.

Phillips is also describing the totality of this dependence as something which is somewhat taboo. I agree with this, but I also think there may be something culturally specific. I remember once going to pick up my older son from nursery school with his baby brother in a sling on my front and one of the other mothers said that she thought carrying a baby like that 'made them dependent'. I wondered what level of independence she thought a baby, only weeks old, was capable of. But we live in a culture where, if there is sufficient space, it is considered normal for new babies to sleep in separate rooms. There are other cultures where children will always be carried until they are capable of independent movement.

Winnicott is also famous for saying 'there is no such thing as a baby'. What he means is that a baby outside a caring relationship will die. This is the other part of the taboo Phillips is referring to. Mothers need to experience primary maternal preoccupation, to fall in love with their babies, in order to provide the constancy and intensity of this care without resentment.

What is specific to me concerns my experience of my father's death when I was eight. He had left one day and I never saw him again. When I became a mother my partner became a father and on an irrational level I had learnt that beloved fathers die. All of us hold this kind of irrational belief, but the content is unique to each of us and, I believe, influences the nature and course of each new mother's postnatal experience.

Adam Phillips referred to the insufficiency of dependence. My individual experience involved my father dying when I was eight. But I think that new parenthood generally evokes mortality: the realization of the vulnerability of the infant; the heightened empathy; the fact that the world is in many parts a dangerous place. What is specific to me gave the experience a certain flavour but did not, I think, alter the content.

While Western Europe is affluent and therefore has low maternal, neonatal and infant mortality rates within the global context, mothers and babies do still die and a zero mortality rate is unachievable. I do not think any woman undergoes pregnancy and childbirth without considering the possibility that either she or her baby might die. The quotation above from the *Guardian* where the pregnant mother is describing her condition as straddling both worlds is, I think, a metaphorical acknowledgement of this. And this is an appropriate thought which gives due regard to the enormity of the phenomenon: the creation of a genetically unique human being. If this implies that I believe the context of childbirth renders 'mad' thoughts normal, then that is correct and I would assert that Winnicott's reference to illness supports me here.

I believe that the end of primary maternal preoccupation occurs when the baby, who is no longer so young, can tolerate separation. However, this is also influenced by the mother's ability to tolerate separation and sometimes this can be pathologically difficult, depending on her own past experiences.

I realize that I am conflating Winnicott's description of primary maternal preoccupation with attachment theory, but to me they are both describing the same phenomenon from different perspectives and this conflation is therefore intellectually economical.

Winnicott is here describing pregnancy, childbirth and the postnatal period from the mother's perspective. He also described birth from an imagined perspective of the baby. He said that in normal childbirth babies feel as though they are initiating the process. Nobody knows exactly how labour is triggered, but it is thought that some mechanism, probably hormonal, within the foeto-placental unit is responsible and so there is a sense in which the baby really does trigger the process. Nevertheless, I think Winnicott was talking about something different. In my view he was contrasting his imagined perspective with one more normally described, whereby the baby is overwhelmed and endangered by the process of birth. Winnicott was suggesting the possibility that since in normal labour the contractions are rhythmic and regular, the baby may come to anticipate and respond to the regularity, may even find the process exhilarating rather than threatening, may even find the regular pressure of the birth canal and the subsequent release pleasurable. Just as this is imaginary and unprovable, so my interpretation is also personal. But the rhetoric of childbirth which is framed in terms of damage and danger is also politically driven and emotive rather than scientific.

The word 'regression' can be used in two senses. Janet Balaskas (1991) means it in one sense when she writes:

> in the hours of labour you will want to withdraw from the normal day-to-day level of things and your attention will naturally turn inwards, as if the whole world contracts to what is happening in your body. In your mind, time takes on a fresh dimension. Hours can pass in what seems like minutes. It is like being in another world... this great opening of the womb happens only a few times in your life. It is a very deep emotional experience which involves a regression to your most basic and primitive feelings. (Balaskas 1991: 91)

What she means here is leaving behind the normal state of everyday consciousness. When she is writing about active birth, she is describing a state of being in labour which will enable the woman to respond instinctively to her body's promptings such that she is more easily able to avoid pharmacological analgesia. If women in labour are to be able to do this, rational thought is an impediment. It is the function of the midwife to take on that aspect for the woman. Regression in this sense means regression from an ostensible state of civilization to a return to the animal. In these circumstances the midwife can be said in psychotherapeutic terms to be holding the boundaries, to be creating a safe space in which the mother can trust that someone else can deal with the practicalities of everyday life. Mothers and other carers do this for young children because they are physically and intellectually incapable of doing it for themselves. In this sense, although the labouring woman is performing a profoundly adult act, the regression she is experiencing is similar to that most often meant when the word is used to mean a return to the infantile. If it is the case that the mother of a new baby relives her own babyhood in order to empathise with and understand her child, and if it is one function of primary maternal preoccupation to be in this state, then on one level all of a midwife's clients will be regressed to some extent.

Bowlby wrote of attachment, which is quite a cold and mechanical word. Winnicott wrote more emotionally from both the mother's and the baby's point of view. Sheila Ernst (1987) also wrote from the point of view of both the mother and the baby, but she used quite an extreme word: 'merging'. Psychotherapists may refer to clients being still in an unhealthy state of merger with the mother. When Sheila Ernst was writing in this way about merging she was deliberately giving a feminist interpretation to what was generally perceived as something pathological. She was implying that the intense closeness of the mother–newborn relationship was not unhealthy, but is in fact the foundation for later mental health. She says that if a child is to achieve a healthy state of separation, there needs to have been an initial total merger. If a mother is merged with her newborn she must, by definition, be in a regressed state. It is possible that the metaphorical holding by the midwife of the mother in labour can make it easier for her to achieve and feel comfortable in this state afterwards.

Some women's experience of labour may be a precipitant of later problems, or a contributor to them. For example, a sense of having been traumatized in labour may exacerbate subsequent problems; a sense of having lost control may be particularly relevant in cases of previous physical or sexual abuse. However, it is also the case that experience of labour can be healing. This is very individual. What may seem objectively intolerable to me may be experienced by the woman as helpful. It may be the mere fact of having been the focus of caring attention for a number of hours, as the mother must focus many subsequent hours of caring attention on her baby, or labour may be experienced as physically cathartic.

Labour tends not to be seen in these terms: it is usually described in terms of the biomedical, and psychotherapists do not have the experience of being with women in labour to inform their discourse. The power of labour to influence the quality of the mother's subsequent relationship with her baby is, I believe, underestimated for these reasons and this underestimation to some extent determines how resources and care are delivered.

I feel that psychology, when it applies itself to childbirth, does not take certain factors into account. I have been a member of the Society for Reproductive and Infant Psychology for 28 years and have seen every one of its journals during that time. Since I qualified as a midwife in 1980 I have done some work in every aspect of women's reproductive life. On the whole, when I read journal articles looking at the psychology of any aspect of this, it seemed to me that two things were seriously underestimated: the power of the phenomenon of labour and the power of the institution. I will deal with the institutional power below.

I think that some midwives take refuge in fragmentation in order specifically to avoid the power of labour. The midwife–mother relationship is therefore attenuated, and it is possible that the mother–baby relationship is also reduced. Certainly Michel Odent thinks that this is the case in many cultures worldwide, including those of the West, when it comes to practices in the third stage of labour which involve separating the mother and baby or hastening the process. He believes that this reduces the level of oxytocin output and therefore the intensity of the immediate attachment (Odent, 2004).

It is obvious how a midwife can provide a powerful quasi-psychotherapeutic holding for a woman in labour, but I maintain also that when, as a community midwife, I was listening to mothers tell their stories of the early days, I was also metaphorically holding them in this state of merger, assuring them that it was normal and healthy and that it was not going to last for ever.

So, I do think that a midwife can be a container in the sense of holding the space for a woman in labour and providing metaphorical holding through the intensity of primary maternal preoccupation, or at least its most intense initial phase. Nevertheless, I maintain that there are powerful institutional pressures militating against midwives adopting this role.

When I was working as a community midwife that level of postnatal support was taken completely for granted; there were many midwives who believed that they were under a legal obligation to visit a new mother daily for ten days. But although this was taken for granted in Britain it was unusual internationally. I remember wondering with some incredulity about the situation in the United States where there was no state-provided postnatal support. It was quite normal at the time for radical midwives in the UK to look with some envy at the Netherlands, where midwives had higher status and were self-employed and there was a home birth rate, at that time, of well over 50 per cent. In the Netherlands the normal pattern of postnatal support then was for a maternity nurse to live in the home for some time and for midwives to take no further part in postnatal care. This system was not as advantageous as it seemed because the maternity nurses, in some cases, supported the mother by bottle feeding the baby. However, postnatal support in the UK was taken so seriously that, when I started training in 1978, I was taught that local authorities were under a legal obligation to provide a home help for the first ten postnatal days if the mother was not adequately supported by her family. I must say that I never knew this to occur and the legal obligation soon evaporated under the pressure of financial constraints.

All this seems very alien now. It is my impression that, in some areas, postnatal visits are limited to one on day seven for neonatal screening and this visit may be made by a maternity care assistant. Maternity care seems very fragmented to me. There are not enough midwives. It is my opinion that best practice, as judged on almost every criterion, is provided by independent midwives and case-holding practices and that continuity of carer is intrinsic to this. If midwives are to provide the parallel process of containment, this continuity allows them to be there at the beginning of primary maternal preoccupation in pregnancy and through the intense climax of labour and birth. And if midwives are to be able to provide this they need to be given their due reward both financially and in terms of status as independent practitioners, equivalent to but very different from obstetric consultants.

When I became a midwife I had the idea that midwifery could be a kind of preventive psychotherapy, that by providing care of the highest standard the midwife could enhance the quality of the mother's relationship with her baby and, because this relationship is the foundation of later mental health, the baby's mental health would inevitably be affected for the better. This idea soon came to seem naive when I realized the extent to which I had underestimated the power of the institutions which dominate childbearing. When I was a student of social psychology our main textbook was *Social Psychology* by Roger Brown (1965). Much of this was concerned with research on conformity and compliance which had been conducted in the aftermath of the Second World War in an attempt to understand how Europe had been in thrall to Fascism in an attempt to prevent the horrors, particularly of Nazism, ever happening again. The tenor of this research demonstrates that people are prone to obedience and compliance if the authority of the institution is sufficiently powerful. This obedience can manifest comparatively easily as behaviour which is abusive.

When Stanley Milgram devised an experiment on obedience (Milgram, 1974), an experimental subject was seated at a table with two stooges, one performing the role of an authoritative scientist wearing a white coat and the other a pretend experimental subject. The real, innocent subject was told that the experiment was an attempt to investigate the role of punishment on learning. The authoritative scientist would give the pretend subject questions and, when he made an error in responding, order the innocent subject to administer an electric shock. In fact, no real electric shocks were administered; both stooges were acting. A significant number of real, innocent subjects would administer electric shocks even when the pretend subject was showing a degree of pain, even when a dial on the table reached a level marked 'danger' in red. The experiment was designed explicitly to test the extent to which ordinary people would obey orders even when this ostensibly involved doing something counter to their principles. The initial experiment, which became very famous, was carried out at a time when the Nazi war criminal Adolf Eichmann was on trial in Israel and questioned whether perpetrators of the Nazi Holocaust were also merely obeying orders. Milgram was sued by some of the real subjects, who claimed they had been traumatized by the experiment and that it was unethical. In spite of the notoriety of this experiment, its results have never been subjectively taken on board in real-life situations where authoritative people administer orders to those lower than them in the hierarchy.

Another example of this was provided by Philip Zimbardo in the Stamford experiment conducted in 1971. Psychology students were allocated at random to one of two categories, that of prison guard or inmate. Within a week those who had been designated inmates were experiencing severe psychological distress as a result of incarceration, while those designated guards had developed abusive behaviour analogous to that which has been demonstrated by Allied forces in the Iraq war.

It may seem an exaggeration to compare medical institutions with prisons, but it is a comparison which has seemed blatant and legitimate to me since I was a student midwife. There is a clear hierarchy: doctor; para-medical staff such as physiotherapists and radiographers; midwives and nurses; students, although the position of medical students may be slightly higher up the hierarchy; and most definitely at the bottom is that of patient. There is an expectation that those higher in the hierarchy instruct those lower. Theoretically, any procedure carried out without informed consent is assault. In practice, true informed consent is rare. I have seen cases of bullying at all levels, including those of women at their most vulnerable, in labour. However much midwives are taught that they should communicate with the women they care for and that their care should be based on informed consent, it seems that they prefer to concede the authority of the obstetricians and institutional procedures. Hierarchy, obedience and fragmentation of care are usually to the psycho-logical benefit of the professional, not the client.

We live in a fragmented and unhealthy society. Within the last year two teenagers have been killed in my neighbourhood, one less than half a mile away, the other known to both my sons as a fellow school student. I think we are in a situation analogous to that of Harlow's monkeys, who could not mother their own young because they had neither been adequately mothered themselves nor been exposed in their kinship groups to other mothers' mothering. I became a midwife because I thought that it might offer a kind of preventive psychother-apy. Then, when I was working in the field, I thought this intention very naive because I was impressed by the power of institutional structures. I do not think that the provision of good-quality postnatal care in the context of continuity of care can allay social breakdown. I do think that the fragmentation and undervaluing of maternity care form another symptom of this social breakdown.

However, I am reluctant completely to ditch my intuition that midwifery could indeed be a preventive psychotherapy. To me, the psychoanalytic theorizing around this indicates that the midwife could be a container, holding the boundaries for the mother to hold her baby metaphorically as well as literally. The fragmentation of care, the low status and the inadequate number of midwives indicate the low status of motherhood generally. In my view this low status and social pathology are not coincidental. But if it were to be the case that midwifery could prop-erly fulfil its function by providing holistic care at this uniquely powerful time of transition, a considerable level of social change would be needed, requiring a higher status to be accorded to both midwifery and mother-hood.

References

AIMS Journal (2007) Issue on Birth Trauma, 19(1).

Balaskas, J. (1991) *New Active Birth*, London: HarperCollins.

Bowlby, J. (1971) *Attachment*, Harmondsworth: Penguin.

Bowlby, J. (1975) *Separation*, Harmondsworth: Penguin.

Bowlby, J. (1981) *Loss*, Harmondsworth: Penguin.

Bowlby, J. (1988) *A Secure Base*, New York: Basic Books.

Brown, R. (1965) S*ocial Psychology*, London: Routledge.

Ernst, S. (1987) Can a daughter be a woman? Women's identity and psychological separation, in Ernst, S. and Maguire, M. (eds), *Living with the Sphinx: Papers from the Women's Therapy Centre*, London, Women's Press.

Freud, S. (1936) *Inhibitions, Symptoms and Anxiety*, London: Hogarth Press.

Guardian (2008) I felt completely out of control, G2 29 Jan., www.guardian.co.uk/lifestyle/2008/jan/29/healthandwellbeing.mentalhealth, accessed March 2010.

Harlow, H. (1958) The nature of love, *American Psychologist* 13: 673–85.

Milgram, S. (1974) *Obedience to Authority: An Experimental View*, London: Tavistock.

Odent, M. (2004) Paper given at Psychoanalysis and Midwifery Conference, London, Freud Society, December.

Phillips, A. (1988) *Winnicott*, London: Fontana Modern Masters.

Schore, A.N. (1994) *Affect Regulation and the Origin of the Self: The Neurobiology of Emotional Development*, Hillsdale, NJ: Lawrence Erlbaum.

Sunderland, M. (2006) *The Science of Parenting*, London: Dorling Kindersley.

Symington, N. (1986) *The Analytic Experience*, London: Free Association Books.

Winnicott, D.W. (1975) Primary maternal preoccupation, in Winnicott, D.W., *Through Paediatrics to Psychoanalysis*, London: Hogarth Press, originally published in *Collected Papers*, 1958.

Zimbardo, www.prisonexp.org/, accessed March 2010.

CHAPTER 14

We Need to Relate

MAVIS KIRKHAM

The midwife–mother relationship lies at the heart of maternity care and this book shows the positive potential of that relationship for all concerned. Nevertheless, there is much about modern maternity care which is experienced as alienating by many midwives and childbearing women; a strange situation for work so fundamentally creative.

The setting and the problem

The midwife is traditionally 'with woman' in the singular, but for many years now the care of individuals has been contained within the more immediate priorities of the hierarchical organization which employs her. There is a real tension between the priorities of providing the best possible care for a known individual and the efficient running of an organization (see Chapter 1). This can create conflicting loyalties for midwives and tremendous headaches for midwifery managers.

There is a lot of fear around birth. We live in a 'risk society' (Beck, 1992) where risk assessment is used as an instrument of social control by instilling fear of not following expert advice, though expert claims to safer care have been used for centuries as a means of 'forging the phantom of incapacity' (Nihell, 1760) in midwives and mothers. Obstetricians and midwives are fearful too (Kirkham and Stapleton, 2001): fearful of litigation and of not doing things right, or of doing them right but not documenting them correctly, or of offending power-holders, be they consultants or senior managers. In hierarchical organizations the response to risks is to manage events more closely and create more rules as to how things should be managed, and thus the opportunities to get things wrong proliferate.

Now I am an old midwife, I am often telephoned by anxious younger colleagues who wish to talk through a clinical incident. It strikes me how many of these conversations focus on worries about not having done the right thing in administrative terms, but they rarely concern the care actually given to the mother. It is amazing how often a midwife can give good care and still worry that she has done the wrong thing or 'missed something' in terms of record keeping or administration. Nevertheless, midwives do worry about not having time to listen to women's concerns (Dykes, 2009).

Centralization and scale

The centralization of maternity services into large hospitals means that most women do not feel that they are at home or on their own territory or even in their own area when having their baby. If services are also fragmented, there is no one with whom the women can link or make a meaningful relationship. If midwives are required to rotate around all departments of a hospital and are continually moved to fill the gaps where staff shortages are greatest, they are unable to develop collegial relationships or a meaningful work context (Ball *et al.*, 2002; Dykes, 2009). Both mothers and midwives find these situations unsettling and unrewarding.

Ruth Deery and Billie Hunter (Chapter 3) describe 'large maternity units where some midwives become obedient technicians in order to cope with whatever the working day throws at them'. Obedient technicians 'have no control over their working environment because they engage in production line work' nor do the mothers on the 'production line' (Dykes, 2006) experience control over their efforts and activities.

There are tensions in large maternity services between the organizational need to craft systems which are efficient across the whole organization and the need of individual midwives to craft their relationships with individual clients to best suit that client's situation and needs (Sennett, 2008).

With the centralization of services, the resulting very large units need to emphasize systems and their management. A great deal of work has been done to improve systems of care in recent years. Usually this work starts from the blockages within the existing fragmented and industrial model of care. Triage is a good example of such an innovation. Originally developed to prioritize battlefield casualties, triage is now accepted practice to filter admissions to large labour wards. Where the labour ward is the mother's only point of contact with the service, 'inappropriate admissions' are inevitable and triage is helpful. It is logical then to develop telephone triage and it is reasonable to expect that 'demand and patient flow is better managed following the introduction of the telephone triage service'

(Cherry *et al.*, 2009: 496). Mothers will benefit from talking to a specialist telephone triage midwife, rather than a busy labour ward midwife who just happened to be dashing past the phone when it rang. Yet how much better if the mother could speak to a midwife she knew and who knew her, where their ongoing relationship informed and was enhanced by that conversation?

How did we move from being with woman to managing 'demand and patient flow'? This has created a situation in which each improvement in the service further fragments a woman's care. How did the word 'patient' slip back into midwifery vocabulary, where it was taboo for a generation? This probably occurred when it came to be followed by the organizational word 'flow'.

The power of the flow

I have been pondering the concept of 'flow' in maternity care for some years now. I was first made aware of this concept when we were evaluating the MIDIRS Informed Choice Leaflets (Kirkham and Stapleton, 2001). The majority of the midwives involved with that large study appeared to 'go with the flow' of obstetric and managerial opinion 'because it made life easier' (Stapleton *et al.*, 2002: 607). This had a divisive effect on relationships, which could be reflected in horizontal violence towards those who did not conform. Midwives certainly ensured that the vast majority of women made what were seen locally as the 'right' choices. A minority of midwives did go against the flow and some excellent care was observed around the facilitation of informed choice. However, this was the work of individuals rather than the strategy in any unit, and these individuals were vulnerable with regard to both the institutional hierarchy and their conforming colleagues.

Midwives have adapted to the power structures within which they have worked. As employees, midwives have received orders from their employers and given orders to their 'patients'. As Mary Cronk (Chapter 4) and Tricia Anderson (Chapter 7) describe, such a situation led midwives to treat women as children. This was not surprising, as that was the treatment they were themselves receiving. The dominance of midwifery by medicine, and more recently by management, has led midwives to cope by internalizing the values of the power-holders, rather than the traditions and values of their own group (Heagarty, 1996; Roberts, 1983). This is the behaviour of an oppressed group (Freire, 1972). In such circumstances there is much pressure to internalize oppressive values and a tendency to act them out on colleagues and clients (Leap, 1997; Stapleton *et al.*, 1998).

Once one is aware of 'flow' in this sense, it is all around, in the institutional weight carried by authoritative knowledge and the accepted rules of standardized practice, as well as the hospital-wide management concept of 'patient flow'. Such a flow, though organizationally smooth, may represent a strong undertow for mothers as they struggle to negotiate their agency (see Chapter 6).

Although I find the power of the organizational flow very worrying, the word can also be used in a positive, individual sense. Individuals have challenged the organizational flow and brought about change. Some individuals have achieved much by their sustained commitment: Nicky Leap has demonstrated what midwives can achieve in London and in Australia and her work has achieved a momentum which endures and grows. Lesley Page's career-long commitment to continuity of care has had a considerable impact on policy and practice in several countries. Alliances of mothers and midwives brought midwifery back from near extinction in New Zealand (see Chapter 12) and hard work by a dedicated body of women has brought real change onto the legislative agenda in Australia at the time of writing (see Hansard Sydney, 2009). Commitment can attract those similarly committed and the flow of practice can change. Independent midwives have kept torches burning and shown what is possible for many years. In New Zealand they are now lead maternity practitioners alongside their medical colleagues and in England independent midwifery care within the NHS could be achieved in the near future (see Chapter 4 and below). Like-minded colleague support is essential and modern communications help; what used to be achieved in national meetings of the Association of Radical Midwives is now achieved daily via the internet. Yet we live in an age when political commitment is lessening and creating a counter-flow takes long, sustained effort.

In a magazine concerning the very different, but still counter-cultural practice of smallholding, I read recently of 'The Flow' as a positive current which we can create and from which we can benefit:

The Flow doesn't seem to work if you wait for it passively; it only works when you are actively pursuing something, seeking opportunities and advice... There is strong evidence in the field of psychology that a positive, outward-looking projection of ideas encourages a more constructive and helpful response from others, a feedback effect that supports and reinforces the advantages of a positive approach. Perhaps The Flow results from the broader projection of a ripple effect, spreading beyond those with whom you are in personal contact to reach and affect a wider audience? (Beat and Beat, 2009: 40)

The ripple effects of positive birthing experiences are discussed in Chapter 6. This quotation also fits my experience as a midwife. Ruth Deery and Billie Hunter explore 'enhancing experiences' and conclude that for midwives' professional experience to be enhancing, a degree of individual autonomy and a 'meaningful relationship' with the client are needed. They conclude that 'there is something in this autonomous use of the self that is pleasurable and satisfying in itself' (Chapter 3). This is exactly what Daniel Goldman described in his book *Emotional Intelligence*:

> Flow is a state of self-forgetfulness... people in flow are so absorbed in the task at hand that they lose all self-consciousness... In this sense moments of flow are egoless. Paradoxically, people in flow exhibit a masterly control of what they are doing, their responses perfectly attuned to the changing demands of the task. And although people perform at their peak while in flow, they are unconcerned with how they are doing... the sheer pleasure of the act itself is what motivates them. (Goleman, 1995: 91)

Such engagement is immensely satisfying for all concerned. It is more complex in midwifery, where it is achieved through a relationship, than in other forms of work. It is the essence of job satisfaction and can have a very positive ripple effect on colleagues. Such flow is the opposite of the worker's experience of bureaucracy (Lipsky, 1980). It requires a degree of autonomy and mutual trust which many midwives rarely experience at work. Yet even in the midst of fragmentation and constant requirements to check rather than listen, such positive flow can appear and when it does it sustains us as midwives.

Relationships and solutions

Relationships and trust

It is clear that mothers and midwives seek to relate well as individuals. Such relationships, grounded in mutual trust, help mothers and increase midwives' job satisfaction; these are the threads which run throughout this book. Where the mother feels safely 'held' by her midwife, this can facilitate the establishment of a positive relationship between the mother and her baby (Chapter 13) and enhance her longer-term confidence as a mother (see Chapters 4 and 6).

Within relationships, trust must rest on common values. This is not to say that it is essential for the midwife and mother to have a common view-point, but the midwife must be aware of, and able to offer respect for and support within, the mother's values and priorities. In this situation, the mother feels that she is acknowledged and valued; she feels safe in the relationship. The midwife can make the woman 'feel special' (Chapters 5 and 12). She can also 'give' (see Chapter 2) what the woman seeks and defines, rather than what the midwife assumes will be best for her.

This is a long way from the professional expert, who knows best, treat-ing the mother like a child (Chapter 4). Even in the most difficult of circumstances, there is integrity in treating each other as adults, whatever the constraints. I have occasionally, and in more than one country, witnessed conversations between midwives and mothers where there was real trust between them as individuals, but where the mother did not trust the maternity services and intended to give birth without professional attendants. Such conversations are respectful and highly educational, though sad. The midwife understands the woman's viewpoint, but feels she cannot accompany the woman on her chosen path for fear of losing her employment or her registration. Thus the boundaries of being 'with woman' are mapped but relationships are kept open.

Listening and being heard

It is fundamental in any relationship that we are heard. Yet so many stud-ies report how women respect midwives' busyness and 'don't like to ask'. Overstretched midwives, working in systems where care is fragmented, see little point in really listening to women whom they will not meet again and are seen by women as 'checking not listening' (Chapter 6; Kirkham and Stapleton, 2001). They have 'no time to care' (Dykes, 2009: 90).

Being heard validates and affirms us. It is undoubtedly what women want, whether they are poor and disadvantaged (Chapter 8), at increased obstetric risk (Chapter 10), Pakistani Muslims (Chapter 9) or midwives themselves (Kirkham *et al.*, 2006). Care which is formulaic, even if it is also smiley (Chapter 6), is organized so as to prevent midwives listening to women, and thereby prevents a relationship, with all its positive poten-tial. So often midwives, giving fragmented care, pressed for time and unheard themselves, dash through their working day.

To stop and ponder would invite trouble; survival meant keeping on top, moving on the surface. To stop was to sink, so like waterboatmen on a pond, staying on top was not to stay anywhere for long. (Davies, 2000: 129)

The waterboatman theory, developed to understand the behaviour of impoverished women, fits midwives in many settings very well. Such 'keeping on top', with attention to prescribed tasks rather than to the concerns of individuals, prevents midwives from hearing women's concerns. It also prevents women from voicing their needs, out of sympathy with the midwife who is 'so busy'. This coping strategy therefore robs midwives of job satisfaction and women of the possibility of being heard and feeling affirmed. It is the opposite of the positive flow described above. Yet the need to cope remains, and such ways of coping are responses to how maternity care is organized.

Reciprocity

Threads of reciprocity and mutuality run throughout this book. Reciprocity is the 'central ingredient' in mutually meaningful relationships (Chapter 3). 'Embracing uncertainty together' (Chapter 2), can ensure that 'the ideal caring relationship is expressed as a mutual process between the midwife and the pregnant woman' (Chapter 10), even when a great deal of medical care is needed. 'Trust needs to be reciprocal' (Chapter 10) in order for the woman to 'feel safe enough to let go' (Chapter 7) and trust her own power to birth her baby or to 'promote a feeling of being in control, even when health professionals guide the process' (Chapter 10).

Reciprocal trust enhances the equality of the partners in a relationship. This is demonstrated in the nature of the New Zealand concept of midwifery partnership. The resulting 'professional friendship', focused on the childbearing woman's needs and so very different from a 'friendly professional' focused on a professional agenda (see Chapter 6), thus makes possible professionalism without dominance (Chapter 12).

Reciprocity and mutuality are words which have been used less in recent years. Perhaps they will fade from our vocabulary, like convalescence and lying-in. Such words make explicit dependence; another word which does not fit comfortably in our modern vocabulary. 'But shame about dependence has a practical consequence. It erodes mutual trust and commitment, and the lack of these social bonds threatens any collective enterprise' (Sennett, 1998: 141). Birth is surely a collective social enterprise. As midwives, we need mothers just as much as they need us. When systems are organized to process patients, rather than to care for individual mothers, we all suffer because we cannot relate.

Within a hierarchical model of maternity care, it is hard to trust mothers when midwives feel themselves to be controlled rather than trusted. Similarly, it is hard to facilitate clients in exercising skills that midwives have not had the opportunity to exercise themselves. Midwives cannot empower women where they themselves feel disempowered.

'To restore trust in others is a reflexive act; it requires less fear of vulnerability in oneself. But this reflexive act has a social context' (Sennett, 1998: 142). The social context of most midwives is one in which reciprocity can lead to mutual disempowerment. Despite policy statements which expect midwives to support women in exercising choice (see Chapter 1), we increasingly lack the opportunity to exercise choice and control or to have experienced facilitation in our work and thereby to have developed the necessary skills. This leaves us very vulnerable and makes us unwilling to give up what power we have. It is noteworthy that strong mutual support among midwives is found in just those situations where midwives have most autonomy and least hierarchical pressures: independent midwifery (van der Kooy, 2009), caseload midwifery (McCourt and Stevens, 2009) and small midwife-led units (Kirkham 2003; Walsh, 2007).

It is a brave midwifery manager who changes the organization of her unit to promote relationships between midwives and mothers, thus increasing her midwives' loyalty to their clients rather than to their employer (Brodie, 1996). She is expected to echo the rest of the hospital's industrial model of care with obedient technicians and midwives who can be continually moved to plug the gaps in the service. Managers too need to feel safe enough to let go of tight control and trust their midwives, but general management gives them little preparation or role models for such reciprocal relationships down the hierarchy.

Balance and integration

There is a thread throughout this book of midwives holding the balance, both within ourselves and within our relationships.

Keeping our own balance

Ruth Deery and Billie Hunter examine midwives balancing engagement and detachment (Chapter 3). Maintaining this balance is a crucial part of the emotional labour of midwifery care in any context. This may be a degree of midwifery detachment in order to facilitate greater involvement by family and friends, as described in Chapter 2, or deciding between self-disclosure and non-disclosure or even fiction in an intense but one-off meeting when caring for a woman in labour, (see Chapter 11), or resorting to formulaic care when undertaking a rushed postnatal visit (see Chapter 9).

Balancing engagement and detachment is essential for our own emotional well-being as midwives and as people. It is also important in order that our clients can exercise autonomy and not feel overdependent on us. The balance is dynamic and changes with time. Our skills in such a balance should develop as we learn and find new mentors and role models. Yet so many of the ways of coping that we see around us, such as waterboatman behaviour (Davies, 2000) or stereotyping women (Kirkham *et al.*, 2002) or fragmented care (Menzies Lyth, 1988) or dissociation (Garrett, 2008), serve to unbalance us in the long term, taking the pleasure out of the job and depriving women of our focused attention and listening. Relationship gives satisfaction and confidence to mothers and midwives; yet most of our coping reactions, whilst saving time and defending us from anxiety, also 'defend' us from relationships and thereby impoverish all concerned.

Colleague support is very important to midwives (Kirkham and Morgan, 2006; Kirkham *et al.*, 2006) and helps us keep our balance through life's ups and downs. Such support can be lacking in stressed and busy workplaces where negative coping skills abound. Skills of mutual support can be taught (e.g. Kirkham, 2004) where their value is appreciated by those who hold the educational agenda. They can also be observed where midwives have some autonomy and are supported in their turn by good relationships with mothers (see above). We can also learn from the new literature on emotion work in midwifery. An excellent starting point for such reading is *Emotions in Midwifery and Reproduction*, edited by Billie Hunter and Ruth Deery (2009), who have both done research in this area.

Holding the balance for women in our care

Midwives balance women's wishes with the requirements of their continuing relationships with colleagues and the smooth running of the organizational unit (Kirkham and Stapleton, 2001; Stapleton *et al.*, 2002). Val Levy (1998, 1999) saw this as a precarious balance, which she portrayed as a midwife walking a tightrope. The midwives she studied used 'protective steering' to protect women in their care, as well as themselves, when choices were made. To do this they had to make assumptions about women:

These assumptions could be revised at a later stage if the midwife gained knowledge of the woman as an individual. Unfortunately, if the midwife and woman only met once (as was probable in the obstetric consultant antenatal clinic) the interaction was unlikely to move beyond the level of stereotype. (Levy, 1999: 107)

The midwives sought to protect these women from a range of potential stressors, including some created by the organizational context of their care, such as limited time and resources (Levy, 1999)

Marie Berg speaks of midwives balancing natural and medical perspectives, keeping the natural perspective open in medically complex situations (Chapter 10). Since 'the proportion of women defined as at high risk is constantly increasing' (Berg, 2002: 54) and identification of obstetric risk is bound to increase feelings of vulnerability:

During obstetrically complicated childbirth it is essential for the women to be recognised and affirmed as genuine subjects. Like women with normal pregnancy and childbirth, they need an emotionally present midwife who sees, supports and inspires self confidence. (Berg, 2002: 54)

Keeping awareness of the balance between what professionals can do and what the woman herself can do becomes more important as medical intervention increases and when women are particularly likely to feel powerless. This is one reason continuity of carer, with the consequent potential for the development of the midwife—mother relationship over time, is seen as particularly important for young and disadvantaged women, as well as those at high obstetric risk (Homer *et al.*, 2008; McCourt and Stevens, 2009)

So much of this book is about keeping options open in the face of pressure to close them or to control women's experience. This requires considerable awareness and skill. Mary Cronk describes how we can craft our use of words to hold conversations with childbearing women as equals, not as overpowering experts (Chapter 4). Since the current default position within health services places power with professionals, the impetus to correct this situation must come from us, as those professionals. Once we start to make moves to correct power imbalances, women will trust us and help us. There are so many examples in this book of women's need for and appreciation of having their voices heard and their concerns acted on.

Holding safe space

Beyond balance there is the work of integration which the skilled midwife can do much to facilitate. Midwives can hold a safe space in which women can forge relationships and can give birth to their babies. This can start with friendship building in antenatal groups where women learn from and grow to support each other (Chapter 2). It becomes vital in labour, where the woman needs to feel safe enough to 'enter an altered state of consciousness' in which the mind can let go and allow the body to be in control (Chapter 7). This can be termed 'regression', in that 'rational thought is an impediment in labour' and 'it is the function of the midwife to take on that aspect for the woman' (Chapter 13). In these circumstances the midwife can be said, in psychotherapeutic terms, to be holding the boundaries: to be creating a safe space in which the mother can trust that someone else can deal with the practicalities of everyday life (Chapter 13).

The merging of the attention of the mother with that of her newborn baby, just as the two become separate people, is crucial for their relationship and the child's development (Chapter 13). This process depends on the mother's experience of being mothered and her environment (Ernst, 1987) and can only happen if the mother feels safe. At and immediately after the birth, the midwife can mother the mother and she has the power to hold this safe space.

Such practice requires considerable skill and knowledge. Meg Taylor suggests that 'midwifery knowledge is that which integrates the hormonal and the emotional' (Chapter 13) and skills resulting from such knowledge are described throughout this book. This area merits research and exploration and calls for research methods with all the sensitivity and flexibility of the practice they are researching. This would mean rethinking research, as the New Zealand midwives have rethought professionalism (Chapter 12), another area of expert power which needs to be reclaimed to meet women's needs.

Holding safe space can also be seen from the viewpoint of social anthropology. In birth the baby crosses the threshold into society and the mother is in a threshold/liminal state in the middle of a rite of passage. Within current systems and power structures, women can feel and be seen as out of place just when they are in such a socially crucial position (Kirkham, 2007a). The midwife is the mother's guardian through the rite of passage to motherhood and it falls to her to create a safe space there.

There is also a physical sense in which midwives can hold a safe space for women. 'Birth territory' can be designed to enhance mothers' feeling of safety and midwives can be guardians of that safe space (Fahy *et al.*, 2008). A safe space is especially important when women feel particularly vulnerable, where they lack support or have experienced trauma. A woman who has been sexually abused (Garrett, 2008) or who has experienced a previous birth as traumatic may need her familiar safe space to give birth. Previous trauma is not usually stated as an indication for home birth, yet those midwives who listen to this need open up safe space in a physical and political sense, challenging the categorization of women on clinical issues alone (Murphy-Lawless, 2009).

The safe space which the midwife–mother relationship can hold promotes the woman's positive relationship with her self and with the new generation. This must be of fundamental social significance; it certainly creates social capital. Yet how often is this work neglected in favour of institutional priorities of paperwork and clearing beds for new admissions?

Hope for the future

If we want to change things we have to be clear about how we see the situation and what we need to change.

The purpose of the relationship

There seem to be two different views on the purpose of the midwife–mother relationship. These are not the separate views of mothers and midwives, but views that spring from the very different discourses of organizations and of women.

From the organizational viewpoint, the midwife–mother relationship is the medium through which the service is provided. The service operates best where the relationship works well, but organizational aims are generalized, laid down and hopefully audited to cover all service users and all eventualities. Thus a service experienced as fragmented by individual women and as frustrating by midwives may be seen as organizationally efficient in terms of staff deployment.

For the service user, the relationship is about feeling safe and able. Many midwives seek to enable their clients to feel safe to 'take up their power' (Chapter 2) and see themselves as 'women who can' (Chapter 5). Midwives also want to feel safe and able in their work.

These two views may be dichotomized as the technocratic and holistic

(Davis-Floyd and Sargent, 1997) or as 'risk versus potential' (Edwards, 2005), but that is to oversimplify the complexity of individual's different views. Fortunately, some wise midwifery managers have shown that these different approaches can be integrated to a considerable extent (Homer et al., 2001, 2008; Leyshon, 2004; Page, 1995), where the midwife–mother relationship and its ongoing development are seen as important and there is a willingness to delegate power to midwives to achieve the potential of that relationship in a way that is appropriate for the individuals involved.

Time and tasks

Within the NHS, midwives feel very pressed for time. Trudy Stevens described time as 'the ultimate control' (Stevens, 2003) for midwives. The tasks which must be completed have increased in number; a trend which is demonstrated very clearly in the growth in antenatal screening procedures. In a business model of care, time is money and tasks must be completed with speed and efficiency. People who are pressed for time cannot relate well. There are two responses to this: we can change the system of care, or we can reduce the tasks which need completing. Both options are promising.

There has been considerable discussion of reducing midwifery tasks with the help of support workers and clerical staff. Delegating work to less skilled staff can help, especially where midwives have some control over which tasks are delegated and do not feel that delegation has a negative impact on their relationship with mothers.

Midwives in England have tended to take on technical tasks delegated to them by doctors. The nature of these tasks has changed over the years. I once taught a midwife, returning to practice, who had not been taught to measure blood pressure in her initial training as this was then a medical task. Now it is a task often undertaken by care assistants. Should we be considering more rapid or wider delegation of technical tasks? I recently spoke with a mother who was booked for a home birth with her midwife in New Zealand. She was happy with her midwifery care, but she complained gently of having to 'go into town' to the lab to have her screening blood samples taken. It was completely accepted there that taking blood was done by laboratory staff at the laboratory. I could not help thinking of the time that community midwives in this country devote to taking blood, transporting blood and associated paperwork. Midwives have been the obvious people to do so many tasks associated with antenatal and postnatal screening. Should we be so obliging in taking on such work? Is screening a separate specialism in its own right? Should we critically review what could be delegated?

Our industrial model of midwifery has a very linear concept of time, as shown in the conveyor belt analogy (Dykes, 2006). This model of time comes from industry, not from birth. Though often treated as inevitable, the model itself carries many risks. Nadine Edwards sees time limits as risky in themselves and examines 'the risk of rushing' (Edwards, 2005: 121).

The mother in labour, or breastfeeding her baby, experiences time as cyclical, lived in response to the activities of her uterus or her baby, not the clock. Similarly, where there is an ongoing relationship between the midwife and the mother, time can be used in response to the mother's needs. When time can be invested in getting to know each other and establishing trust, issues will be revealed when the mother feels safe enough to raise them. This is very different from the endless list of questions which must be asked on booking, some so intrusive that I wonder how many women answer them truthfully. In an ongoing relationship time will be invested in preparation for labour, building the women's confidence in her body and her supporters. Where time is thus used responsively, more time may not be needed, but both parties will need flexibility to respond to each other.

Trudy Stevens examined caseload midwifery and time:

This necessitated a deconstruction of the 'modern' way of compartmentalising time, returning to a more 'traditional' way of conceiving and using it... The different way of using their time enabled midwives to meet mothers on a level that acknowledged and facilitated the physiological timing of childbirth. Nevertheless, this change conflicted with the institutional concepts of time and the way time was used by others, generating tensions. (Stevens, 2003: 290)

Such tensions are common when only part of a midwifery service changes and expectations are unchanged. So many schemes have failed because midwives have been given too large a caseload or expected to work to the same timescale as their colleagues within the industrial model. Nevertheless, research has shown the potential of such a way of working (e.g. McCourt and Stevens, 2009) and where change is on a larger scale, expectations are also likely to change (Homer *et al.*, 2008). A flexible response from management can help midwives model a flexible response to mothers, whose babies will live in cyclical not linear time.

One phrase which is really useful for new mothers is 'watch your baby, not the clock'. Wouldn't it be useful if midwives could do the same thing and 'watch the woman, not the clock' (Fielder, 2009)?

Scale

The midwife–mother relationship works best where mother and midwife can get to know each other over time, rather than relationships being many and fleeting. The relationship between a community midwife and a woman booked for a home birth is often cited as ideal. Yet the 'special' relationship with the community midwife (Chapter 5) can continue in hospital, if the midwife follows the woman rather than staffing the conveyor belt. If this is an organizational priority, it is possible to keep relationships on a human scale with one-to-one care, even within large hospitals (Homer *et al.*, 2008).

Colleague relationships are very important for midwives (Kirkham and Morgan, 2006; Kirkham *et al.*, 2006). Having a small and supportive group of colleagues is one reason for the success of birth centre care from the midwife's point of view (Kirkham, 2003; Walsh, 2007). Good support and supervision (Jones, 2000) mean that midwives feel they are in a safe setting in which they can develop their practice. With really good management support, it is possible to keep relationships meaningful and manageable for the midwife as well as the mother, even within a large hospital (Homer *et al.*, 2008; Stevens, 2003). This involves much reorganization and rethinking and is a real management challenge, but we know that it can be done. Surely we owe this to ourselves, as midwives, as well as to the women who need hospital care.

It is possible to move back to being with women. Trudy Stevens' work demonstrates this (Stevens, 2003), as do changes in midwifery care in New Zealand and Australia. There is now plenty of research about what midwifery care can achieve in small-scale settings where relationships can develop, be they caseholding projects, birth centres or independent midwifery. This research can provide a secure basis for us to be clear and proud about what we do well as midwives.

Emotion work

'Parallel to the obvious intellectual and technical art of midwifery... lays the equally important emotional art.' This is what Arlie Hochschild describes as 'mastery of the complex art of relating to the entire personality and soul – not just the body – of a birthing mother' (Hochschild, 2009: viii).

If midwives' emotion work is to extend beyond efficient processing of clients, it calls for the involvement of the self. In analysing the adaptations which midwives had to make in order to provide care for a caseload of women, Trudy Stevens reported:

> it was apparent that particular structures that had become separated in 'modern' society became fused again. The role and person of the midwife became one, and the professional:client dichotomy became a relationship of mutuality where the expertise of both midwife and mother were valued. Such fusion presented a radical alteration to the way caseload midwives worked. (Stevens, 2003: 290)

Such fusion can only occur where those involved have some autonomy and feel safe in their relationship. Chris Bewley reports the painful experiences of childless midwives in a conventional hospital setting (Chapter 11) and warns of the danger of self-disclosure in such a setting. Yet this is not without irony in the context of the midwife's licence to intrude into the body and being of her client.

It requires considerable skill and support to be emotionally available to mothers. This is only practicable when we know who we are required to be available to and can judge the nature of their needs over time. Just as mothers need to feel safe to give birth, midwives need safe, skilled supervision to learn appropriate skills.

We know that continuing support can have a positive impact on the outcomes of care (Hodnett *et al.*, 2007). The emotional skills involved in such support are subtle, varied and need to be sustained. It is the midwife's attention which enables the woman to feel that she is heard and validated. The nature of the midwife's presence, especially during labour, can be experienced as enabling or diminishing depending on whether she is 'emotionally present' (Berg, 2002: 54) or just 'checking' (Edwards, 2005).

Midwives' emotion work with mothers can facilitate the development of their social networks and the support resources available to new mothers within a community. This enhances social capital, which is defined as 'the connections amongst individuals – social networks and the norms of reciprocity and trustworthiness that arise from them' (Putnam, 2000: 42). In the crucial social resource of such capital, trust is fundamental and it has been taken as a marker of social capital in surveys (Knack and Keefer, 2000). This two-way trust echoes throughout this book. The potential of midwifery to enhance social capital has been underestimated, despite the work of many midwives and their involvement in community development (e.g. Dykes, 2003). As well as enhancement of the social capital of the communities within which midwives work, the social capital of midwifery as a movement merits our greater attention (Brodie, 2003).

Where the midwife can integrate her technical skills and her emotional skills in her work, this can be very satisfying. 'The positive psychological benefits this may hold for both parties, and particularly the possibility of offering a protective mechanism against undue stress and 'burnout' for midwives has been posited' (Stevens, 2003: 237).

Other models of maternity care

The birth of new members of a society is seen as so important that there is usually a 'right' way of doing birth which fits the values of the society concerned. 'We find that within any given system, birth practices appear packaged into a relatively uniform, systematic, standardised, ritualised, even morally required routine' (Jordan, 1980: 2). Brigitte Jordan's statement was a revelation to me when I first read it, for it explained the actions of all those who were unwilling to change and inclined to belittle and witch-hunt those they saw as deviant, whatever their own position with regard to maternity services.

But can such rigidity be appropriate in a modern society which valorizes choice and flexibility? Those of us within maternity services have had to be flexible in accommodating unprecedented change in recent years. Yet despite official rhetoric (see Chapter 1), the flexibility to accommodate alternative models of care seems difficult to achieve, at least in the UK.

One model of care which holds out great hope is that put forward by Independent Midwives UK (van der Kooy, 2009 and www.independent-midwives.org.uk). This model would enable independent midwives to provide care for individual women contracted through the NHS. This would mean that any woman could access independent midwifery care without having to pay for it privately, independent midwives would have access to NHS facilities for their clients, and insurance for independent midwives would be available through the NHS.

This model builds on the existing policy for choice and high-quality care and the structure of the marketplace in health care with a policy of encouraging plurality of providers, 'and the growth of the third [voluntary] sector and social enterprises as valid sources of healthcare providers is established. Payments based on standardised tariffs also provide a mechanism whereby there is a level playing field' (van der Kooy, 2009:

525). This model thus builds on market options in care which have been widely used in some areas of health care but not, as yet, in maternity care.

This model would enable women to choose a continuing relationship with a midwife without sacrificing NHS benefits. It would also enable midwives to determine their own workload and spend time with women 'rather than meeting the institution's needs. Time is the key and there can be no shortcuts without compromising quality of care' (van der Kooy, 2009: 524). The availability of such a model is also likely to have a positive impact on mainstream services.

Political change

Wider political change is clearly needed. There is ample evidence that the current market values underpinning public services create considerable problems (Edwards, 2008; Pollock, 2004). If services are motivated by a desire to cut costs, rather than a desire for excellence, it is inevitable that staffing is cut or client–staff contact is reduced in time or grade/cost of staff. To achieve this, staff use of time is more and more strictly controlled. Such is efficiency. In such a situation, management, far from striving for excellence, tends to fear it (Page, 1997) and we hear the terrible arguments for closing birth centres or innovative services on grounds of 'equity', meaning the lowest common denominator of service provision. These patterns of response cannot be appropriate for a service based on and offered through relationships. Nor do they attend to all that relationships can achieve, for all parties, as shown so vividly throughout this book. As midwives, we can achieve so much. Are we sufficiently proud and public about these achievements?

Whenever I speak to multi-professional audiences about our set of studies, including *Why Do Midwives Leave?* and *Why Midwives Stay* (Ball *et al.*, 2002; Kirkham *et al.*, 2006), I am told that the frustrating situation of midwives is 'just the same' in other public service professions. It may be that 'guardian' organizations, dedicated to pubic service (Jacobs, 1992), should run on very different principles from those of commercial organizations, since their concern is with social, not financial, capital. It may be that the hierarchical structures of the modern NHS are out of place in today's world (Fairtlough, 2005) or that the market values underpinning the organization of the modern NHS are out of date in the real marketplace. These issues need discussion across the public services.

In the conclusion to the first edition of this book I wrote:

There are striking parallels between the experiences and the needs of midwives and mothers, yet so often they meet in settings where both lack power and midwives' fear and professional allegiance do not allow them to identify with women. It is my hope that naming the issues creates the possibility for debate. Describing what is been done creates the possibility that more *can* be done. Thus we continue to nibble at the monolith of hierarchical organisations and the professional paradigm.

The problem lies in our reluctance as midwives to take up our power and form relationships and alliances, and in our fears of moving the power towards women despite the benefits described by the midwives who do this. (Kirkham 2000: 249)

Much has happened since then, some of it described in this edition. There are precedents for doing far more that nibbling at monoliths. Alternatives are being created: alternative ways of working (e.g. McCourt and Stevens, 2009; Milan, 2005; van der Kooy, 2009) and alternative ways of seeing our work (e.g. Hunter and Deery, 2009; Kirkham, 2007b; Murphy-Lawless, 1998). As midwives in relationships with mothers, we have the power to improve the health and well-being of families and communities. For our own sakes, as well as theirs, we need to use that power.

References

Ball, L., Curtis, P. and Kirkham, M. (2002) *Why Do Midwives Leave?* London: Royal College of Midwives.

Beat, A. and Beat, R. (2009) School for smallholders, Part 7, The Flow. *Country Smallholding* August: 37–40.

Beck, U. (1992) *Risk Society: Towards a New Modernity,* London: Sage.

Berg, M. (2002) *Genuine Caring in Caring for the Genuine: Childbearing and High Risk as Experienced by Women and Midwives,* Uppsala, Sweden: Acta Universitatis Upsaliensis.

Brodie, P. (1996) *Australian Team Midwives in Transition,* Oslo: International Confederation of Midwives, 23rd Triennial Conference.

Brodie, P. (2003) The Invisibility of Midwifery – Will Developing Social Capital Make a Difference? Professional Doctorate in Midwifery thesis, University of Technology, Sydney.

Cherry, A., Friel, R., Dowden, B., Ashton, K., Evans, R., Pugh, Y. and Evans, Y. (2009) Managing demand: Telephone triage in acute maternity services, *British Journal of Midwifery* 17(8): 496–500.

Davies, J. (2000) Being with women who are economically without, in Kirkham, M. (ed.), *The Midwife–Mother Relationship,* Basingstoke: Macmillan.

Davis-Floyd, R.E. and Sargent, C.F. (1997) *Childbirth and Authoritative Knowledge,* Berkeley, CA: University of California Press.

Dykes, F. (2003) *Infant Feeding Initiative: A Report Evaluating the Breastfeeding Practice Projects 1999–2002,* London: Department of Health.

Dykes, F. (2006) *Breastfeeding in Hospital: Mothers, Midwives and the Production Line*, London: Routledge.

Dykes, F. (2009) 'No time to care': Midwifery work on postnatal wards in England, in Hunter, B. and Deery, R. (eds), *Emotions in Midwifery and Reproduction*, Basingstoke: Palgrave.

Edwards, N.P. (2005) *Birthing Autonomy: Women's Experiences of Planning Home Births*, London: Routledge.

Edwards, N. (2008) Safety in birth: The contextual conundrums faced by women in a 'risk society', driven by neoliberal policies, *MIDIRS Midwifery Digest* 18(4): 463–70.

Ernst, S. (1987) Can a daughter be a woman? Women's identity and psychological separation, in Ernst, S. and Maguire, M. (eds), *Living with the Sphinx: Papers from the Women's Therapy Centre*, London: Women's Press.

Fahy, K., Foureur, K. and Hastie, C. (eds) (2008) *Birth Territory and Midwifery Guardianship*, Sydney: Books for Midwives.

Fairtlough, G. (2005) *The Three Ways of Getting Things Done: Hierarchy, Heterarchy and Responsible Autonomy in Organisations*, Bridport: Triarchy Press.

Fielder, A. (2009) Personal communication.

Freire, P. (1972) *The Pedagogy of the Oppressed*, Harmondsworth: Penguin.

Garrett, E.F. (2008) The childbearing experiences of survivors of childhood sexual abuse, PhD thesis, Sheffield Hallam University.

Goleman, D. (1995) *Emotional Intelligence*, New York: Bantam Books.

Hansard (2009) Commonweath of Australia, House of Representatives, Votes and Proceedings Wed June 24th 2009, Sydney Australia, Hansard.

Heagarty, B.V. (1996) Reassessing the guilty: The Midwives Act and the control of English midwives in the early 20th century, in Kirkham, M. (ed.), *Supervision of Midwives*, Hales: Books for Midwives Press.

Hochschild, A.R. (2009) Foreword, in Hunter, B. and Deery, R. (eds), *Emotions in Midwifery and Reproduction*, Basingstoke: Palgrave.

Hodnett, E.D., Gates, S., Hofmyr, G.J. and Sakala, C. (2007) Continuous support for women during childbirth, *Cochrane Database of Systematic Reviews* Issue 2. Art. No: CD003766 DOI: 10.1002/14651858. CD003766. pub2.

Homer, C., Brodie, P. and Leap, N. (2001) *Establishing Models of Continuity of Midwifery Care in Australia: A Resource for Midwives*, Sydney: University of Technology Sydney, Centre for Family Health and Midwifery.

Homer, C., Brodie, P. and Leap, N. (2008) *Midwifery Continuity of Care*, Sydney: Churchill Livingstone/Elsevier.

Hunter, B. and Deery, R. (eds) (2009) *Emotions in Midwifery and Reproduction*, Basingstoke: Palgrave.

Jacobs, J. (1992) *Systems of Survival: A Dialogue on the Moral Foundations of Commerce and Politics*, London: Hodder and Stoughton.

Jones, O. (2000) Supervision in a midwife managed birth centre, in Kirkham, M. (ed.), *Developments in the Supervision of Midwives*, Manchester: Books for Midwives.

Jordan, B. (1980) *Birth in Four Cultures*, Montreal: Eden Press.

Kirkham, M. (ed.) (2000) *The Midwife–Mother Relationship*, Basingstoke: Macmillan.

Kirkham, M. (ed.) (2003) *Birth Centres: A Social Model for Maternity Care*, Oxford: Elsevier.

Kirkham, M. (2004) Midwives: Praise and beyond, *Practicing Midwife* 7(2): 20–21.

Kirkham, M. (ed.) (2007a) *Exploring the Dirty Side of Women's Health*, London: Routledge.

Kirkham, M. (2007b) Traumatised midwives, *AIMS Journal* 19(1): 12–13.

Kirkham, M. and Morgan, R.K. (2006) *Why Midwives Return and their Subsequent Experience*, London: Department of Health (www.nhsemployers.org and www.rcm.org).

Kirkham, M. and Stapleton, H. (eds) (2001) *Informed Choice in Maternity Care: An Evaluation of Evidence Based Leaflets*, York: NHS Centre for Reviews and Dissemination.

Kirkham, M., Morgan, R.K. and Davies, C. (2006) *Why Midwives Stay*, London: Department of Health (www.nhsemployers.org and www.rcm.org).

Kirkham, M., Stapleton, H., Curtis, P. and Thomas, G. (2002) Stereotyping as a professional defence mechanism, *British Journal of Midwifery* 10(9): 509–13.

Knack, S. and Keefer, P. (2000) Does social capital have an economic pay-off? *Quarterly Journal of Economics* 112(4): 1251–85.

Leap, N. (1997) Making sense of 'horizontal violence' in midwifery, *British Journal of Midwifery* 5(11): 689.

Levy, V. (1998) Facilitating and making informed choices during pregnancy, PhD thesis, University of Sheffield.

Levy, V. (1999) Protective steering: A grounded theory study of the processes by which midwives facilitate informed choices during pregnancy, *Journal of Advanced Nursing* 29(1): 104–12.

Leyshon, L. (2004) Integrating caseloads across a whole service: The Torbay model, *MIDIRS Midwifery Digest* 14(1, Supplement 1): S9–S11.

Lipsky, M. (1980) *Street-Level Bureaucracy: Dilemmas of the Individual in Public Services*, New York, Russel Sage Foundation.

McCourt, C. and Stevens, T. (2009) Relationship and reciprocity in caseload midwifery, in Hunter, B. and Deery, R. (eds), *Emotions in Midwifery and Reproduction*, Basingstoke: Palgrave.

Menzies Lyth, I. (1988) *Containing Anxiety in Institutions: Selected Essays Vol 1*, London: Free Association Books.

Milan, M. (2005) Independent midwifery compared with other caseload practice, *MIDIRS Midwifery Digest* 15(4): 439–49.

Murphy-Lawless, J. (1998) *Reading Birth and Death: A History of Obstetric Thinking*, Cork: Cork University Press.

Murphy-Lawless, J. (2009) Personal communication.

Nihell, E. (1760) *A Treatise on the Art of Midwifery: Setting Forth Various Abuses Therein, Especially as to the Practice of Instruments*, London: Haymarket.

Page, L. (ed.) (1995) *Effective Group Practice in Midwifery: Working with Women*, Oxford: Blackwell.

Page, L. (1997) Misplaced values: In fear of excellence, *British Journal of Midwifery* 5(11): 652–4.

Pollock, A.M. (2004) *NHS plc*, London: Verso.

Putnam, R. (2000) *Bowling Alone: The Collapse and Revival of American Community*, New York: Simon and Schuster.

Roberts, S.J. (1983) Oppressed group behaviour: Implications for nursing, *Advances in Nursing Science* July: 21–30.

Sennett, R. (1998) *The Corrosion of Character: The Personal Consequences of Work in the New Capitalism*, New York: Norton.

Sennett, R. (2008) *The Craftsman*, New York: Yale University Press.

Stapleton, H., Duerden, J. and Kirkham, M. (1998) *Evaluation of the Impact of the Supervision of Midwives on Professional Practice and the Quality of Midwifery Care*, London: ENB.

Stapleton, H., Kirkham, M., Thomas, G. and Curtis, P. (2002) Midwives in the middle: Balance and vulnerability, *British Journal of Midwifery* 10(10): 607–11.

Stephens, T.A. (2003) Midwife to mid wif: A study of caseload midwifery, PhD thesis, Thames Valley University.

van der Kooy, B. (2009) Choice for women and choice for midwives – making it happen, *British Journal of Midwifery* 17(9): 524–5.

Walsh, D. (2007) *Improving Maternity Services, Small is Beautiful – Lessons from a Birth Centre*, London: Radcliffe Publishing.

Index

273